Physiological Effects of Food Carbohydrates

Physiological Effects of Food Carbohydrates

**Allene Jeanes and
John Hodge,** *Editors*

A symposium co-sponsored by
the Division of Carbohydrate
Chemistry and the Division
of Agricultural and Food
Chemistry at the 168th
Meeting of the American
Chemical Society,
Atlantic City, N. J.,
Sept. 11–12, 1974.

ACS SYMPOSIUM SERIES **15**

AMERICAN CHEMICAL SOCIETY

WASHINGTON, D. C.   1975

Library of Congress CIP Data

Physiological effects of food carbohydrates

(ACS symposium series; 15)

Includes bibliographical references and index.

1. Carbohydrates—Physiological effect—Congresses. 2.
Carbohydrate metabolism—Congresses.
I. Jeanes, Allene Rosalind, 1906-. II. Hodge,
John E., 1914- . III. American Chemical Society.
Division of Carbohydrate Chemistry. IV. American
Chemical Society. Division of Agricultural and Food
Chemistry. V. Series: American Chemical Society. ACS
symposium series; 15. [DNLM: 1. Carbohydrates—
Metabolism—Congresses. QU75 A512p 1974]

QP701.P48   612'.396   75-14071
ISBN 0-8412-0246-X   ACSMC8 15 1-355 (1975)

ACS Symposium Series

Robert F. Gould, *Series Editor*

FOREWORD

The ACS SYMPOSIUM SERIES was founded in 1974 to provide a medium for publishing symposia quickly in book form. The format of the SERIES parallels that of its predecessor, ADVANCES IN CHEMISTRY SERIES, except that in order to save time the papers are not typeset but are reproduced as they are submitted by the authors in camera-ready form. As a further means of saving time, the papers are not edited or reviewed except by the symposium chairman, who becomes editor of the book. Papers published in the ACS SYMPOSIUM SERIES are original contributions not published elsewhere in whole or major part and include reports of research as well as reviews since symposia may embrace both types of presentation.

CONTENTS

PREFACE

Significant progress has been made in evaluating the physiological effects that have been attributed to food carbohydrates. Because the findings are related to the structure, enzymology, and complexing interactions of carbohydrates, as well as to improved compositions of processed foods, this symposium was organized in the interests of the Division of Carbohydrate Chemistry and the Division of Agricultural and Food Chemistry.

Some common disorders definitely associated with dietary carbohydrates are diabetes, stress responses resulting from hypoglycemia, dental caries, eye cataracts, flatulence, and fermentative diarrhea. The postulated role of sugar in the development of atherosclerosis and coronary heart disease has been impugned and debated, but, more importantly, it is being carefully investigated. Investigations center on underlying causes of carbohydrate-induced disorders—e.g., altered enzyme activity in the digestive tract and elevated insulin, cholesterol, and triglyceride levels in serum. Numerous studies show differences according to the type of carbohydrate ingested.

Because refined sugars and starches have been referred to as "empty calories," one might wonder whether carbohydrate is needed at all in the diet. Some popular reducing diets contain little carbohydrate. The Food and Nutrition Board of the National Research Council, National Academy of Sciences, has stated in the 1974 edition of "Recommended Dietary Allowances":

Carbohydrates can be made in the body from some amino acids and the glycerol moiety of fats; there is therefore no specific requirement for this nutrient in the diet. However, it is desirable to include some preformed carbohydrate in the diet to avoid ketosis, excessive breakdown of body protein, loss of cations, especially sodium, and involuntary dehydration. Fifty to 100 g of digestible carbohydrate a day will offset the undesirable metabolic responses associated with high fat diets and fasting.

The topics of this symposium are related to improved carbohydrate and mineral balance in foods of the future. As food supplies for expanding populations become more critical, the more abundant and economical carbohydrates should be used to maximum advantage to spare the less abundant proteins and fats. However, to establish the optimum ratio of carbohydrates to fats, the physiological effects of their combinations should be delineated more clearly. It now appears that indigestible, as well as digestible, carbohydrate should be considered in formulating processed foods. The postulated benefits of dietary fiber (largely indigestible polysaccharides) in aiding the elimination of toxins and in reducing serum cholesterol are discussed. Other advantages that might accrue from ingesting or infusing certain types of carbohydrate in place of other types are cited here. Disadvantages in refining high-carbohydrate cereals and sugar to the point of near depletion of essential mineral content are viewed from a physiological basis.

During this century significant changes have taken place in the types of carbohydrate that are made available in our food supplies. U.S. Department of Agriculture statistics show that we are being exposed more to refined sugars and less to starch and dietary fiber as the proportions of fat (mainly) and protein increase in prepared foods. Among the refined sugars, the proportion of intact sucrose is decreasing relative to D-fructose, D-glucose, and the maltose and maltooligosaccharides of starch hydrolyzates. The increasing incorporation of starch sirups, including those that contain D-fructose produced by glucose isomerase, is expected to accentuate this trend. The level of lactose, ingested mainly from milk and dairy products rather than from added lactose, has remained about constant.

Critics declare that consumers now have less control over their carbohydrate intake than their forebears had because the compositions of prepared convenience foods and beverages vary significantly from those of natural foods. Expanding urban populations dictate an increasing supply of stable processed foods; therefore, the benefits of adding sugars and modified polysaccharides to improve the stability and acceptance of prepared foods should be weighed against adverse nutritional effects. Although processing practices have been viewed with alarm in some sectors, we really cannot know whether the changes in carbohydrate composition are innocuous until the physiological effects of the additives have been defined under conditions of normal use. This symposium and others like it attest to the activity of scientists in different disciplines who are supplying answers to the questions raised about the healthfulness of refined sugars and gums.

Some of the subjects selected for this symposium were critically reviewed in the International Conference on Sugars in Nutrition held at the Vanderbilt University School of Medicine in 1972 ("Sugars in Nutrition," H. L. Sipple and K. W. McNutt, Eds., Academic Press, New York, 1974). However, more recent experimental results and additional information on the physiology of dietary and infused sugars are presented here, and mostly by different authorities. Parts A and B of this symposium might therefore be regarded as a supplement to "Sugars in Nutrition." Part C covers physiological effects of polysaccharides, which were not covered in the Vanderbilt conference, including some food additive gums and dietary fiber. This information also can be expanded by reference to the Symposium on Fiber in Human Nutrition held by the Nutrition Society at the University of Edinburgh School of Medicine (*Proc. Nutr. Soc.* (1973) **32**, 123-167). Another symposium publication, "Molecular Structure and Function of Food Carbohydrate" (G. G. Birch and L. F. Green, Eds., Wiley, New York, 1973), contains several papers that are related to the topics of this symposium.

JOHN E. HODGE

Northern Regional Research Laboratory
Agricultural Research Service, USDA
Peoria, Ill.
December 1974

Part A

Physiological Effects of Ingested and Infused Carbohydrates: Introduction

WILLIS A. GORTNER

National Program Staff, Agricultural Research Service, U.S. Department of Agriculture, Beltsville, Md. 20705

This timely symposium was organized by Dr. Allene Jeanes and Mr. John Hodge of the Northern Regional Research Center, Agricultural Research Service, U.S. Department of Agriculture, Peoria, Illinois. To them should go full credit for developing the program and for selecting the authoritative specialists who will present the papers.

As chemists or as food technologists, we have a keen interest in the emergence of recommendations for dietary carbohydrates and identification of the forms of carbohydrate that may be useful in meeting the requirements for man. Presently there is no accepted minimum requirement or maximum tolerance for either total carbohydrate or for any of the individual carbohydrates in the diet. Yet, considerable evidence has accumulated recently showing that both the quantity and the kind of dietary carbohydrate markedly affect metabolic processes. These processes will be considered in depth in some of the papers on this symposium.

Carbohydrate supplies a large proportion of man's caloric needs. In underdeveloped countries as much as 80% of the total calorie intake is in the form of carbohydrates. In the developed countries, the proportion is smaller but still substantial. In the United States in 1973, carbohydrate furnished nearly half of the calories in the daily food supply.

The nature of the carbohydrate has also changed over the years. There has been a steady decline in the per capita consumption of starch. Where starch formerly accounted for more than two-thirds of the intake of carbohydrates, it now accounts for less than half the total. The simple sugars, especially sucrose, now provide more than half of the available carbohydrates. Even the nature and amount of dietary fiber has been changing, and this fiber has been gaining increasing recognition as an important part of the diet, although it is essentially indigestible carbohydrate.

Hopefully, this symposium will give us a better understanding of what and how carbohydrates should be regulated through diet, and some of the health benefits that might be achieved.

1

1

The Physiology of the Intestinal Absorption of Sugars

ROBERT K. CRANE

College of Medicine and Dentistry of New Jersey, Rutgers Medical School, Department of Physiology, Piscataway, N. J. 08854

This review has to do with the physiology of the intestinal absorption of sugars and should properly begin with a brief discussion of the components of the physiological system which carries out this indispensable task.

The small intestine where the absorption of sugars takes place is a tube connecting to the stomach at its upper end and to the large intestine at its lower. In the human adult the tube is about 280 cm (9 feet) in length and an average 4 cm (1-1/2 inches) in internal diameter. The area of the inner surface of the tube is much greater than implied by these two measurements because the inner surface is heavily folded and everywhere on the folds there are to be found numerous projections called villi (1). Villi are readily seen under a microscope of low power and there are perhaps as many as 25,000,000 villi in all. As indicated in Figure 1, each villus is covered by a sheet of absorptive epithelial cells punctuated at intervals by the so-called goblet cells which supply protective mucous. Between the villi are to be found crypts within which the cells are produced and from which they migrate outward along the surface of a villus during a short 3-4 days of active life before being extruded into the lumen of the gut where they disintegrate and are digested.

The villus is the working unit of the small intestine. It is on this structure that the inner ends of the absorptive cells are brought into close proximity to the blood and lymph which must pick up absorbed nutrients and carry them to the other parts of the body. The outer ends of the absorptive cells are in contact with the contents of the intestine and are specialized to perform their necessary work. The outer end of each cell is a "brush border" made up of closely packed, parallel cylindrical processes called microvilli. The limiting plasma membrane of the cell follows the contours of the microvilli. Just beneath the brush border along the sides of the cells are to be found specialized junctional structures by means of which the absorptive cells are held together into a more or less continuous sheet.

2

Expanding our horizon to include the whole of the intestinal surface while retaining our view of its microscopic appearance it is clear that, so far as concerns digestion and absorption, the collective brush borders of the epithelial sheet form a junctional barrier between the outside of the body and the inside through which nutrients must pass in order to reach the circulation and enter metabolism. The collective brush borders separate the digestive functions of the intestinal lumen contributed by the secreted enzymes of the pancreas from the metabolic functions contributed by the cells. The brush borders also contribute digestive functions of their own as well as the selectivity, energy transduction and other properties of absorption anticipated for a cell membrane occupying this particular location.

The brush border membrane acts as a bilayer lipoidal matrix composed of the fatty chains of phospholipids and glycosphingolipids interspersed with cholesterol (2) and perforated here and there by aqueous channels through which water and small molecules may pass by diffusion. Lipid soluble molecules of most any size diffuse readily across the matrix of the membrane. However, the membrane is a substantial barrier to the rapid diffusion of large, highly water soluble molecules like the hexoses because these do not enter the matrix and the dimensional properties of the aqueous channels are too small, being equivalent only to those of pores of 4-5 Å in radius (3), (4). There are also aqueous channels between the cells because the junctional complexes of the intestinal epithelium are not tight (5). However, these channels are also too small for the rapid passage of hexoses.

Those hexoses which do get across the brush border membrane rapidly and in quantity; and this group naturally includes the major dietary hexoses, glucose, galactose, and fructose, do so because they fit the specificity requirements and are able to bind to membrane transport carriers (6). The actual mode of operation of carriers is currently unknown. However, their apparent mode of operation, insofar as we can know it from kinetics, is most easily described as like that of a ferryboat, capable of shuttling water soluble molecules across the lipoidal matrix. Carrier function is diagrammed in Figure 2 where the upper part is an operational model and the lower part is a kinetic model of a simple so-called facilitated diffusion type of carrier to which constants may be assigned as indicated. The assumptions are few and simple. Substrate interacts with the binding site of a carrier on either side of the membrane and is translocated in association with the carrier. The binding site of the carrier can translocate whether or not it carries substrate. All interactions are usually assumed to be symmetrical and equilibrium is then achieved at equal transmembrane concentrations or activities. For the most part, fructose crosses the brush border membrane by means of a carrier with these properties (7, 8, 9).

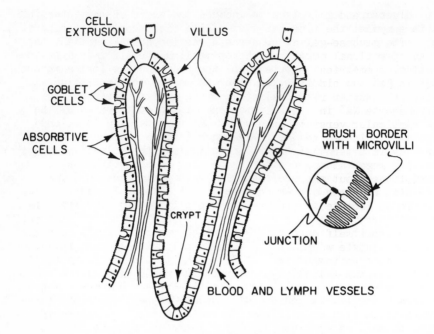

Figure 1. Schematic of features of villus architecture and the mucosal lining of the small intestine

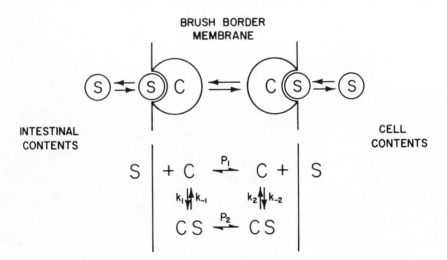

Figure 2. Schematic of a facilitated diffusion (monofunctional) carrier. P is the permeability coefficient.

Glucose and galactose, however, use a carrier which though it is somewhat the same is also somewhat and importantly different. The glucose-galactose carrier, depicted in Figure 3 both as an operational model and as a kinetic model, is an equilibrating, symmetrical carrier like the fructose carrier except that it has two binding sites instead of one.   The glucose-galactose carrier requires Na^+ for its efficient operation and cotransports Na^+ in a ternary complex along with the sugar (6). The particular version of the Na^+-dependent carrier shown in Figure 3 indicates that the binding site can translocate either empty or in a ternary complex with both of its substrates, but not with sugar alone.   There are other versions with other assumptions about the requirements for translocation but the essential features are very similar (10).

In an isolated system, a carrier with two binding sites is an equilibrating carrier like the carrier with one binding site. The carrier itself can serve only to dissipate gradients and the stationary state would find equal concentrations of sugar and equal concentrations of Na^+ on the two sides of the membranes. In the cellular system, however, the Na^+-dependent glucose-galactose carrier is able to transduce metabolic energy and to achieve "uphill" or against the gradient transport by coupling to the transcellular flux of Na^+. The system in the intestine seems to work as suggested by the diagram in Figure 4. Metabolic energy in the form of ATP is put into a sodium pump in the basolateral membranes of the absorptive cells to drive a transcellular flux of Na^+ from the brush border end to the basolateral end (12).   The glucose-galactose carrier couples sugar entry to this flux by being a route for the entry of sodium ion at the brush border membrane and achieves an "uphill" cellular accumulation of sugar at the expense of the "downhill" flux of Na^+.

Intact di- and higher saccharides do not get across the brush border membrane in quantity and we thus infer that the needed carriers do not exist (13).   Tiny amounts of dietary di- and oligosaccharides are sometimes found in the urine of individuals under study but these tiny amounts are attributable to diffusion of these large compounds through regions of the intestine where the normal barrier has been broken down by injury or by disease.

Recently our laboratory has identified a route of cellular entry of monosaccharides in addition to that provided by the Na^+-dependent carriers of Figures 3 and 4 (14, 15). This new route to be briefly described later is related to the activity of those hydrolases which are an intrinsic part of the brush border membrane.   As is discussed at further length by Dr. Gary Cray in this Symposium and as is shown in Table I, there are imbedded in the outer surface of the brush border membrane a substantial list of bond-specific hydrolytic or transfer activities.   The

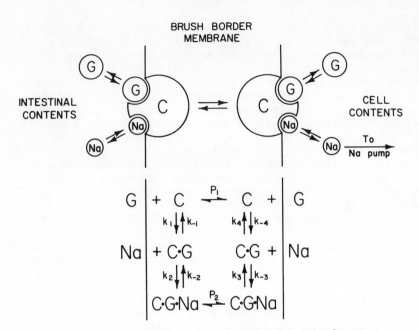

Figure 3. *Schematic of a sodium-dependent bifunctional carrier*

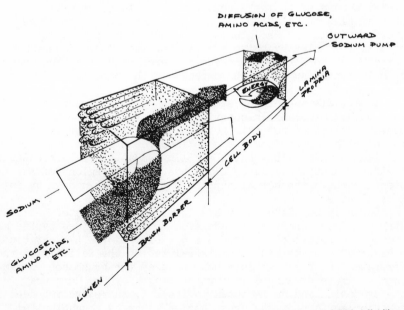

American Journal of Clinical Nutrition

Figure 4. *Schematic of energy transduction between the baso-lateral sodium pump and brush border Na⁺-dependent carriers by means of the Na⁺ through flux* (11)

TABLE I

BRUSH BORDER ENZYME ACTIVITIES*

Oligopeptidase
γ-glutamyl transpeptidase
Enterokinase
Glucoamylase (oligosaccharidase)
Maltase
Sucrase
Isomaltase (α-dextrinase)
Lactase
Trehalase
Phlorizin Hydrolase (glycosylceramidase)
Alkaline Phosphatase

*as of 1974 according to Crane (16).

saccharidases among these enzymes; namely, glucoamylase (which is
highly active against oligosaccharides) maltase, sucrase, isomaltase, (which Gray would prefer to call α-dextrinase after the
natural substrate found as a product of pancreatic amylase
action) lactase, trehalase, and phlorizin hydrolase share the
work of polysaccharide digestion with pancreatic amylase as
suggested in Figure 5.

Digestive-Sequence

Polysaccharides

Pancreatic Amylase   ↕

Oligosaccharides
and Disaccharides

Brush Border Saccharidases   ↕

Monosaccharides

Figure 5. Sequential roles in carbohydrate digestion of pancreatic amylase and brush border saccharidases

    In the adult, pancreatic amylase splits amylose only as far
as maltotriose and maltose (17) and amylopectin to maltotriose,
maltose and α-dextrins (18). The brush border saccharidases
then take over to cleave free glucose from these products. The
brush border enzymes also contribute directly the digestive

capacity of the intestine for dietary disaccharides.

A good deal of work has made it clear that the brush border membrane is a digestive-absorptive surface on which the monosaccharide substrates for the carriers are formed by the action of di- and oligosaccharidases, if they are not provided in free form in the diet (19). There is a close proximity at the brush border membrane between the sequential processes of digestion and absorption and because of this only a relatively small amount of monosaccharide accumulates in the lumen during the digestion of a disaccharide. In Figure 6, taken from Gray and Santiago (20), it is seen that only 10 percent of the glucose formed by brush border hydrolysis of sucrose over a 30 cm segment of intestine was found in the lumen; 90 percent having been absorbed. The experience with lactose and maltose was similar. Fructose was less well absorbed than glucose formed at the same time from sucrose because its different transport system is less efficient at equal concentrations. Galactose was less well absorbed than glucose formed at the same time from lactose because it has to compete with that glucose for the same transport system and has a lower affinity for it.

Overall, it is clear that the absorption of the monosaccharide products of disaccharide digestion is efficient. In part, as already mentioned, this may be explained by the close functional proximity of the membrane digestive enzymes to the membrane transport systems; a proximity that we have labeled "kinetic advantage" (19). Also in part this may be explained by a function of the disaccharidases as a route for the direct translocation of some of their products without the intervention of the normal carrier mechanisms, as recently documented in publications from our laboratory (14, 15) and fully corroborated by Diedrich (21). However, there is no reliable evidence to support the idea that the absorption of the monosaccharide products of disaccharides can be substantially more efficient than the absorption of the free monosaccharides themselves. For the past 15 years, a concept has been floating about to the effect that there may be an advantage for absorption to feed sugars in the form of disaccharides rather than as free monosaccharides. This concept got its start with some in vitro experiments of Chain and his colleagues (22). Our studies (19) did nothing to detract from the idea and direct in vivo experimental support for a small effect seemed to be provided by human studies carried out by Ian MacDonald (23). The most recent work on humans does not support the idea. In fact, it is possible that the idea has finally been laid to rest by the careful studies of Cook (24) who has found absolutely no difference in the portal blood levels of fructose and glucose whether it is sucrose that is placed in the lumen of the intestine or whether it is an equimolar mixture of glucose and fructose.

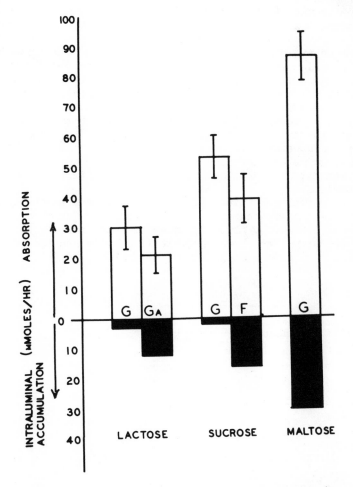

Figure 6. Role of monosaccharides released by the digestion of disaccharides over a 30-cm infusion-to-collection distance in human intestine (20)

The usefulness to the organism of the direct translocation of monosaccharides by brush border digestive hydrolases is currently a physiological puzzle and, for this reason, the data base for this new transport pathway will not be developed here to any great extent. Suffice it to say that in vitro studies carried out under conditions where the normal carrier mechanisms for glucose transport are either saturated with substrate and thus operating at a maximal rate or completely inhibited by the omission of Na$^+$ have demonstrated an additional component of glucose entry into the cells when any disaccharide substrate of a brush border enzyme is provided. In the case of sucrose, fructose as well as glucose enters and accumulates in the cells. Moreover, the components of translocation contributed by the individual enzymes are additive when more than one disaccharide is used. Clearly, these systems for direct translocation increase the total capacity of the intestine for carbohydrate absorption substantially over the capacity contributed by the monosaccharide carrier mechanisms. However, the circumstances under which this additional capacity may fulfill a need are far from obvious.

The reason for this, which is probably not generally appreciated, is that the capacity of the intestine for absorption of the monosaccharides, glucose, galactose and fructose is already truly enormous. As shown in Table II, Holdsworth and Dawson (25)

TABLE II

THE CAPACITY OF THE GUT TO ABSORB SUGARS

Measured: Glucose $= \dfrac{0.4 \text{ g}}{\text{min. x 30 cm}}$

Fructose = 0.9 x glucose

Calculated: Glucose $= \dfrac{0.4}{\text{min. x 30 cm}} \times \dfrac{1440 \text{ min}}{\text{day}} \times 280$ cm = 5374 g/day

Fructose = 5374 x 0.9 = 4837 g/day

THUS

Total Daily Capacity = 10,211 g > 22 lb. > 50,000 cal.

measured the absorptive capacity over a 30 cm segment of intestine in normal humans. At perfusate sugar concentrations of 5 g/100 ml they obtained the measured values of 0.4 g/min/30 cm for glucose and 90 percent of that value for fructose. From these it may be calculated that the total daily capacity is 10,211 g of a mixture of glucose and fructose; an amount equivalent to over 22 pounds of sugar and more than 50,000 calories. Although not all parts of the intestine have the same capacity as the part studied by Holdsworth and Dawson, the extrapolated maximal rate was nearly twice that of the value assumed in Table II; namely 0.73 g/min/30 cm and the total capacity calculated is probably a reasonable compromise. Galactose, tested alone, was absorbed even more rapidly than glucose.

Such a capacity for sugar absorption is ten times more than would be needed to provide for even the most unreasonable individual caloric requirements since foods in addition to sugars are generally also eaten and its great size indicates that control of sugar absorption is not exerted at the level of the processes of digestion and absorption at the brush border membrane. Control is exerted by a negative feedback mechanism involving receptors in the upper intestine and the motility of the stomach.

The relationships between the stomach and the intestines are diagrammed in Figure 7. The digestive features above the stomach and of the stomach itself are not included because it is a matter of fact that the really indispensable function of the stomach is to serve as a reservoir for foodstuffs and to provide for their release in small increments into the small intestine through the intermittent opening of the pyloric valve. The small intestine digests and absorbs these increments as they are received but its ability to do so depends upon certain physiological limitations. Perhaps most important is the fact that the mucosal surface of the small intestine is osmoresponsive. That is to say, when the contents of the stomach are released into the upper small intestine water shifts between the extracellular fluid spaces of the body and the lumen of the intestine so as to balance the osmotic activities across the mucosal membrane (26). Normally, the process is grossly unremarkable and goes unnoticed. Under abnormal circumstances, however, such as following surgery of the stomach so extensive as to eliminate its reservoir function, the simple act of eating may lead to sudden and excessive hyperosmolarity in the upper intestine with consequent water shifts large enough to result in the physiological response known as the "dumping dyndrome" wherein there can be serious vasomotor disturbances including sweating, nausea, diarrhea, a fall in blood pressure and weakness (27).

Similarly, the large intestine is also osmoresponsive (28) but it cannot absorb sugars. Thus when, due to disease or surgery, the small intestinal capacity for sugar digestion or absorption is so greatly reduced that a substantial amount of unabsorbed sugar enters the large intestine, diarrhea will ensue owing to the osmotic properties of the sugar itself as well as to any increase in osmotically active molecules through bacterial breakdown of the sugar to lactic and other acids (28). It takes only 54 grams of glucose to produce one liter of the osmotic equivalent of the extracellular fluids and, thus, at least one liter of excess excretion.

Under normal circumstances the system is under control and such untoward effects do not happen. Foodstuffs in general, fats, especially, but proteins also as well as carbohydrates, when they enter the intestine through the pyloric valve elicit responses which slow gastric emptying. The case of sugars is shown in Figure 8 by a summation of many studies carried out by J. N. Hunt and his colleagues.

An initial "meal" of 750 ml of a solution of citrate was placed by tube into the stomach. Most of the "meal" was delivered to the intestine over the next 20 minutes. The volume delivered in the same span of time was reduced by the addition of glucose and the degree to which the delivered volume was reduced increased as the glucose concentration increased. Clearly, receptors in the lining of the small intestine respond to the entering glucose in proportion to its concentration and act to reduce gastric motility presumably by hormonal mechanisms. The receptors for glucose are osmoreceptors and they are sugar specific. Fructose generally did not elicit an inhibitory response at low concentrations. Clear responses to fructose required concentrations of about 300 millimoles/liter and more. Sucrose, or a mixture of glucose and fructose, as might be expected, were intermediate in their effects.

Once the process of stomach emptying starts the stomach delivers its contents at a rate roughly proportional to their nutritive density (kcal/ml) (J. N. Hunt, personal communication) and in a predictable and exponential fashion until the stomach is very nearly empty. During this process, monosaccharides, in the diet or produced by digestion, are moving into and down the intestine and are being absorbed by the carrier mechanisms earlier mentioned; fructose by means of a facilitated diffusion carrier, glucose and galactose by means of a Na^+-dependent cotransport carrier. It may be asked, why? What is the value to the economy of the organism that these particular mechanisms are used and that different mechanisms are used for different kinds of sugar. An answer may be that the needs are best matched in this way.

The fundamental difference between the two carrier systems is that the one, the Na^+-dependent carrier, can be energized to produce active (against the concentration gradient) transport whereas the other, the facilitated diffusion carrier cannot. This difference would seem to match the energy demands of the respective absorptive problems.

In the case of fructose, fructose levels in the blood during its absorption are low, being only one-tenth those of glucose during its absorption, (10-15 mg % as against 150-200 mg %) and fructose is rapidly metabolized reducing the late- or post-absorptive blood fructose to very low levels. Consequently, there is no large stable blood-to-intestinal lumen gradient of fructose concentration and there may simply be no need for

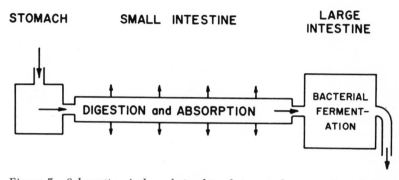

Figure 7. Schematic of the relationships between the stomach and the
intestines

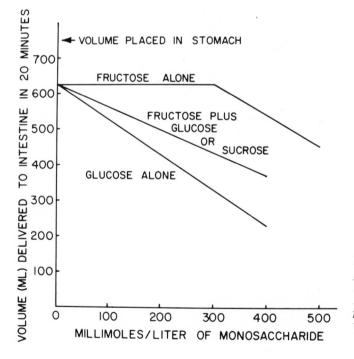

Figure 8. Effect of carbohydrate content on the rate of stomach emptying of a test meal. Drawn from data published in graphic form by Hunt and Knox (29).

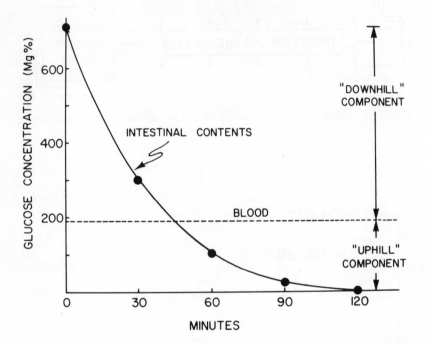

Figure 9. Time course of glucose absorption from a loop of rabbit intestine, in vivo. *Drawn from data published in graphic form by Bárány and Sperber* (30).

fructose to be absorbed by an energized transport system. Hence, the facilitated diffusion carrier suffices. The case is different for glucose. The blood in health always contains appreciable (80-90 mg %) glucose and one may be certain that a quantitatively important part of the absorption of a load of glucose will require the participation of an energized carrier because that part of absorption will necessarily be "uphill" from the lumen to the blood.

What takes place in the intestine following a load of glucose is well illustrated by the experiments of Barany and Sperber (30) with live rabbits as shown in Figure 9. These workers placed a certain volume of a concentrated glucose solution into a closed loop of the rabbit's intestine and sampled the contents of the loop at the intervals thereafter. Initially the concentration of glucose in the intestine was higher than glucose in the blood. Consequently, absorption during this period took place down the concentration gradient and net transfer of sugar from the intestine to the blood stream would require no energy input other than diffusional. This is the "downhill" component. Later, as absorption progressed, the concentration of glucose in the intestine became lower than in the blood. Continued absorption consequently took place "uphill" against the concentration gradient and would require the input of energy other than diffusional.

At the outset, one might suppose that two different carriers are used; one for the downhill component and another for the uphill. However, this is not the case. The evidence says that the same carriers are used for both components. If these carriers were to have the requirement for the consumption of metabolic energy in the uphill mode built into the biochemical mechanisms they would be wasteful when operating in the downhill mode.

In Table III are compared four types of membrane transport which are either known or have been proposed to occur in animal cells. These are:

(1) Facilitated diffusion which for present purposes is viewed as having the characteristics of a symmetrical biochemical reaction in which the stationary state achieved will be a 1/1 equilibrium between fructose inside and fructose outside the cell. Facilitated diffusion can operate only "downhill". (2) Vectorial biochemical reactions of the kind envisaged in the phosphorylation-dephosphorylation hypothesis of the 1930's - 1950's (31) wherein it was proposed that the energy for accumulation was delivered to the substrate, glucose, by the transfer of phosphate from ATP with subsequent hydrolysis to release free sugar. Roseman and his colleagues and Kaback have studied systems in bacterial membranes which are of this general type except that phosphorylated sugar and not free sugar is accumulated (32). The asymmetry of the biochemical reactions in such systems is obvious. (3) Covalently energized carriers which are like the

TABLE III

Reactions Involved in and Energy Utilization by Various
Hypothetical Types of Membrane Transport

Descriptive Name	Reaction Involved	Stationary State	Downhill or Uphill Transport Capability	Is Bond Energy Consumed in Downhill Mode
(1) Symmetrical Biochemical Reaction (Facilitated Diffusion)	C + Fo ↔ C·F ↔ C + Fi	[Fi] = [Fo]	Downhill only	no
(2) Vectorial Biochemical Reaction	C + Go + ATP ↔ C·G6P + ADP; C·G6P + HOH ↔ C + Gi + P	[Gi] > [Go]	both	yes
(3) Covalently Energized Carrier	C + ATP ↔ C∼P + ADP; C∼P + Go + HOH ↔ C + Gi + P	[Gi] > [Go]	both	yes
(4) Cotransport Energized Carrier	C + Nao ↔ C·Na; C·Na + Go ↔ C·Na·G; C·Na·G ↔ C·Na + Gi; C·Na ↔ C + Nai ↔ to pump	[Gi] > [Go] ; [Nai] < [Nao]	both	no

C = carrier, F = fructose, G = glucose, P = phosphate, o = outside, i = inside.

vectorial biochemical reactions in that they are fundamentally asymmetrical but which differ in that the energy for accumulation is delivered to the carrier rather than to the substrate. Perhaps the best example of a covalently energized carrier is the cell membrane sodium pump which expresses itself as an Na^+-K^+ activated ATPase (33). (4) Cotransport energized carriers of the kind already described above. In the absence of a Na^+ flux the reactions of these carriers are symmetrical. In the presence of a Na^+ flux the reactions are, as indicated, asymmetrical. As a consequence of this duality the cotransport energized system is the only one of the four which is not only capable of both uphill as well as downhill transport but which also does not have an absolute requirement to utilize bond energy in the downhill mode. The cotransport energized system is capable of adjusting energy use to energy need and is thus conservative. The ability of the intestine to absorb such enormous quantities of foodstuff as calculated above is what one might expect of an organ which evolved its functions under conditions of limited food supply where stress would be expected on developing a system with the ability to capture every last available molecule. Under the same conditions there would seem to be an advantage to a transport mechanism which did not waste this precious food in providing energy merely to satisfy the needs of the mechanism and not the needs of the work.

Summary

The following points can be reiterated in summary.

1. Sugar is absorbed in the form of monosaccharides by means of specific brush border membrane carriers which are in close functional proximity to the brush border digestive hydrolases or by means of an hydrolase-related direct translocation.

2. There is normally no advantage for absorption to provide sugar in the form of disaccharide.

3. The total capacity of the small intestine for sugar absorption is enormous.

4. The rate of carbohydrate absorption is controlled by negative feed-back to stomach emptying from sugar-specific osmoreceptors located in the upper intestine. The receptors are less responsive to fructose than to glucose.

5. The absorption of glucose and galactose can take place both up as well as down a concentration gradient from intestine to blood. The same carriers are used in both the downhill and the uphill modes.

6. The carriers for glucose and galactose are energized by the cotransport of Na^+ thus providing a possible advantage for energy conservation in that bond energy need not be consumed in the downhill mode.

Acknowledgments

The work of the author cited in this review was supported by grants from the National Science Foundation and the National Institute of Arthritis, Metabolism and Digestive Diseases.
Mr. R. Milton prepared the illustrations.

Literature Cited

1. Bloom, W. and Fawcett, D. W. "A Textbook of Histology", 9th Edition, pp. 560-568, W. B. Saunders Co., Philadelphia, 1968.
2. Forstner, G. and Wherrett, J. R. Biochim. Biophys. Acta. (1973) 306, 446-459.
3. Lindemann, B. and Solomon, A. K. J. Gen. Physiol. (1962) 45, 801-810.
4. Fordtran, J. S., Rector, F. C., Jr., Ewton, M. F., Soter, N. and Kinney, J. J. Clinical Invest. (1965) 44, 1935-1944.
5. Frömter, E. and Diamond, J. Nature New Biology (1972) 235, 9-13.
6. Crane, R. K. in Code, C. F. Editor "Handbook of Physiology, Section 6. Alimentary Canal, Volume 3. Intestinal Absorption," pp. 1323-1351, American Physiological Society, Washington, 1968.
7. Schultz, S. G. and Strecker, C. K. Biochim. Biophys. Acta. (1970) 211, 586-588.
8. Gracey, M., Burke, V. and Oshin, A. Biochim. Biophys. Acta. (1972) 266, 397-406.
9. Honegger, P. and Semenza, G. Biochim. Biophys. Acta. (1973) 318, 390-410.
10. Schultz, S. G. and Curran, P. F. Physiol. Revs. (1970) 50, 637-718.
11. Crane, R. K. Amer. J. Clinical Nutrition (1969) 22, 242-249.
12. Diamond, J. M. Federation Proc. (1971) 30, 6-13.
13. Crane, R. K. in M. Florkin and E. Stotz, Editors, "Comprehensive Biochemistry, Vol. 17, Carbohydrate Metabolism", pp. 1-14, Elsevier, Amsterdam, 1969.
14. Malathi, P., Ramaswamy, K., Caspary, W. F. and Crane, R. K. (1973) Biochim. Biophys. Acta. 307, 613-622.
15. Ramaswamy, K., Malathi, P., Caspary, W. F. and Crane, R. K. (1974) Biochim. Biophys. Acta. 345, 39-48.
16. Crane, R. K. in T. Z. Csaky, Editor, "Intestinal Absorption and Malabsorption", Raven, Press, New York, in press.
17. Messer, M. and Kerry, K. R. (1967) Biochim. Biophys. Acta. 132, 432-443.
18. Walker, G. J. and Whelan, W. J. (1960) Biochem. J. 76, 257-263.
19. Crane, R. K. in K. B. Warren, Editor, Symposia of the International Society for Cell Biology, Vol. 5, Intracellular Transport, pp. 71-102, Academic Press, New York, 1966.

20. Gray, G. M. and Santiago, N. A. (1966) Gastroenterology 51, 489-498.
21. Diedrich, D. F. and Hanke, D. W. in T. Z. Csaky, Editor, Intestinal Absorption and Malabsorption", Raven Press, New York, in press.
22. Chain, E. B., Mansford, K. R. L. and Pocchiari, F. (1960) J. Physiol. 154, 39-51.
23. MacDonald, I. and Turner, L. J. (1968) The Lancet 1, 841-843.
24. Cook, G. C. (1970) Clinical Sci. 38, 687-697.
25. Holdsworth, C. D. and Dawson, A. M. (1964) Clinical Sci. 27, 371-379.
26. Code, C. F., Bass, P., McClary, G. B., Jr., Newnum, R. L. and Orvis, A. L. (1960) Amer. J. Physiol. 199, 281-288.
27. MacDonald, J. M., Webster, M.M., Jr., Tennyson, C. H. and Drapanas, T. (1969) Amer. J. Surgery 117, 204-213.
28. Phillips, S. F. (1972) Gastroenterology 63, 495-518.
29. Hunt, J. N. and Knox, M. T. in Code, C. F., Editor, Handbook of Physiology, Section 6: Alimentary Canal, Vol. 4, Motility, pp. 1917-1935, American Physiological Society, Washington, 1968.
30. Bárány, E. and Sperber, E. (1939) Skand. Arch. Physiol. 81, 290-299.
31. Crane, R. K. (1960) Physiol. Revs. 40, 789-825.
32. Kaback, H. R. in Tosteson, D. C., Editor, The Molecular Basis of Membrane Function, pp. 421-444, Prentice-Hall, Inc., Englewood Cliffs, 1969.
33. Caldwell, P. C. in Bittar, E. E., Editor, Membranes and Ion Transport, Vol. 1, pp. 433-461, Wiley-Interscience, New York, 1970.

2

Metabolic Effects of Dietary Carbohydrates—A Review

SHELDON REISER

U.S. Department of Agriculture, ARS, Nutrition Institute,
Carbohydrate Nutrition Laboratory, Beltsville, Md. 20705

Many environmental changes have been characteristic of
societies described as "Western", "urbanized" or "affluent."
Among these changes are a decrease in physical activity, an
increase in mental stress and changes in dietary patterns. The
changes in dietary patterns of carbohydrate intake that have
been developing in the United States are shown in Figure 1 (1).
The share of total carbohydrate in the U.S. diet provided by
sugars as compared to starch has risen from about 32% around
the turn of the century until today sugars, predominantly
sucrose, contribute more than 50% of the total carbohydrate.
While the average per capita consumption of flours and cereals
has dropped from 300 lbs/year in 1909 to 141 lbs/year in 1970,
the consumption of refined sugar and other sweeteners has increased from 87 to 126 lbs/year (1,2). These are average
figures. Experts estimate that the sugar consumption by the
young, that is between 6-20 years of age, probably ranges from
140 to 150 lbs/year (2). The metabolic implications of high
sucrose intake in the young will be discussed later.
    These affluent societies are also characterized by an in-
crease in the incidence of heart disease and diabetes. Diabetes
and heart disease represent two of the most critical health problems in the U.S. today. Diabetes now affects about 5 million
Americans and results in over 35,000 deaths annually. By 1980,
it is estimated that more than 10% of all Americans will have
diabetes or the inherited trait of diabetes (3). One out of every four adults in the U.S. between 18-79 years of age has been
diagnosed as having or suspected of having heart disease (4). A
close relationship between heart disease and diabetes is indicated by the findings that diabetics have a much higher risk of
developing heart disease than the general population (5,6) and
that 25% or more of patients with vascular disease are diabetic
(7).
    One of the most intriguing aspects of this changing pattern
of carbohydrate consumption in urbanized cultures is the relationship between the increased intake of refined carbohydrates

such as sucrose and the etiology of various diseases. In recent years several controversial hypotheses have implicated·the increased ingestion of sucrose, as compared to the more complex carbohydrates, as an important factor in the etiology of coronary heart disease (8-10) and diabetes (10,11). It is recognized that many environmental factors, including dietary factors, as well as genetic factors influence these diseases and thus the unequivocal role of one of these factors independent of the others is difficult to evaluate. However, in view of the controversy surrounding dietary carbohydrate, it is the purpose of this review to describe some of the metabolic effects observed after feeding sucrose to experimental animals and man and to evaluate the relationship between these metabolic changes and the disease states.

An area of considerable controversy is the interpretation of retrospective or epidemiological studies that attempt to prove the increased incidence of a disease by correlation with the increased intake of a dietary constituent. Although retrospective studies do not permit definitive conclusions to be drawn as to the causal significance of the correlations detected, they are useful in identifying trends and in suggesting specific problem areas worthy of further study. Many retrospective studies have indicated a correlation between sucrose intake and heart disease (8,10,12-15), but I would like to concentrate primarily on the data gathered by an international cooperative study on the relationship between dietary factors and deaths from heart disease in 37 countries, published by Masironi in 1970 (16). Table 1 summarizes these results. Mortality data from heart disease (arteriosclerotic and degenerative) were taken from "World Health Statistics Annuals" and various age and sex groups were defined. Dietary data were taken from the "Food balance sheets" published by the Food and Agriculture Organization. From these correlation coefficients it can be seen that while sucrose is somewhat less strongly correlated with death rates than is fat, there is nonetheless a strong positive correlation. Since the intake of dietary calories, fat and sucrose are similarly correlated, these results are still open to various interpretations. Although on the average dietary sucrose comprises well over 50% of the simple sugars of the diet, it appears to be much more strongly correlated with heart disease deaths than the total of all the simple dietary sugars which also include lactose, fructose and glucose. This suggests that sucrose has a specific action on heart disease not shared by these other sugars. It is also apparent that a strong inverse relationship exists between the amount of complex carbohydrate in the diet and deaths from heart disease. This relationship supports the contention of Burkitt (17) and Trowell (18) that dietary fiber may exert an important preventative action against the incidence of heart disease.

The question then arises as to what metabolic properties of dietary sucrose or its component monosaccharides can mediate

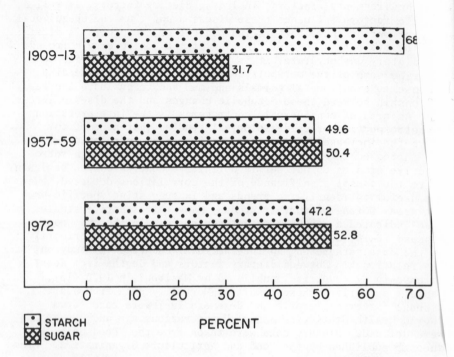

Figure I.   Carbohydrate from starch and sugar. Carbohydrate consumption in the
United States during the indicated years is based on food disappearing into consumption channels. Carbohydrate in foods such as milk, fruit, and sweeteners was
assumed to be present mainly as sugar, and carbohydrate in foods such as grain
products and vegetables was assumed to be present mainly as starch. Adapted from
Ref. 1.

Table 1

Correlation coefficients between death rates from heart disease and dietary factors for 37 countries during the 1960's

Age-sex	Total fat	Sucrose	Simple sugars	Complex carbohydrates
Males, 55-64 years	0.74	0.66	0.31	-0.74
Females, 55-64 years	0.55	0.64	0.33	-0.59
Males, 45-54 years	0.70	0.64	0.32	-0.71
Both sexes, all ages	0.84	0.56	0.24	-0.72
Both sexes, all ages (1940's-1950's)	0.70	0.75	0.52	-0.63

Adapted from (16)

Death rates per 100,000 population for arteriosclerotic and degenerative heart disease were taken from "World Health Statistics Annuals" (World Health Organization, 1958, 1968) and the various groups defined by age and sex. Dietary data were taken in from "Food balance sheets" published by the Food and Agriculture Organization (1949, 1966).

an increased incidence of vascular complications, heart disease
and diabetes. Since a fundamental difference between dietary
starch and sucrose resides in the nature of the monosaccharide
units comprising the respective molecules, much of the interest
in dietary sucrose has focused on the metabolic effects of
fructose. Studies with humans and experimental animals have
established that diets containing sucrose or fructose produce
larger increases in blood lipids (19-23), especially the triglyceride fraction (24-28), and in hepatic lipogenic enzymes
(29-35) than diets containing an equivalent amount of glucose
or glucose polymers. The magnitude and duration of the hyperlipemia is controlled by factors such as amount of sugar fed,
age and sex of the subject, the nature of the other dietary
ingredients and genetic predisposition. Younger subjects and
premenopausal females show less increase than older subjects
and males (25,26). An important factor in this sucrose effect
appears to be the amount and nature of the dietary fat. On low
fat diets, i.e., less than 5%, the increase in triglyceride
synthesis from carbohydrate is a necessary and expected physiological process. Table 2, adapted from the work of Macdonald
(36), shows that when young men were fed a diet containing 60%
carbohydrate, 30% fat and 9% protein for 5 days, the magnitude
of the triglyceridemia was dependent on the nature of both the
carbohydrate and the fat. Sucrose significantly increased
blood triglycerides only when the dietary fat was cream and
not when it was sunflower oil. In contrast, glucose did not
increase the triglycerides with either fat. The effect of
sunflower oil may be due to acceleration in the removal of
endogenous triglycerides since Nestel and Barter (37) have
shown that subjects consuming diets rich in polyunsaturated
fat have faster clearance rates than subjects fed saturated
fat. These results also might explain apparent contradictions
found in the literature as to the effect of dietary sucrose on
serum lipids in that unsaturated fatty acids may mask this
effect. Work from Yudkin's laboratory (Table 3, (38)) shows
that sucrose produces a larger increase in serum triglycerides
and cholesterol than does starch in rats fed an atherogenic
diet containing 16% hydrogenated coconut oil and 1% cholesterol
for 100 days. The carbohydrate comprised 47% of the diet. By
180 days, the levels of the blood lipids had fallen, but there
was still the same relative increase in cholesterol and triglyceride levels produced by the sucrose as compared to starch.
These results again indicate that sucrose together with other
dietary factors can produce a combination that is potentially
more detrimental to the health of the consumer than either of
the factors alone.

The major effect of dietary sucrose on lipid metabolism
involves the triglycerides. The risk factor involved in elevated levels of blood triglyceride has recently been confirmed
by a joint statement on Diet and Coronary Disease from the

Table 2

Effect of dietary carbohydrate and lipid on fasting blood triglycerides in young men after 5 days on diet

Diet	Triglycerides
	mg/100 ml
Control	78 ± 5 $P < 0.025$
Sucrose-cream	95 ± 6
Sucrose-sunflower oil	69 ± 4
Glucose-cream	71 ± 9
Glucose-sunflower oil	75 ± 7

Adapted from (36)

The diets contained approximately 9% of the calories as protein (calcium caseinate), 60% of the calories as carbohydrate (either sucrose or glucose) and 30% of the calories as fat (either cream or sunflower oil). Each value represents the mean $\pm$ S.E.M. from 5 subjects.

Table 3

Effect of an atherogenic diet containing starch or sucrose on blood lipids in rats

Duration of experiment	Carbohydrate	Triglycerides		Cholesterol	
days		mg/100 ml		mg/100 ml	
100	starch	144		577	
	sucrose	262	P < 0.001	787	P < 0.02
180	starch	114		392	
	sucrose	195	P < 0.001	517	P < 0.001

Adapted from (38)

Adult rats were fed a diet consisting of 47 parts carbohydrate (either starch or sucrose), 25 parts casein, 16 parts hydrogenated coconut oil, 5 parts mineral salts, 5 parts cellulose, vitamins, 1 part cholesterol and 1 part cholic acid. Each value represents the mean values from at least 4 rats.

National Academy of Science, National Research Council and the
American Medical Association Councils on Food and Nutrition
(39). In addition a recent prospective study of the occurrence
of new events of heart disease in 3000 Scandinavian men showed
that a high fasting plasma triglyceride level was as important
a risk factor as a high cholesterol level and was independent
of the level of plasma cholesterol (40). The physiological
significance of some of the studies relating sucrose intake
to increased triglycerides has been questioned because of the
comparatively large quantities of sucrose used. Table 4,
adapted from work by Mukherjee and coworkers (41), shows that
on diets containing refined sugar at levels consistent with
those consumed in many areas of the world, i.e., 12%, but
lower than the sucrose levels in the U.S. diet, sucrose, as
compared to starch or glucose, increased the levels of blood
triglyceride, blood cholesterol and liver triglyceride in rats
after 30 days. Fructose acted similarly to sucrose but failed
to increase blood cholesterol levels. Glucose, as compared
with starch, tended to decrease triglyceride levels and increase cholesterol levels. While efforts to show similar
effects of low levels of dietary sucrose on triglyceride levels
in humans have not been equally successful (42), it has been
consistently shown that when there is a greatly reduced dietary
intake of sucrose by humans, triglyceride levels decrease (43-
45). The fall in serum triglyceride is greater for those
subjects with higher initial levels than for those with lower
initial levels.

The importance of the increase in blood triglycerides by
dietary sucrose has been questioned because, in many cases, the
effect is only transitory and, after a period of adaptation,
triglycerides return to normal (46). In general, these events
can be explained on the basis that dietary fructose or sucrose
induces an increase in liver lipogenesis so that the influx of
triglycerides into the plasma exceeds the removal capacity.
Contributing to this triglyceridemia is the decreased activity
of adipose tissue lipoprotein lipase or clearing factor observed
after the feeding of sucrose or fructose as compared to glucose
(27). This adaptation still involves an increased throughput
of dietary sucrose as triglyceride in the normal person with
the potential danger that a defect or breakdown in this adaptation might produce triglyceridemia. More important, there
are segments of the population that appear to have a genetic
predisposition that results in an inability to adapt to changes
in dietary carbohydrate and who show a large and permanent increase in blood triglycerides as a result of an increase in the
intake of sucrose. This type of hyperlipemia has been described
as carbohydrate-induced or Type IV by Fredrickson, Levy and
Lees (47). Carbohydrate-induced hyperlipemia has been shown
to be associated with abnormal glucose tolerance, diabetes and
heart disease. Wood et al., (48) have estimated that 8.6% of

Table 4

Effect of dietary sugars on serum and liver lipids in rats

Dietary carbohydrate	Serum triglyceride	Serum cholesterol	Liver triglyceride
	mg/100 ml	mg/100 ml	mg/g
64% starch	59.4 $\pm$ 2.5	37.0 $\pm$ 1.7	11.80 $\pm$ 0.07
12% glucose 52% starch	25.5 $\pm$ 4.3	46.3 $\pm$ 1.4	8.30 $\pm$ 1.91
12% fructose 52% starch	97.2 $\pm$ 1.7	43.2 $\pm$ 5.3	20.30 $\pm$ 0.25
12% sucrose 52% starch	95.0 $\pm$ 1.8	98.7 $\pm$ 6.9	15.80 $\pm$ 0.50

Adapted from (41)

Each value represents the average of 8 experiments carried out in duplicate $\pm$ S.E.M.

free-living volunteers in California, aged 25-79, showed the
Type IV lipoproteinemia pattern, 4.8% in women and 13% in men.
Numerous studies have demonstrated that in patients with
carbohydrate-induced lipemia, sucrose produced much larger
increases in blood triglycerides than starch (49-56). Figure
II summarizes studies from Kuo's laboratory (54) on the effect
of dietary sucrose on the levels of blood triglycerides in Type
IV hyperlipemic patients. A self-selected diet produced a
marked triglyceridemia, 120 mg/100 ml being considered about
normal. A diet containing the 60% carbohydrate primarily as
sucrose increased the triglycerides further while a 60% starch
diet dramatically lowered the triglycerides. Each dietary
period was of 3 weeks duration. Table 5, adapted from the
work of Little and Antar (55,56), shows the pattern of blood
triglycerides in patients with either Type II (fat sensitive)
or Type III, IV and V lipemias as a function of the nature of
the dietary carbohydrate, starch or sucrose, and the nature of
fat, saturated or unsaturated. The Type III, IV and V patients
exhibited higher levels of triglycerides, characteristic of
these types of lipemias, and showed a much larger increase in
triglyceride due to sucrose than the Type II patients. In
contrast to the sucrose-induced increase of triglycerides in
normal subjects, the nature of the fat, saturated or unsaturated,
did not effect the magnitude of the sucrose increase. However,
the blood triglyceride levels were lower in diets containing
unsaturated than in those containing saturated fats. From these
results it is apparent that dietary sucrose is an important environmental factor in the expression of carbohydrate-sensitivity
in genetically susceptible subjects.

In order to determine the primary biochemical defect characterizing the interaction between diet and genetic expression,
the carbohydrate-sensitive BHE[a] strain of rat has been used
extensively by scientists at the Nutrition Institrue of the U.S.
Department of Agriculture (57-71). BHE rats have been shown to
gain more body weight and accumulate more carcass and liver lipid
(60,61,63,66), have increased activities of hepatic lipogenic
enzymes (64,71) and have higher levels of blood lipids (63,71)
than other strains of rats fed the same high carbohydrate diet.
Studies by Berdanier and coworkers (68) have demonstrated that
the BHE rat exhibits a marked hyperinsulinemia early in life as
compared to similarly fed Wistar rats (Figure III). Fifty days
of age corresponds to about 5-7 years of age in a human. By
100 days of age the insulin levels had decreased dramatically.
The importance of this early hyperinsulinemia was confirmed by
tests with other rat strains. Wistar rats made hyperinsulinemic

---

[a] The BHE strain results from a cross between the Pennsylvania
State College strain and the Osborne-Mendel (also called Yale)
strains. BHE animals are currently available from Flow
Laboratories, Dublin, Virginia.

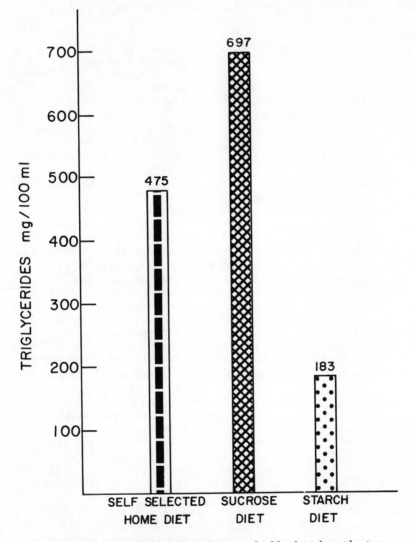

Figure II.   Effect of dietary carbohydrate on the blood triglycerides in type IV hyperlipemia patients. Each value represents the mean serum triglyceride level observed in six hyperglyceridemic patients during the consumption of a home diet and when an equivalent amount of carbohydrate was supplied primarily as sucrose or starch. Adapted from Ref. 54.

Table 5

Blood triglycerides in Type II and Type III, IV and V hyperlipemia patients as a function of the nature of the dietary carbohydrate and fat

Patient	Fat	Carbohydrate	Blood triglyceride (mg/100 ml)	sucrose increase %
Type II	saturated	starch	109	
		sucrose	123	13
Type III, IV and V	saturated	starch	251	
		sucrose	392	51
Type III, IV and V	unsaturated	starch	190	
		sucrose	324	70

Adapted from (55, 56)

The hyperlipemic patients were classified as to Type according to Fredrickson et al. (47). Each value represents the mean from at least 5 patients.

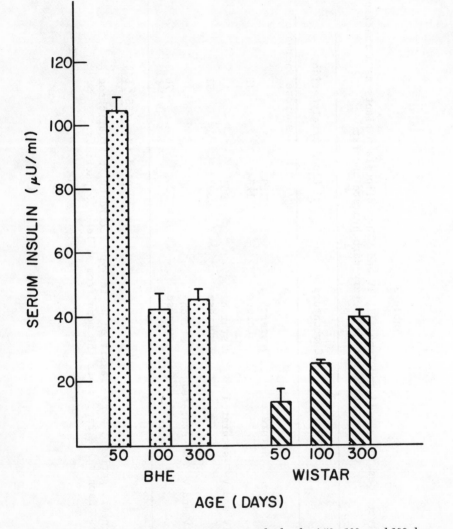

Figure III. Fasting serum immunoreactive insulin levels of 50-, 100-, and 300-day old BHE and Wistar rats. Each value represents the mean and the S.E.M. from at least 10 rats. Adapted from Ref. 68.

at an early age by the injection of insulin or by feeding tol-
butamide, developed a pattern of increased hepatic lipogenic
enzyme activity similar to that observed in BHE rats. It was
also found that feeding sucrose to the BHE rats from weanling
to 50 days of age appeared to exert long-lasting metabolic
effects on parameters such as serum lipids and insulin even
after the sugar had not been fed for 100 days (72). These
findings taken together with the pattern of very high sucrose
intake by the young suggest that the conditions for the induction of the metabolism characterizing carbohydrate-sensitivity
is optimal at an early age. Figure IV shows that adipose tissue
from BHE rats exhibited a much smaller sensitivity to insulin,
as measured by CO_2 release from glucose, than did adipose from
Wistar rats (73). With increasing age, tissue sensitivity of
both strains was reduced but the strain difference persisted.
These results suggest that the hyperinsulinemia observed in the
BHE rat occurs as a consequence of the reduced tissue sensitivity
to insulin and that normalization of serum insulin levels may
represent a gradual depletion of pancreatic insulin stores.
This conclusion was supported by finding that at 50 days the
pancreas from BHE rats contained slightly more total insulin
than Wistar rats but at 150 days this situation was reversed
(73). In a related study, Vrána and coworkers (74) demonstrated
a decreased adipose tissue sensitivity of sucrose-fed as compared
to starch-fed Wistar rats (Table 6). These results show that
while insulin did not significantly increase glucose incorporation into lipid in the sucrose-fed rats even at 1000 μUnits
insulin/ml, starch-fed rats incorporated 2.7 times as much
glucose into lipid due to insulin. Rats fed equal amounts of
starch and sucrose gave intermediate insulin responses.

    Longitudinal studies of the events resulting from the
carbohydrate sensitivity have shown that BHE rats developed
a glucose intolerance as a function of age and at 425 days of
age showed symptoms of arteriosclerosis of the coronary vessels
(71). Therefore, the relationship between heart disease and
diabetes might be attributed to a common metabolic defect that
produces a hyperinsulinemic response to a sucrose stress,
especially in those individuals genetically predisposed toward
carbohydrate sensitivity. In this connection it has been reported that high sucrose intake produced hyperinsulinism in
about 1/3 of the human subjects tested and that the increase
was greater in patients with peripheral vascular disease than
in normal subjects (75).

    Many of the findings relating dietary sucrose to diabetes
have come from the work of Dr. Aharon Cohen in Israel (10,33,51
76-90). Retrospective studies linking diabetes to sucrose have
been based on the emergence of diabetes as a serious health
problem in specific ethnic groups that have recently undergone
changes in their traditional dietary patterns characterized by
an increased intake of refined carbohydrate at the expense of

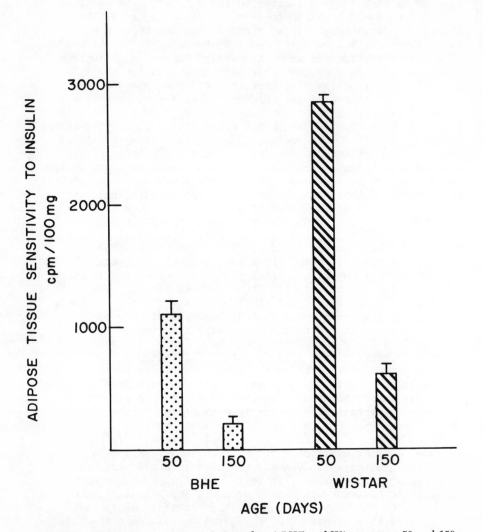

Figure IV.   Adipose tissue sensitivity to insulin of BHE and Wistar rats at 50 and 150 days of age. Tissue sensitivity is expressed as the difference in counts per minute between the basal- and insulin-stimulated CO_2 release from radioactive glucose by slices of epididyml fat pads. Each value represents the mean ± S.E.M from 24 rats. Adapted from Ref. 73.

Table 6

Effect of dietary sucrose on the insulin sensitivity of rat adipose tissue as measured
by incorporation of glucose into lipid

| Dietary Carbohydrate | Insulin concentration (μUnits/ml) | | |
| | 0 | 1000 | insulin increase |
	cpm/mg protein		
Starch	2371	6290	2.7
Starch + sucrose	1905	3640	1.9
Sucrose	2019	2240	1.1

Adapted from (74)

Adult rats were fed diets containing 20% calories as protein, 10% calories as fat
and 70% calories as carbohydrate, either starch and/or sucrose as indicated. Each
value represents the mean values from 6 rats.

crude, unrefined carbohydrate (11). These retrospective studies
are typified by results obtained with the Yemenite Jews. In a
survey of the prevalence of diabetes in Israel during 1958-1959
it was found that of the 5000 Yemenites examined who had been
living in Israel for less than 10 years, only 3 cases of diabetes were found (76). In contrast, among Yemenites who had
lived in Israel for more than 25 years the incidence of diabetes was 2.9%, or even more than that of Jews coming from
Western countries. On analyzing the different environmental
factors that might have caused this increase, the daily dietary
patterns of the Yemenites in Yemen and in Israel were compared
(Table 7) (10). The total caloric intake was only slightly
less in the Yemen than in Israel. Two outstanding differences
in the type of food consumed were apparent. First, in the
Yemen the fats consumed were mainly of animal origin. Vegetable
oil was rarely used. In Israel the settled Yemenites consumed
similar amounts of total animal fat together with margarine
and, in addition, about 30 grams of vegetable oil. Second,
in the Yemen the carbohydrate consumed was mainly starch with
almost no sucrose used. In Israel there was a tenfold increase
in dietary sucrose. It was concluded, therefore, that if diet
were an environmental factor in the etiology of diabetes in
this ethnic group, the most likely dietary suspect was sucrose.

The hypothesis that sucrose is an etiological factor in
diabetes has been tested in genetically selected rats (84).
These rats were bred on the basis of glucose tolerance tests.
Animals showing the highest rise in blood sugar, called the
"Upward selection," were mated and rats with the lowest rise
in blood glucose values, or "Downward selection," were mated.
The blood glucose values of these animals 60 minutes after an
intragastric glucose load in both the Upward and Downward
selected lines, as a function of generation and dietary carb-
hydrate, are shown in Figure V (89). In succeeding generations
of the Upward line fed sucrose the level of blood glucose rose
to high values and a considerable number of the animals developed a diabetic-like syndrome with high fasting blood glucose
and spontaneous glucosuria. This effect could be shown with
as little as 25% of the dietary carbohydrate as sucrose. In
contrast, the sibling Upward strain fed starch did not show a
rise in blood glucose. In the offspring of the Downward selected line, blood glucose did not rise in rats fed either the
sucrose or the starch diet. The diabetes appearing in the
sucrose-fed Upward selected line showed other symptoms of human
adult-onset diabetes such as initial increased fasting plasma
insulin levels, peripheral insulin resistance and retinal and
renal vascular complications (89). These results show the need
for interaction between genetic and dietary factors for the
expression of the diabetic syndrome to become evident.

A prominent explanation for the increased diabetogenic and
lipogenic capacity of dietary sucrose as opposed to dietary

Table 7

Daily food intake pattern of Yemenites living in Yemen as compared to Yemenites living in Israel

Groups	Calories	Protein	Fat		Carbohydrates	
			Animal + Margarine	Oil	Total	Sucrose
		g	g	g	g	g
Yemenites; new immigrants	2237	80	43	14	351	6
Yemenites; old settlers	2559	86	51	30	372	63

Adapted from (10)

Each value represents the average daily food intake from 20 families.

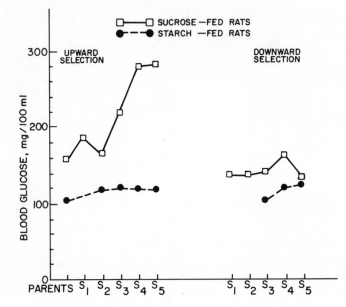

Figure V. Blood glucose values at 60 minutes after a gastric glucose load in genetically selected sucrose- and starch-fed rats. The Upward selection represents the progeny resulting from the mating of males and females with highest blood glucose values following a glucose tolerance test. The Downward selection represents the progeny resulting from the mating of males and females with the lowest blood glucose values following a glucose tolerance test. Each rat was given an intragastric glucose load of 350 mg/100 g body weight. Each point represents the mean from at least 12 rats. Adapted from Ref. 89.

starch is based on differences in the rates of intestinal
digestion and absorption of the component monosaccharides
(78,81,91,92). The feeding of diets high in sucrose has been
shown to produce an adaptive increase in the activity of intestinal sucrase (93-96) while starch feeding does not appear to
influence the activity or rate of release of pancreatic amylase.
A more rapid and efficient absorption of glucose from sucrose-
fed than from starch-fed subjects, as already suggested by work
from Crane's laboratory (97,98), would produce increases in
postprandial blood glucose with a resulting strong stimulation
of the insulin response. Such stimulation, when repeated,
might produce a chronic hyperinsulinemia which eventually
could impair the insulin producing system and produce diabetic-
like symptoms. The initial period of chronic hyperinsulinemia
could signal a pattern of enzyme inductions which could direct
the pathways of carbohydrate metabolism toward increased lipogenesis, thus explaining the increased activity of the lipogenic
enzymes found after sucrose feeding. In addition to these
factors, fructose metabolism in the liver may also contribute
to a reduced glucose tolerance in sucrose-fed animals by increasing the levels of glucose 6-phosphatase activity (33).
This enzyme is required to form blood glucose. Fructose-fed
rats have also shown deficient hepatic utilization of glucose
(99).

If dietary sucrose is an etiological factor in any disease,
an understanding of the specific metabolic characteristics of
fructose may provide information as to the mechanisms that may
be involved. There are marked differences in the metabolism
of absorbed fructose in the small intestines of various species.
These differences appear to be of fundamental importance in
determining the subsequent metabolic fate of fructose. In the
rat (100) and in man (101) fructose is poorly metabolized and
appears in the portal blood primarily as fructose together with
a small amount of lactate. In contrast, in the small intestine
of the guinea pig fructose is mainly converted to glucose (102).
The physiological importance of this difference in intestinal
metabolism can be seen in the failure of fructose feeding to
induce hypertriglyceridemia in guinea pigs as it does in rats
and man (27). It is, therefore, possible to correlate the
hypertriglyceridemic effect of fructose feeding with the
appearance of unchanged fructose in the circulation. Studies
using both humans (103) and rats (104) have shown that fructose
infusion results in a dramatic decrease of hepatic adenine
nucleotides, especially ATP. Glucose infusion did not produce
comparable decreases in the nucleotide levels (103). These
results suggest that fructose may act as an "ATP sink" in the
liver. Since the clearing of blood triglycerides by the liver
has been reported to be an active process (46,105), a decreased
level of hepatic ATP may prevent normal clearing (106) thereby
contributing to increased levels of blood triglycerides. The

fatty livers found in sucrose-fed rats could also be explained on the basis of a decreased ATP-dependent synthesis of the phospholipids required to mobilize liver lipid.

In Conclusion: During this review, the metabolic effects of dietary sucrose reported by numerous investigators and the implications of these results as they pertain to the health and well-being of humans and experimental animals have been described. In some studies, particularly with humans, these effects have not been consistently observed or when observed have been interpreted differently. However, the results of the studies described in this review are consistent with the following: (1) Although sucrose alone has not as yet been shown to be an important risk factor in the etiology of heart disease and diabetes in the majority of the population, sucrose together with other environmental factors may produce a combination that is more lipogenic or diabetogenic than any of the factors alone. (2) Sucrose alone may be a very important etiological factor in heart disease and diabetes in that segment of the population described as "carbohydrate sensitive." It is apparent that much more work on this problem is required, especially in early identification of carbohydrate-sensitive individuals. These findings, however, indicate that a reversal of the present trend of increased consumption of refined sugar to an increased consumption of the more complex and natural forms of carbohydrates should be encouraged.

Questions:

Q. Did the Yemenites have different dietary fiber intake in Yemen and in Israel?

A. Since the daily carbohydrate intake of the Yemenites was very similar in the Yemen and in Israel and since the sucrose intake had increased so dramatically in Israel, it is safe to assume that the intake of dietary fiber was less in Israel than in the Yemen. However, actual fiber contents in these diets were not reported.

Q. Are there studies currently underway to identify carbohydrate-sensitive individuals?

A. We are currently trying to fund a cooperative study with Dr. Cohen in Israel that we believe can establish parameters for the identification of carbohydrate-sensitivity. These studies are a continuation of the survey of the Yemenites who migrated to Israel prior to 1958 and who exhibited practically no diabetes at that time. We plan to measure various blood hormones and blood lipids in a sample of this population and to correlate the levels of these parameters with the incidence of symptoms of diabetes and heart disease, the level of dietary sugar and the familial clustering of the subjects. We hope to determine whether the affected individuals will have had a high intake of sugar, whether they were genetically related and whether they showed specific increases in the blood parameters tested.

Literature Cited:
1. Page, L. & Friend, B. "Sugars in Nutrition," edited by
    Sipple, H. & McNutt, J., p. 93. Nutrition Foundation
    Monograph Series, Academic Press, New York, 1974.
2. "Hearings before the Select Committee on Nutrition and
    Human Needs of the United States Senate, Part 2 - Sugar
    in diet, diabetes and heart diseases," p. 147, U.S.
    Government Printing Office, Washington, D.C., 1973.
3. "Hearings before the Select Committee on Nutrition and
    Human Needs of the United States Senate, Part 2 - Sugar in
    diet, diabetes and heart diseases," p. 146, U.S. Government
    Printing Office, Washington, D.C., 1973.
4. Weir, C. E., "An Evaluation of Research in the United
    States on Human Nutrition, Report No. 2, Benefits from
    Nutrition Research," p. 16, U.S. Department of Agriculture,
    Washington, D.C., 1971.
5. Ostrander, L. D., "Early Diabetes," edited by Camerini-
    Davalos, R. & Cole, H. S., p.365, Academic Press, New York,
    1970.
6. Keen, H., "Early Diabetes," edited by Camerini-Davalos, R.
    & Cole, H. S., p. 437, Academic Press, New York, 1970.
7. Wahlberg, F. & Thomasson, B., "Carbohydrate Metabolism and
    its Disorders," Vol. 2, edited by Dickens, E., Whelan,
    J. J. & Randle, P. J., p. 188, Academic Press, New York,
    1968.
8. Yudkin, J., Lancet, (1957), ii, 155.
9. Michaels, L., Brit. Heart J., (1966), 28, 258.
10. Cohen, A. M., Bavly, S. & Poznanski, R., Lancet, (1966),
    ii, 1399.
11. Cleave, T. L. & Campbell, G. D., "Diabetes, Coronary
    Thrombosis, and the Saccharine Disease," p. 15, John Wright
    & Sons, Ltd., Bristol, 1969.
12. Antar, M. A., Ohlson, M. A. & Hodges, R. E., Am. J. Clin.
    Nutr., (1964), 14, 169.
13. Osancova, K., Hejda, S. & Zvolankova, K., Lancet, (1965),
    i, 494.
14. Lopez, A., Krehl, W. A., Hodges, R. E. & Good, E. I., Am.
    J. Clin. Nutr., (1966), 19, 361.
15. Yudkin, J. & Morland, J., Am. J. Clin. Nutr., (1967), 20,
    503.
16. Masironi, R., Bull. Wld. Hlth. Org., (1970), 42, 103.
17. Burkitt, D. P., Walker, A. R. P. & Painter, N. S., JAMA,
    (1974), 229,1068.
18. Trowell, H., Am. J. Clin. Nutr., (1973), 25, 926.
19. Winitz, M., Graff, J. & Sudman, D. A., Arch. Biochem.
    Biophys., (1964), 108, 576.
20. Hodges, R. E. & Krehl, W. A., Am. J. Clin. Nutr., (1965),
    17, 334.
21. Macdonald, I. & Roberts, J. B., Metabolism, (1965), 14, 991.

22. Dalderup, L. M., Nesser, W. & Keller, A. H. M., Voeding, (1968), 29, 245.
23. Naismith, D. J., "Sugar. Chemical, Biological and Nutritional Aspects of Sucrose," edited by Yudkin, J., Edelman, J. & Haugh, L., p. 123, Butterworth's, London, 1971.
24. Macdonald, I. & Braithwaite, D. M., Clin. Sci., (1964), 27, 23.
25. Macdonald, I., Clin. Sci., (1965), 29, 193.
26. Macdonald, I., Am. J. Clin. Nutr., (1966), 18, 369.
27. Bar-On, H. & Stein, Y., J. Nutr., (1968), 94, 95.
28. Szanto, S. & Yudkin, J., Postgrad. Med. J., (1969), 45, 602.
29. Nikkila, E. A. & Ojala, K., Life Sci., (1965), 4, 937.
30. Fábry, P., Poledrie, R., Kazdová, L. & Braun, T., Nutr. Diet., (1968), 10, 81.
31. Naismith, D. J., Proc. Nutr. Soc., (1971), 30, 259.
32. Pereira, J. N. & Jangaard, N., Metabolism, (1971), 20, 392.
33. Cohen, A., Briller, S. & Shafrir, E., Biochim. Biophys. Acts, (1972), 279, 129.
34. Chevalier, M. M., Wiley, J. H. & Leveille, G. A., J. Nutr. (1972), 102, 337.
35. Michaelis, O. E., IV & Szepesi, B., J. Nutr., (1973), 103, 697.
36. Macdonald, I., Am. J. Clin. Nutr., (1967), 20, 345.
37. Nestel, P. J. & Barter, P. J., Am. J. Clin. Nutr., (1973), 241.
38. Qureshi, R. U., Akinyanju, P. A. & Yudkin, J. Nutr. Metabol., (1970), 12, 347.
39. Nutr. Reviews, (1972), 30, 223.
40. Carlson, L. A. & Böttiger, L. E., Lancet, (1972), i, 865.
41. Mukherjee, S., Basu, M. & Trivedi, K., J. Atheroscler Res. (1969), 10, 261.
42. Truswell, A. S., "Sugar and Human Health," edited by Stewart, S. C., p. 50, The International Sugar Research Foundation, Bethesda, Md., 1972.
43. Rifkind, B. M., Lawson, D. H. & Gale, M., Lancet, (1966), ii, 1379.
44. Mann, J. I., Truswell, A. S., Hendricks, D. A. & Manning, E., Lancet, (1970), i, 870.
45. Roberts, A. M., Proc. Nutr. Soc., (1971), 30, 71A.
46. Ahrens, R. A., Am. J. Clin. Nutr., (1974), 27, 403.
47. Fredrickson, D. S., Levy, R. I. & Lees, R. S., New Eng. J. Med., (1967), 276, 34, 94, 148, 215, 273.
48. Wood, P. D. S., Stern, M. P., Silver, A., Reaven, G. M. & von der Groeben, J., Circulation, (1972), XLV, 114.
49. Kaufmann, N. A., Gutman, A., Barzilai, D., Eshchar, J., Blondheim, S. H. & Stein, Y., Israel J. Med. Sci., (1965), 1, 389.

50. Kuo, P. T. & Bassett, D. R., Ann. Intern. Med., (1965), 62, 1199.
51. Cohen, A. M., Kaufmann, N. A. & Poznanski, R., Brit. Med. J., (1966), 1, 339.
52. Kaufmann, N. A., Poznanski, R., Blondheim, S. H. & Stein, Y., Am. J. Clin. Nutr., (1966), 18, 261.
53. Kaufmann, N. A., Poznanski, R., Blondheim, S. H. & Stein, Y., Israel J. Med. Sci., (1966), 2, 715.
54. Kuo, P. T., Feng, L., Cohen, N. N., Fitts, W. T., Jr. & Miller, L. D., Am. J. Clin. Nutr., (1967), 20, 116.
55. Little, J. A., Birchwood, B. L., Simmons, D. A., Antar, M. A., Kallos, A., Buckley, G. C. & Csima, A. Atherosclerosis, (1970), 11, 173.
56. Antar, M. A., Little, J. A., Lucas, C., Buckley, G. C. & Csima, A., Atherosclerosis, (1970), 11, 191.
57. Marshall, M. W. & Womack, M., J. Nutr., (1954), 52, 51.
58. Womack, M. & Marshall, M. W., J. Nutr., (1955), 57, 193.
59. Marshall, M. W., Hildebrand, H. W., Dupont, J. L. & Womack, M., J. Nutr., (1959), 69, 371.
60. Marshall, M. W. & Hildebrand, H. E., J. Nutr., (1963), 79, 227.
61. Adams, M., Home Econ. Res. Rept., No. 24, USDA, (1964).
62. Durand, A. M. A., Fisher, M. & Adams, M., Arch. Path., (1964), 77, 268.
63. Taylor, D. C., Conway, E. S., Schuster, E. M. & Adams, M., J. Nutr., (1967), 91, 275.
64. Chang, M. L. W., Schuster, E. M., Lee, J. A., Snodgrass, C. & Benton, D. A., J. Nutr., (1968), 96, 368.
65. Durand, A. M. A., Fisher, M. & Adams, M., Arch. Path. (1968), 85, 318.
66. Marshall, M. W., Womack, M., Hildebrand, H. & Munson, A. W., Proc. Soc. Exp. Biol. Med., (1969), 132, 227.
67. Berdanier, C. D., Szepesi, B., Moser, P. & Diachenko, S., Proc. Soc. Exp. Biol. Med., (1971), 137, 668.
68. Berdanier, C. D., Marshall, M. W. & Moser, P., Life Sci., (1971), 10, 105.
69. Marshall, M. W., Durand, A. M. A. & Adams, M., Fourth International Symposium of ICLA., p. 383. Nat. Acad. Sci., Washington, D. C., 1971.
70. Chang, M. L. W., Lee, J. A. & Simmons, N., Proc. Soc. Exp. Biol. Med., (1971), 138, 742.
71. Berdanier, C. D., J. Nutr., (1974), 104, 1246.
72. Moser, P. B. & Berdanier, C. D., J. Nutr., (1974), 104, 687.
73. Berdanier, C. D., Diabetologia, (1974), 10, 1.
74. Vrána, A., Slabochová, Z., Kazdova, L. & Fábry, P., Nutr. Rep. Int., (1971), 3, 31.
75. Yudkin, J., Szanto, S. & Kakkar, V. V., Postgrad. Med. J., (1969), 45, 608.
76. Cohen, A. M., Metabolism, (1961), 10, 50.
77. Cohen, A. M., Am. Heart J., (1963), 65, 291.

78. Cohen, A. M. & Teitelbaum, A., Am. J. Physiol., (1964), 206, 105.
79. Cohen, A. M., Teitelbaum, A., Balogh, M. & Groen, J. J., Am. J. Clin. Nutr., (1966), 19, 59.
80. Cohen, A. M., Am. J. Clin. Nutr., (1967), 20, 126.
81. Cohen, A. M., Life Sci., (1968), 7, 23.
82. Cohen, A. M. & Rosenmann, E., Diabetologia, (1971), 7, 25.
83. Rosenmann, E., Teitelbaum, A. & Cohen, A. M., Diabetes, (1971), 20, 803.
84. Cohen, A. M., Teitelbaum, A. & Saliternik, R., Metabolism, (1972), 21, 235.
85. Yanko, L., Michaelson, I. C. & Cohen, A. M., Israel J. Med. Sci., (1972), 8, 1633.
86. Cohen, A. M., Acta Med. Scand. Suppl., (1972), 542, 173.
87. Cohen, A. M., Michaelson, I. C. & Yanko, L., Am. J. Ophth., (1972), 73, 863.
88. Shafrir, E., Teitelbaum, A. & Cohen, A. M., Israel J. Med. Sci., (1972), 8, 990.
89. Cohen, A. M., "Hearings before the Select Committee on Nutrition and Human Needs of the United States Senate, Part 2 - Sugar in diet, diabetes and heart diseases," p. 167, U.S. Government Printing Office, Washington, D.C. 1973.
90. Rosenmann, E., Palti, Z., Teitelbaum, A. & Cohen, A. M., Metabolism, (1974), 23, 343.
91. Crossley, J. N. & Macdonald, I., Nutr. Metabol., (1970), 12, 171.
92. Jourdan, M. H., Nutr. Metabol., (1972), 14, 28.
93. Blair, D. G., Yakimets, W. & Tuba, J., Can. J. Biochem. Physiol., (1963), 41, 917.
94. Deren, J. & Zamcheck, N., Fed. Proc., (1965), 24, 203.
95. Deren, J. J., Broitman, S. A. & Zamcheck, N., J. Clin. Invest., (1967), 46, 186.
96. Reddy, B. S., Pleasants, J. R. & Wostmann, B. S., J. Nutr., (1968), 95, 413.
97. Malathi, P., Ramaswamy, K., Caspary, W. F. & Crane, R. K., Biochim. Biophys. Acta, (1973), 307, 613.
98. Ramaswamy, K., Malathi, P., Caspary, W. F & Crane, R. K., Biochim. Biophys. Acta, (1974), 345, 39.
99. Hill, R., Baker, N. & Chaikoff, I. L., J. Biol. Chem., (1954), 209, 705.
100. Mavrias, D. A. & Mayer, R. J., Biochim. Biophys. Acta, (1973), 291, 531.
101. Cook, G. C., Clin. Sci., (1969), 37, 675.
102. Mavrias, D. A. & Mayer, R. J., Biochim. Biophys. Acta, (1973), 291, 538.
103. Bode, C., Schumacher, H., Goebell, H., Zelder, O. & Pelzel, H., Hormone Metab. Res., (1971), 3, 289.
104. Woods, H. F., Eggleston, L. V. & Krebs, H. A., Biochem. J., (1970), 119, 501.

105. Havel, R. J., Proceedings of the Second International
     Symposium on Atherosclerosis, p. 210, edited by Jones,
     R. J., New York, Springer Verlag, 1970.
106. Schotz, M. C., Arnesjö, B. & Olivecrona, T., Biochim.
     Biophys. Acta, (1966), 125, 485.

3

Factors Influencing Adipose Tissue Response to Food Carbohydrates[1]

DALE R. ROMSOS and GILBERT A. LEVEILLE

Food Science and Human Nutrition, Michigan State University,
East Lansing, Mich. 48824

Interest has been renewed on the influence of dietary carbohydrates in human nutrition. Not only is the quantity of carbohydrate in the diet changing but the types of carbohydrate consumed by the Western World has also changed during the past 50 years. These changes, in some cases, have been implicated as a contributing factor to numerous diseases. For example, sucrose has been implicated as a major factor in the development of cardiovascular disease (1). However, it should be pointed out that not all researchers are in agreement on this point (2, 3). In this review we will discuss our efforts to understand the role of dietary carbohydrate in the control of adipose tissue fatty acid synthesis. Since the metabolic response of one organ, in some cases, influences metabolism in another organ, our studies have involved lipid metabolism in liver as well as in adipose tissue.

Dietary Factors Influencing Adipose Tissue Response to Carbohydrates

Studies concerning the influence of the quantity of carbohydrate in the diet on adipose tissue fatty acid synthesis are complex since modification of one dietary variable imposes a change on another dietary variable. Frequently dietary carbohydrate and fat are interchanged in studies on the influence of diet on lipid metabolism. If the carbohydrate content of the diet is modified without a concomitant change in another nutrient, the nutrient:energy ratio of the diet is changed. Generally a reduction in the carbohydrate content of the diet will depress fatty acid synthesis in adipose tissue preparations of both rats and pigs; however, there are exceptions.

---

[1] Supported by Grant HL-14677 from the National Institute of Health, U.S. Public Health Service. Journal Article No. 7023 Michigan Agriculture Experiment Station.

These exceptions may aid in our understanding of the control of lipid metabolism in adipose tissue. Substitution of medium-chain-triglycerides (MCT) for dietary glucose did not influence adipose tissue lipogenesis in the rat even though the carbohydrate content of the diet was decreased (4) (Table 1). Lipogenesis in pig adipose tissue was depressed less by the addition of 10% MCT to the diet than by the addition of lard or corn oil (5) (Table 1). Similarly, replacement of dietary glucose with 1,3-butanediol (BD) did not depress adipose tissue lipogenesis in the rat or pig (6, 7) (Table 2). Thus, it is apparent that the role of carbohydrate content of the diet in the regulation of adipose tissue metabolism is complex and involves its relationship with other dietary ingredients. Both MCT and BD have marked influences on hepatic metabolism (4,6, 8). Their metabolism elevates circulating ketone body levels. Preferential oxidation of ketone bodies by muscle would spare glucose for use in adipose tissue.

TABLE 1.   IN VITRO FATTY ACID SYNTHESIS IN ADIPOSE TISSUE FROM RATS AND PIGS FED MEDIUM-CHAIN TRIGLYCERIDES[1]

	Diet	
Species	Control	MCT
Rat	1143 + 63	1170 + 72
Pig	659 + 46	526 + 28

[1]From (4) and (5). Diets fed for 3 weeks. Rat - 12% MCT. Pig - 10% MCT. Fatty acid synthesis expressed as nmoles glucose-U-^{14}C incorporated into fatty acids/100 mg tissue/ 2 hr.

TABLE 2.   IN VITRO FATTY ACID SYNTHESIS IN ADIPOSE TISSUE FROM RATS AND PIGS FED BUTANEDIOL[1]

	Diet	
Species	Control	17% BD energy
Rat	844 + 77	700 + 72
Pig	184 + 28	250 + 29

[1]From (6) and (7). Diets fed for 3 weeks. Results expressed as nanomoles glucose-U-^{14}C incorporated into fatty acids/100 mg tissue/2 hr.

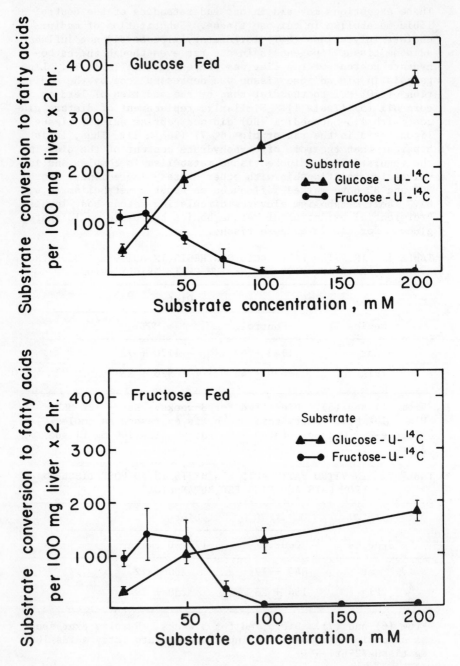

Biochimica et Biophysica Acta

Figure 1. In vitro *conversion of glucose–U–*[14]*C and fructose–U–*[14]*C to fatty acids in liver slices from glucose- or fructose-fed rats* (19)

Pattern of food intake also alters adipose tissue lipid metabolism. The capacity of adipose tissue preparations from meal-fed rats or pigs to convert carbohydrate to fatty acids is increased dramatically (9,10). Thus, it is apparent that factors which alter the pattern of carbohydrate intake may also influence lipid metabolism in adipose tissue. The remainder of our discussion will center on the influence of dietary fructose on adipose tissue metabolism.

Intestinal Transport and Peripheral Fructose Levels

Virtually all species studied can absorb and utilize fructose. However, it is important to recognize that the intestine has species-specific influences on fructose metabolism. In the guinea pig and hamster fructose is largely converted to glucose during transfer across the intestinal wall whereas in other species, including man, the laboratory rat, and the chick, fructose is absorbed largely unchanged (11). The chick absorbed approximately 85% of a fructose-^{14}C dose unchanged (11). In the rat at least, fructose absorption appears to occur via an active carrier-mediated mechanism (12,13). Thus, it is apparent that in a consideration of the influence of dietary fructose on adipose tissue metabolism one must be aware of the species-specific response of the intestine to fructose.

Feeding diets containing fructose to species that absorb fructose intact increases the portal vein concentration of fructose markedly; however, peripheral circulating levels of fructose are elevated to a much lesser extent (14). This has been taken to indicate that hepatic metabolism of fructose is extensive.

Dietary Fructose and Hepatic and Adipose Tissue Lipogenesis

It is clear that substituting fructose for glucose in the diet of rats leads to changes in lipid metabolism. To increase our understanding of the influence of dietary carbohydrates on metabolism we have examined hepatic and adipose tissue responses to dietary fructose. It is generally accepted that feeding fructose to rats increases the rate of fatty acid synthesis in the liver; however, results from in vitro estimates of hepatic fatty acid synthesis are not all in agreement (15,16,17,18).

We examined the influence of substrate source and concentration on hepatic lipogenesis in rats fed glucose or fructose-containing diet (Figure 1). Glucose-^{14}C conversion to fatty acids increased as the concentration of substrate increased, probably related to the ability of high levels of glucose to saturate glucokinase and thus increase acetyl CoA formation. Fructose-^{14}C conversion to hepatic fatty acids was higher than glucose-^{14}C conversion to fatty acids when the substrate concentration was 10 mM; however as substrate concentration was increased, hepatic conversion of fructose to fatty acids was markedly decreased. This decrease in fructose conversion to fatty acids when the fructose level in the incubation media exceeded 50 mM was probably related to the rapid phosphorylation of fructose and the subsequent decrease in ATP levels. We measured ATP levels in liver slices and observed that ATP levels were depressed by more than 50% when the media contained 100 mM fructose rather than 100 mM glucose (19).

We then examined in vivo adenine nucleotide levels in liver from rats fed glucose or fructose. ATP levels were elevated in livers of rats fed fructose (Table 3). Whether this increase in hepatic ATP level would allow rats consuming a large dose of fructose, such as might occur in meal-fed animals, to more effectively dispose of this dose under in vivo conditions remains to be established.

TABLE 3. EFFECT OF DIETARY FRUCTOSE AND GLUCOSE ON LIVER
ADENINE NUCLEOTIDE LEVELS IN VIVO[1]

	Dietary Carbohydrate	
μm/liver	Glucose	Fructose
ATP	25	39
ADP	9	11
AMP	6	5

[1]From (19). Diets were fed for 3 weeks.

Various techniques have been employed to obtain in vivo estimates of fatty acid synthesis in rats fed various carbohydrates. Oral, intraperitoneal or intravenous administration of a tracer dose of labeled substrate is complicated by possible differences in rates of substrate absorption, by intestinal metabolism of the substrate or by possible isotope-dilution effects at the tissue level. We elected to utilize ^{3}H-labeled water as a tool to obtain total rates of fatty acid synthesis, largely independent of the source of acetyl groups which are incorporated into fatty acids. It is clear that the in vivo rate of fatty acid synthesis in liver of fructose fed rats was higher than observed in glucose fed animals (Table 4).

TABLE 4.   EFFECT OF DIETARY CARBOHYDRATE ON IN VIVO FATTY
ACID SYNTHESIS[1]

	Dietary Carbohydrate	
Tissue	Glucose	Fructose
Liver	47 ± 6	80 ± 13
Extra Hepatic	14 ± 1	7 ± 1

[1]From (19). Results expressed as dpm x 10^2 per gram.

Recognizing that dietary fructose elevated the rate of
hepatic lipogenesis, we examined lipid metabolism in adipose
tissue, the predominant lipogenic organ in the rat, of rats fed
fructose. In epididymal adipose tissue, fatty acid synthesis
from fructose-^{14}C was lower than observed from glucose-^{14}C re-
gardless of dietary carbohydrate fed (Table 5). Further,
dietary fructose depressed lipogenesis from both substrates.
These results suggested to us that the relative importance of
the adipose tissue to fatty acid synthesis may be decreased in
fructose-fed rats. Estimates of the in vivo rate of fatty acid
synthesis obtained with tritiated water also indicated that the
extra hepatic rate of fatty acid synthesis was decreased in rats
fed fructose (Table 4). Although the total rate of fatty acid
synthesis in rats fed fructose was unchanged, the relative importance of the liver was increased and that of the extra hepatic tissues decreased when fructose, rather than glucose, was
fed to rats.

TABLE 5.   INFLUENCE OF DIETARY CARBOHYDRATE SOURCE ON IN VITRO
FATTY ACID SYNTHESIS IN RAT ADIPOSE TISSUE[1]

	Dietary Carbohydrate	
Substrate	Glucose	Fructose
Glucose-U-[14]C	540 ± 61	271 ± 57
Fructose-U-[14]C	191 ± 19	87 ± 26

[1]From (19). Results expressed as nmoles substrate converted to
fatty acids per 100 mg tissue per 2 hrs.

Several factors are probably involved in this shift in metabolism in the presence of dietary fructose. Froesch (20) has recently reviewed fructose metabolism in adipose tissue. He noted that fructose transport into the adipocyte appears to be mediated by a carrier with a relatively high apparent K_m for fructose; thus significant transport of fructose occurs only when blood fructose levels are high. Further, insulin does not stimulate fructose uptake by rat adipose tissue. Since adipose tissue lacks fructokinase, hexokinase is probably involved in the phosphorylation of fructose in this tissue. Physiologically, fructose-^{14}C conversion to fatty acids in rat adipose tissue probably occurs only after prior hepatic conversion of fructose-^{14}C to glucose-[14]C.

One of the key control points in the conversion of dietary carbohydrate to fatty acids in rat adipose tissue is at the level of glucose entry into the adipocyte, an insulin dependent process. Thus, various dietary carbohydrates might influence fatty acid synthesis in adipose tissue via their effect on circulating insulin levels. Bruckdorfer et al (21) have demonstrated that rats fed fructose have lower circulating insulin levels than do rats fed glucose. Also, an oral dose of fructose does not increase plasma insulin levels in fasted rats whereas a comparable glucose load doubled plasma insulin levels. Results of these studies suggest that the rapid metabolism of fructose by the liver coupled with lower circulating insulin levels in fructose fed rats contribute to the decreased rate of fatty acid synthesis observed in these rats.

Conclusions and Speculation

Dietary carbohydrates do influence adipose tissue fatty acid synthesis in rats and pigs. One of the key control points in the conversion of dietary carbohydrates to fatty acids is at the level of glucose entry into the adipocyte, an insulin dependent process. A reduction in carbohydrate intake generally would be expected to depress insulin secretion; however if compounds readily converted to ketones, such as MCT or BD, are substituted for the carbohydrate portion of the diet insulin, secretion might not decrease since ketones also stimulate insulin release. Meal-eating also increases insulin release and glucose stimulates a greater insulin release than does fructose. If the adipocyte maintains its sensitivity to insulin, these dietary conditions would be expected to increase glucose entry into the cell thereby stimulating fatty acid synthesis. The role of dietary factors in maintaining insulin sensitivity of the adipocyte are not clear.

Literature Cited

1. Yudkin, J. Proc. Nutr. Soc. (1972) 31, 331-337.
2. Walker, A. R. P. Atherosclerosis (1971) 14, 137-152.
3. Keys, A. Atherosclerosis (1971) 14, 193-202.
4. Wiley, J. H., and Leveille, G. A. J. Nutr. (1973) 103, 829-835.
5. Allee, G. L., Romsos, D. R., Leveille, G. A. and Baker, D. H. Proc. Soc. Exp. Biol. Med. (1972) 139, 422-427.
6. Romsos, D. R., Sasse, C. and Leveille, G. A. J. Nutr. (1974) 104, 202-209.
7. Romsos, D. R., Belo, P. S., Miller, E. R. and Leveille, G. A. J. Nutr. (1974) Submitted.
8. Romsos, D. R., Belo, P. S. and Leveille, G. A. J. Nutr. (1974) 104, In press.
9. Leveille, G. A. J. Nutr. (1967) 91, 25-34.
10. Allee, G. L., Romsos, D. R., Leveille, G. A. and Baker, D. H. J. Nutr. (1972) 102, 1115-1122.
11. Leveille, G. A., Akinbami, T. K. and Ikediobi, C. O. Proc. Soc. Exp. Biol. Med. (1970) 135, 483-486.
12. Macrae, A. R. and Neudoerffer, T. S. Biochim. Biophys. Acta (1972) 288, 137-144.
13. Gracey, M., Burke, V. and Oshin, A. Biochim. Biophys. Acta (1972) 266, 397-406.
14. Topping, D. L. and Mayes, P. A. Nutr. Metabol. (1971) 13, 331-338.
15. Chevalier, M. M., Wiley, J. H. and Leveille, G. A. J. Nutr. (1972) 102, 337-342.
16. Zakim, D., Pardini, R. S., Herman, R. H. and Sauberlich, H. E. Biochim. Biophys. Acta (1967) 144, 242-251.
17. Kritchevsky, D. and Tepper, S. A. Med. Exp. (1969) 19, 329-341.
18. Bender, A. E. and Thadoni, P. V. Nutr. Metabol. (1970) 12, 22-39.
19. Romsos, D. R., and Leveille, G. A. Biochim. Biophys. Acta (1974) 360, 1-11.
20. Froesch, E. R. Acta Med. Scand. (1972) Suppl. 542, 37-46.
21. Bruckdorfer, K. R., Khan, I. H., and Yudkin, J. Biochem. J. (1972) 129, 439-445.

4

Benefits of Dietary Fructose in Alleviating the Human Stress Response

J. DANIEL PALM

Department of Biology, St. Olaf College, Northfield, Minn.

The structural characteristics which distinguish fructose from glucose result in differential physiological properties. For some uses glucose is the sugar of choice. For other situations fructose has distinct advantages. It has recently been found that when pure fructose is exchanged for most other carbohydrates in a good high-protein low-carbohydrate diet, it deserves a reputation of being "nature's tranquilizer", or the ideal "crave-control" food, and the answer to most of the problems associated with hypoglycemia.

Hypoglycemia is not a distinct disease. The name of the disorder indicates a deficiency of sugar in the blood sufficient to maintain the nervous system control. It is a physiological disorder that is commonly found in persons with diagnoses of schizophrenia, alcoholism, migraine headaches, hyperactivity, severe overweight and many other disorders. Hypoglycemia is a stress which normally results in a response which raises the blood sugar concentration. Everyone experiences some hypoglycemia each day. It is hypoglycemia which triggers the morning and afternoon treks to the coffee and sweet-roll counter. It causes students, and sometimes others, to fall asleep during classes and conferences. It is hypoglycemia that causes the tremor of the hands and the recognition of hunger when meals are delayed. Hypoglycemia appears to be the most repetitive stress for all members of society. For some unfortunate persons hypoglycemia is not a temporary condition which is rapidly corrected by normal homeostatic responses. In some it persists because insufficient adrenalin is released to convert the liver glycogen to glucose. Such persons remain physiologically and emotionally depressed. In others hypoglycemia persists despite the mobilization of massive amounts of adrenalin which normally increases the blood sugar concentration. The persons with this variety of hypoglycemia develop various symptoms of hypomania. The association of hypoglycemia with both physical and emotional disorders deserves attention.

Ever since hypoglycemia was recognized as a consequence of the injection of excessive amounts of insulin in diabetic patients,

it has been known that most cases of hypoglycemia do not result
from hyperinsulinism. Nor is hypoglycemia due to a deficiency of
carbohydrates in the diet. (1) Most cases are functional hypo-
glycemias which are triggered by dietary carbohydrates without any
evidence of over-mobilization of insulin. For this reason, Conn,
a quarter of a century ago, introduced a high-protein low-carbohydrate diet for hypoglycemics to provide for gluconeogenesis from
the proteins and for a lessening of the chances for insulin release by dietary carbohydrates. (2) Until now this has been the
dietary regimen of preference for hypoglycemics although it did
not resolve all of the problems for these persons. A diet that
relies primarily on proteins for the energy and substrate requirements of the brain is not only expensive and somewhat unpalatable
but it runs the risk of gout and other problems of excretion of
the metabolic end-products of protein utilization. (3) Unfortunately, the brain cannot utilize fats for all of its requirements.
The alternative is to provide a sugar which will not induce insulin release but yet provides for the requirements of the nervous
system. Glucose causes insulin release. Insulin causes the storage of excess sugar as glycogen in the liver and so lowers the
blood sugar concentration. Pure fructose does not cause insulin
release. (4) Although fructose has long been used by diabetics
in Europe its use has not been promoted in the United States where
insulin therapy and dietary balance programs are predominant.
(5, 6)

Although an extensive literature on fructose metabolism in
the human as well as in experimental animals has accumulated, most
studies have been conducted using challenge doses by dietary or
injection routes without regard for the abnormalacy of these conditions. (7, 8) Unfortunately, several studies have been reported as studies of fructose which were actually studies of sucrose
in comparison to glucose, liquid glucose, and starch. (9, 10)
Yet the differences found as a result of such diets were attributed to the fructose component of the sucrose without any attempt
to study the effects of pure fructose. Such conclusions seem
wholly unjustified. Several studies have demonstrated that insulin can promote the storage of fructose as glycogen. (11, 12).
If the diet includes insulin-inducing carbohydrates, the metabolic
advantages of fructose may be expected to be diminished.

Glucose is actively transported from the gut so that its concentration rises rapidly after dietary intake. Fructose is passively moved through the cells by diffusion. (13) There is insufficient evidence to support the contention that any significant
amount of fructose is regularly converted to glucose either in the
gut or in hepatic cells. (14) Since sugars are primarily absorbed by cells in the upper digestive tract, the ingestion of large
amounts of fructose at any one time can lead, in some persons, to
increased water retention in the large bowel and the onset of
diarrhea. (15) A simple precaution against such an event is to
provide the dietary fructose in smaller amounts to decrease the

likelihood of fructose passing into the lower digestive tract.

It is well known that excess carbohydrates, those which exceed the immediate demand for cellular energy, are stored either as glycogen or fat. When fructose is provided in a diet in exchange for insulin-inducing carbohydrates, it would be expected that all excess fructose must be converted to fat. There are some studies with experimental animals which support this general recognition. (16, 17) This has led to a concern that an exchange of fructose for glucose would result in a rise in plasma triglycerides and cholesterol.

Stress conditions cause the physiological stress responses. Hypoglycemia is a stress. Normally it is corrected by the changes which result from the stress response. The pioneer work by Hans Selye on the General Stress Response is well known and the interrelationships to many disorders have been established. (18, 19) All stress conditions, whether they come from the emotions, physical trauma, toxicity, or physiological deficiency, are detected by cells of the nervous system and communicated to the hypothalamus of the brain. These cells directly stimulate sympathetic nerves to secrete noradrenalin. The hypothalamic cells also secrete release factors into the blood of the portal vessels which supply the pituitary. When the pituitary is stimulated by these release factors it secretes ACTH (adrenocorticotrophic hormone) to cause the adrenal cortex to elaborate specific hormones. The steroid hormones of the adrenal cortex have several effects. They cause the mobilization of both fat and proteins for cellular use and cause the release of adrenalin from the adrenal medulla. It is this adrenalin, in addition to its other actions, which initiates the changes required to convert liver glycogen to glucose which can be supplied to the brain. It is primarily this portion of the stress response that is related to carbohydrate metabolism.

Only recently has it been possible to study in detail the relationship between stress and the sympathetic nervous system hormones. It has only been in the past few years that all of the metabolic products of the sympathetic hormones have been known. (20) In just over one decade, von Euler received a Nobel Prize for his discovery of noradrenalin as the primary transmitter of the peripheral sympathetic nerve cells. Axelrod was awarded a Nobel Prize for his discovery of the enzyme COMT (catechol-O-methyl transferase) which catalyzes the methylation of the sympathetic hormones and thus deactivates these molecules. Sutherland was then the recipient of a Nobel Prize for his discovery of cyclic AMP (3'5' AMP) and its relationship to the conversion of glycogen to glucose under the influence of adrenalin. Many other investigators have provided other insights and methodologies for the analysis of the metabolism of these hormones. (21, 22) All of this information was necessary before other ideas about stress and the stress response could be tested.

It is a part of our general dogma that stress contributes to such varied disorders as coronary thrombosis, hypertension, peptic

ulcers and gall stones in addition to a variety of nervous disorders. A simplistic, layman's description concludes that schizophrenia is a disorder of orientation and behavior which develops
when a person is exposed to stress which exceeds his ability to
cope. The common depressants which are used to decrease the
symptomatology of schizophrenia suppress the activity of the sympathetic system. (23) Conversely, adrenalin and the drugs which
mimic the sympathetic hormones are known to exacerbate the symptoms of schizophrenia. (24) Many psychiatrists believe that the
origins of schizophrenia relate to an inappropriate perception of
stress so that these persons over-respond to stresses which would
not disrupt the lives of most persons. (25) Yet these practi-
tioners also recognize the physiological regulations and implications of the stress responses.

The recognition of the involvement of stress in the etiology
of schizophrenia adds another orientation to the study of stress-
related disorders. The inclusion of a concept of stress initiation of behavioral changes and the acceptance of the possibility
of an inheritable component of schizophrenia has led to a search
for metabolic defects in the regulation of the hormones which are
associated with the sympathetic system. Many of the concepts
about the general stress response can now be extended to behavioral disorders and studied as biochemical problems.

The complete pathways and products of the enzymatic deactivation of the catecholamine hormones, noradrenalin and adrenalin, are
known. After the mobilization of these hormones of the stress response the metabolic products accumulate in the urine. The urine
thus serves as a repository of evidence of the stress response.
It is apparent that a deficiency in any one of the enzymes involved in the deactivation of the hormones would result in the absence
of particular end-products in the collected urine. (26) When
early morning urine samples from a group of institutionalized but
non-medicated schizophrenics were tested by gas chromatographic
separation of the components and flame ionization detection of
each molecular variety, all of the normal end-products of noradrenalin and adrenalin were found in each of the urines. (27)
This demonstrated that schizophrenics as a group are not characteristically deficient in any of the enzymes which are normally
involved in the deactivation of the sympathetic system hormones.
The data did provide one enigma. The night-time accumulation of
these products in the urine appeared to be much greater than had
been found in the samples obtained from a control population. The
magnitude of the accumulation of these catecholamine products provided the basis for a hypothesis that these schizophrenic patients
were responding to stress conditions even during their periods of
sleep which probably involve physiological stress factors. It was
then discovered that the records of many of these patients contained information about glucose tolerance tests which had all
been indicative of hypoglycemia.

The simultaneous findings of hypoglycemia and the exceedingly

high values of the sympathetic system products appear initially to
be logically inconsistent. Normally adrenalin initiates the conversion of glycogen to glucose. The presence of large amounts of
catecholamine products in the urine indicates high sympathetic
system activity which would be expected to be associated with an
abundance of blood sugar. This discovery of the hypoglycemia associated with evidences of hyperactivity of the sympathetic system
led to another hypothesis. It is proposed that among schizophrenics an initiating stress condition is a deficiency of blood sugar
which requires the mobilization of adrenalin which for some reason
is unable to effectively raise the blood sugar level to the required level and the stress response is continued. The focus of
this hypothesis is that since all stresses are additive the stress
of hypoglycemia should be seen as a sufficient, if not required,
stress to precipitate schizophrenic behavior.

Some of the symptoms of schizophrenics seem to be related
directly to the deficiency of sugar for neural system control
while other symptoms appear to be more related to the high concentration of active sympathetic system hormones. Such a hypothesis
reconciles the hypoglycemia with the presence of high catecholamine products in the urine and suggests a basis for the biologic
component of schizophrenia.

Unfortunately the diet of most institutionalized schizophrenics is preponderantly carbohydrate and contains a paucity of proteins. Such a diet is disasterous for a person with tendencies to
functional hypoglycemia. The depressive drugs which are commonly
used to control the behavior of the schizophrenics interfere with
the normal abilities for raising the blood sugar concentration.
Therefore, a test program among institutionalized schizophrenics
to evaluate the effectiveness of a program to externally regulate
the blood sugar level by exchanging fructose for the normal insulin-inducing carbohydrates is virtually impossible.

It is the behavioral characteristics which distinguish the
schizophrenic from the alcoholic, the hyperactive or hypomanic,
and the crave-eater who becomes obese. These are also stress-
induced disorders in which the behavior often appears to accomo-
date or compensate for the stress factors. The alcoholic has
learned that alcohol depresses the perception of stress even if he
does not recognize that alcohol does not supply the brain with the
sugar it needs. The hyperactive feels better adjusted if he can
increase his activity and by this means accomplish some increase
in blood sugar. He might just take a brisk walk to get more adrenalin and more sugar rather than actually be "burning off" energy. Too much blood sugar makes a person sluggish, not active.
The stress-eater consumes candies, pastries, and fruits and thus
keeps the blood sugar high enough to temporarily avoid the stress
response. In these persons the effectiveness of the insulin control of the sugar storage system predicates a reinitiation of the
functional hypoglycemia and a return of the stress.

If the same reasoning is extended to schizophrenia it can be

suggested that this behavior compensates for a deficiency of
blood sugar regulation even if it isolates the person from effective social interactions.

Since hypoglycemia is a common characteristic of all of these
disorders in which behaviors may compensate for the deficiency in
regulation of the blood sugar levels, the investigations of the
effectiveness of fructose in providing sugar for the brain without
precipitating insulin release and the return of the hypoglycemia
can be done on persons who have no known problems in blood sugar
regulation. Several questions remain concerning the applicability
of fructose exchange diets. If fructose is given in small amounts
in hourly intervals does an appreciable amount get converted to
glucose which could initiate the insulin release? If fructose is
exchanged for most of the other carbohydrates in a diet does it
promote the accumulation of plasma triglycerides and plasma cholesterol? If fructose is used in a dietary program to prevent hypoglycemia is there a demonstrable change in the accumulation of
the enzymatic products of the sympathetic system hormones since it
is logical to assume that the magnitude of the stress condition
will be mirrored in the magnitude of the measured stress response?
Three different investigative programs have been conducted to
answer these questions.

Experiments

Blood absorption curves of sugars were determined from blood
samples obtained from experimental subjects every five minutes after ingestion of the sugars. The sugar concentrations were measured using a Beckman Glucose Analyzer. Determinations were made
on three separate days for each of the subjects. One day 50 grams
of sucrose syrup was ingested after four consecutive samples showed the blood glucose concentration to be nearly stable at 90 mg./
100 ml. of blood. Another day 25 grams of glucose was ingested.
The third test utilized 25 grams of fructose. Least-squares fit-
ted lines were computed from the data obtained from the blood glucose concentrations. Figure 1 illustrates a typical set of glucose concentration curves from these experiments. Pure glucose
entered the blood stream more rapidly than glucose obtained from
sucrose (slope = $1.54 \pm$ S.D. 0.0656 versus a slope of $0.983 \pm$ S.D.
0.555) although the practicality of this difference is negligible.
Although it is necessary to digest the sucrose to glucose and
fructose before its absorption, the delay imposed on the absorption of glucose from sucrose is essentially inconsequential. When
the blood glucose determinations were made following the ingestion
of 25 grams of fructose, the slope of the line was not found to be
significantly different from the normal variation of the blood
glucose as a function of the stress response to the hypoglycemia
together with the stress of the sample collection. The only bit
of value of this data is to show that fructose is not converted to
glucose in any significant amounts in reasonable dietary exchange

programs.

In order to determine if an exchange of 100 grams of pure
fructose for most of the other carbohydrates of a normal diet
would affect the concentration of plasma triglycerides and cholesterol these substances were measured from plasma obtained from 17
healthy persons who were not following any dietary regimens.
These persons were then asked to continue their regular eating
habits but to exchange 100 grams of fructose for most of the insulin-inducing carbohydrates for a period of three days. The
plasma cholesterol and plasma triglycerides were measured at the
end of this three day diet program. Table 1 and Figures 2, 3 illustrate the levels of these lipid substances. There is no evidence of consistent change in these substances as the result of
the fructose provided in 8-10 grams each hour.

A project to test the effectiveness of dietary fructose to
regulate the blood sugar concentration utilized the urinary accumulation of catecholamine metabolites to quantify the stress
response initiated by hypoglycemia. For this test 24 hour urine
were collected from 20 normal, healthy adults who followed the
high-protein low-carbohydrate diet with fructose one day and with
other carbohydrates another day. Initially it was intended to
utilize a high pressure liquid chromatographic automated system
to determine all of the catecholamine metabolites in the urine.
Technical difficulties encountered in screening some contaminants
which obscured the definitive separation of the catecholamine
metabolites prevents the inclusion of this data at this time.
The total catecholamines (noradrenalin and adrenalin) and the
methylated intermediates (normetadrenalin and metadrenalin) were
determined using the Bio-Rad Catecholamine Test Kits. Figure 4
demonstrates the relationships of these compounds. VMA was determined from the same samples at two independent commercial medical
laboratories. One of the laboratories used the Pisano, Crout,
and Abraham method (28) while the other used the method of Gitlow,
et al (29). Both the control and the diet test day samples of
urine were determined by the same laboratory at the same time.

The urines were collected in glass jugs containing 15 ml.
conc. HCl. Care was taken to insure all of the bottles were fit-
ted with teflon cover inserts to eliminate contamination of the
samples by cork or paper products. All of the catecholamine
urine samples were hydrolyzed at pH 0.5 for 20 minutes in capped
tubes placed in boiling water. The Bio-Rad system of analysis was
modified slightly to provide an internal standard for each sample
and thus reduce the problems of fluorescence quenching and to increase the reliability of determination of all of the products.
Catecholamines were eluted from the disposable columns with 10 ml.
of 4.0 N. boric acid. The eluate was divided into four equal portions. Portion 1 remained as the control. Portion 2 was the unknown sample. Portion 3 was spiked with 1 ug of noradrenalin
standard. Portion 4 was spiked with 2 ug of noradrenalin standard.
All portions were brought to the same volume with glass distilled

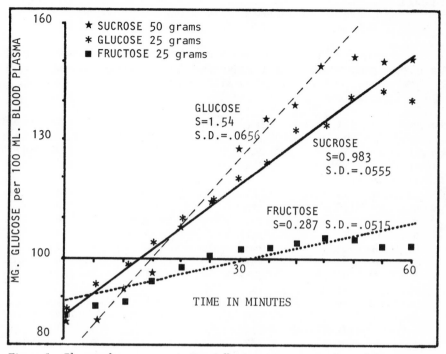

Figure 1. *Plasma glucose concentration following ingestion of three different sugars*

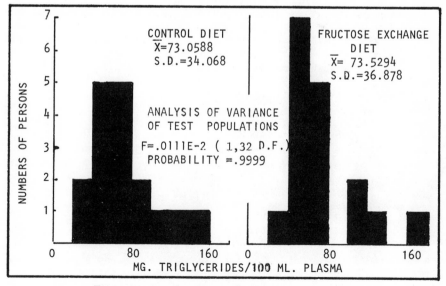

Figure 2. *Distributions of plasma triglyceride levels*

Table 1.   Effect of Diet on Plasma Cholesterol and Plasma Triglycerides. Diet Program
Exchanged 100 grams Fructose for 100 grams of Other Carbohydrates

SUBJECT CODE	CONTROL DIET CHOLESTEROL mg./100 ml. plasma	FRUCTOSE DIET CHOLESTEROL mg./100 ml. plasma	CONTROL DIET TRIGLYCERIDES mg./100 ml. plasma	FRUCTOSE DIET TRIGLYCERIDES mg./100 ml. plasma
CB	217	181	137	178
LJ	197	205	91	129
IJ	256	243	114	61
MJ	214	216	61	57
GJ	158	183	53	38
JD	193	214	68	78
KK	197	222	151	106
OM	170	195	56	43
JK	186	187	53	49
IN	222	246	46	59
DJ	170	187	76	41
GB	190	235	50	55
GK	232	232	79	70
IM	138	163	35	67
AC	127	148	27	43
SK	173	170	61	73
VO	301	363	84	103

$\bar{X}$= 196.529 $\bar{X}$= 211.176 $\bar{X}$= 73.0588 $\bar{X}$= 73.5294
S.E.= 10.3174   S.E.=11.7584   S.E.=8.2629   S.E.=8.94432
S.D.=42.5399   S.D.=48.481   S.D.=34.0688   S.D.=36.8784

F=.876673 (1,32 D.F.)   F=.150008E-2 (1,32 D.F.)

Probability=.99999   Probability=.99999

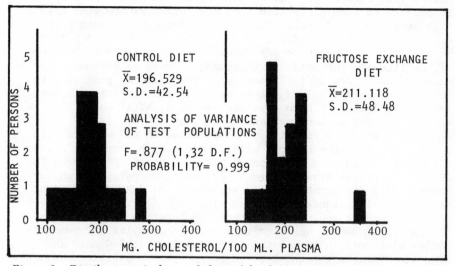

Figure 3.   Distributions of plasma cholesterol levels as a function of dietary program

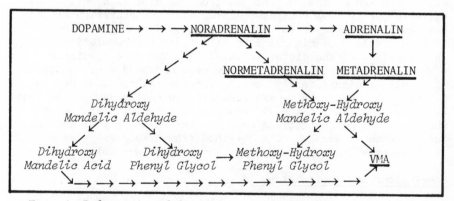

Figure 4.   Pathways of metabolic conversions of catecholamine excretion products

water. The fluorescence of Portions 2,3, and 4 were measured in
comparison to that of Portion 1 with a Turner Fluorometer with a
high sensitivity adapter. The three fluorescence readings for
each urine sample were fed into a computer to determine a least-
squares line of the three determinations, to print out the slope
of the line and the point of intercept as well as determine the
standard deviation of the intercept. The computer program then
multiplied the determined values by the amount of urine in the
initial 24 hour sample to give the amount of total catecholamines
excreted in the 24 hour period.

The 0-methyl derivatives, normetadrenalin and metadrenalin
were eluted from the columns with 10 ml. 4.0. N. ammonium hydrox-
ide after the columns had been washed with distilled water. The
10 ml. eluate was divided into 4 portions; control, unknown, unknown + 3 ug of normetadrenalin standard, and unknown + 9 ug of
normetadrenalin standard. The samples were diluted to equal volumes and read at 360 nm on a Beckman DU Spectrophotometer. The
absorbance at 350 nm was used to screen the samples for contamination which may influence the determinations at 360 nm. The
same computer program which was used for the computations of catecholamine concentrations was also used to determine the values of
the methylated derivatives of the catecholamines.

In all 20 cases the measured concentration of the total catecholamines excreted was higher on the day of the control diet than
on the day of the fructose exchange diet. The data obtained from
the two test sets (Table 2) shows that the decrease in catecholamine excretion on the day of the fructose diet is significantly
different at the 99% confidence interval. The excretion of the
0-methylated derivates (metadrenalin) showed no significant
changes (Table 3). Figures 5, 6 illustrate the population shift
as a function of the dietary change. The VMA concentrations
(Table 4) while not higher in every case on the day of the control
diet, differ significantly between the control and test day to
demonstrate a decrease in VMA accumulation on the day of the fructose exchange diet at the 95% confidence interval. In the cases
where the VMA concentrations were greater on the day of the fructose diet these samples were obtained from female subjects who
were menstruating on the day that this sample was collected.

Conclusions and Implications

The exchange of fructose for other dietary carbohydrates
(100 grams exchanged for most of the insulin-inducing carbohydrates of the control diet) maintains a sufficiency of blood sugar to prevent the stress of hypoglycemia. This conclusion is
justified by the significant decrease in the urinary accumulation
of total catecholamines and VMA on the day of the fructose diet.

The implications of these findings have wide application and
significance. General experience among the hundreds of persons
who have regularly used fructose in exchange for glucose in quasi-

Table 2.   Daily Excretion of Urinary Catecholamines

SUBJECT	CONTROL DIET VOLUME ml/24 h.	FRUCTOSE DIET VOLUME ml/24 h.	CONTROL DIET CATECHOL. ug/24 h.	S.D.	FRUCTOSE DIET CATECHOL. ug/24 h.	S.D.
RC	1700	1800	159.4	1.04	132.0	0.52
YJ	1725	1600	87.0	0.59	80.7	0.53
QL	1610	1400	152.5	0.78	104.7	0.78
RJ	1820	2365	282.0	1.68	75.7	0.45
RS	1280	900	175.5	1.46	68.9	1.16
QB	1445	600	125.5	0.89	69.8	1.16
QR	1900	755	154.6	1.15	129.4	1.06
FL	2460	1780	156.9	0.38	83.6	0.36
AE	1230	1360	86.4	0.62	73.4	0.42
UJ	2005	1310	103.9	0.59	72.0	0.82
AW	815	1550	210.6	1.34	75.1	0.33
CB	1420	1700	116.9	0.57	40.9	0.47
SB	1550	1810	236.6	1.55	158.9	0.55
OB	1610	1965	94.2	0.67	74.9	0.54
GB	1020	1230	65.3	1.14	61.5	0.60
HB	710	690	70.5	1.27	45.3	0.76
IB	1800	1810	136.4	0.38	105.7	0.33
QG	1710	1030	195.4	1.20	96.9	1.61
QV	1910	2320	217.8	0.68	125.3	0.27
UC	850	1080	100.8	0.64	73.4	1.17

$\overline{X}$= 146.41 $\overline{X}$= 87.4
S.E.=13.26   S.E.=6.77
S.D.=59.32   S.D.=30.2786

F=15.6986 (1,38 D.F.)

Probability=0.00055

Table 3.   Daily Excretion of Urinary Catecholamine Metholated Products

SUBJECT	CONTROL DIET METADR. ug/24 h.	S.D.	FRUCTOSE DIET METADR. ug/24 h.	S.D.
RC	1526.5	9.29	1731.5	5.09
YJ	1351.0	8.46	1365.0	9.07
QL	2192.0	7.74	1491.5	10.87
RJ	1571.2	8.96	2165.8	9.65
RS	1369.8	10.75	1847.6	20.80
QB	991.4	6.95	973.0	17.58
QR	1012.0	5.46	945.1	6.61
FL	2190.1	4.85	1552.7	4.45
AE	2098.8	8.57	2018.7	7.78
UJ	1247.6	6.27	1242.0	9.75
AW	2005.8	12.87	1894.8	6.16
CB	1564.3	5.60	1683.4	5.04
SB	2722.9	17.61	2456.0	6.87
OB	1459.1	9.38	1266.0	6.49
GB	814.4	8.34	712.5	6.10
HB	581.0	8.45	432.8	6.68
IB	2367.0	7.18	1627.4	4.63
QG	1747.2	10.80	1232.4	12.18
QV	1648.9	4.64	993.5	2.41
UC	1917.0	12.06	1502.9	14.36

$\overline{X}$= 1618.9 $\overline{X}$= 1456.7
S.E.=122.66   S.E.=112.21
S.D.=548.537   S.D.=501.809

F=0.951672 (1,38 D.F.)

Probability=.99999

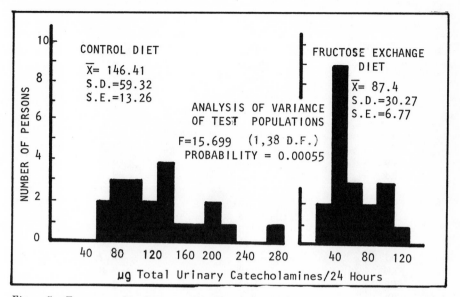

Figure 5.   *Frequency distributions of total urinary catecholamines excreted during day of dietary exchange program*

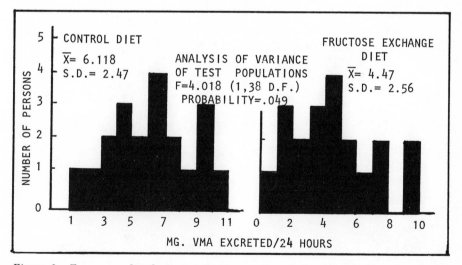

Figure 6.   *Frequency distribution of VMA excretion during day of dietary exchange*

Table 4. Daily Excretion of Urinary VMA

SUBJECT	CONTROL DIET VMA mg/ 24 h.	FRUCTOSE DIET VMA mg/ 24 h.
RC	10.2	7.3
YJ	9.7	9.1
QL	6.0	5.5
RJ	7.6	9.6
RS	4.6	4.1
QB	5.6	2.9
QR	1.8	0.1
FL	9.3	1.6
AE	6.4	4.4
UJ	7.9	6.2
AW	4.3	3.8
CB	5.1	3.6
SB	9.1	5.7
OB	8.0	4.6
GB	3.1	1.8
HB	2.3	1.3
IB	3.8	3.3
QG	6.0	4.3
QV	4.1	2.6
UC	6.4	7.6

$\overline{X}$= 6.118 $\overline{X}$= 4.47

S.E.= .553   S.E.= .572

S.D.=2.473   S.E.=2.5584

F=4.01786 (1,38 D.F.)

Probability=0.0494

clinical test programs during the past two years has indicated
that 100 grams of fructose per day together with the elimination
of insulin-inducing carbohydrates in the diet completely elimin-
ates the hunger, fatigue and anxiety that accompany most weight
reduction diets. The same amount of fructose can completely
eliminate the insatiable demand for alcohol among alcoholics.
Such an exchange of sugars can reduce or eliminate migraine headaches for persons who are prone to such problems. The provision
of fructose does not make angels out of all hyperactive children
but the general experience has shown them to be much more manage-
able.

It is necessary to remember that fructose is not a drug. It
is only a food that in itself is deficient in vitamins, amino
acids, and minerals. Fructose does not change behavior. It al-
lows a person to change the behavior if the stress problem disorder involves the regulation of blood sugar. The logic for the use
of fructose in this manner is completely consistent with all of
the known properties of glucose and fructose metabolism. The ex-
tension of the ideas into clinical applications and tests will be
left to the physicians and psychologists to determine the extent
of the advantages of such a program. The immediate inclusion of
this dietary program can be expected to be beneficial for persons
with cerebral hemorrhage or coronary damage which depress the rhyth-
micity of adrenal cortical steroid hormones and who therefore are
kept in physiological as well as psychological depression and are
unable to manage their blood glucose regulation sufficiently.

Fortunately fructose can be purchased in many good food
stores. The advantages of its use can be recognized by anyone
who follows the simple exchange of fructose for the majority of
the glucose of a good diet. To insure some glycogen is kept
available the inclusion of glucose in the form of toast, cereal,
and fruits for the first meal of the day is advisable for most
persons.

It is apparent that the exchange of fructose for other carbohydrates is advantageous to many who have no recognized pathology. Fructose provides distinct advantage to the athlete since
it will not induce insulin release. If other sugars are consumed
before strenuous activity the presence of the insulin and the release of adrenalin prevents either of these hormones from accom-
plishing their normal function of blood sugar regulation. Among
those persons who drink alcoholic beverages the provision of fructose will prevent hypoglycemia as well as in others, but it has
the added advantage of preventing the necessity of the stress response steroid release of fats into the blood. When fats are released they compete for the same enzymes as those used to metabolize the alcohol. If the fats and the alcohol are not completely
metabolized they are converted to ketones which can cause nausea
and headaches. Fructose has been used to prevent colic in small
babies. The list can go on and on.

Although fructose does not promote dental plaque as effectively as glucose the hourly intake of fructose in candies, hot and cold beverages, salad dressings, and jello-like deserts will result in cavities unless there is an increase in dental care. A small portion of the population is deficient in the enzymes necessary to utilize fructose. This hereditary condition of fructose intolerance prevents these persons from eliminating hypoglycemia by exchanging fructose for other carbohydrates. Such persons have a dislike for candies and sweetened foods although they can usually eat fruits without discomfort.

Acknowledgements

The author wishes to give particular recognition to Mr. John B. Hawley, Jr., a Minneapolis industrialist, for his financial support of this research. Thanks are also extended to my assistant, Ms. Marcia Dietz, for her valuable help and to my colleagues, Duane Olson and Stewart Hendrickson, for their continued support. The help provided to the research by Paul Westhoff, Ms. Barbara Hanson and John Swanson is also appreciated.

Literature Cited

1. Hearn, W.R., E. J. Webel, R.W. Randolph, and N.E. Parks, Proc. Soc. Exp. Biol. (1961) 107, 515.
2. Conn, J.W. and H.S. Seltzer, Amer. J. Med., (1955) 19, 460.
3. Talbott, J.H., "Gout", Grune & Stratton, New York (1964).
4. Aitken, J.M. and M.G. Dunningan, Brit. Med. J. (1969) 3, 276.
5. Craig, J.W., W.R. Drucker, M.Owens et al., Proc. Soc. Exp. Biol. (1951) 78, 698.
6. Roch-Norlund, A.E., E. Hultman, and L.H. Nilsson, in "Symposium on Clinical and Metabolic Aspects of Fructose", E.A. Nikkila and J.K. Huttunen eds., Acta Medica Scandinavica, Suppl. (1972) 542.
7. Woods, H.F., L.V. Eggleston and H.A. Krebs, Biochem J. (1970) 119.
8. Yu, D.T. and M.S. Phillips, J. Ultrastructure Res. (1971) 36 222.
9. Yudkin, J. Edelman and L.Hough (eds.) "Sugar", Butterworths, London (1971).
10. Yudkin, J. and J. Roddy, Lancet (1964) 2, 6.
11. Weinstein, J.J. and J. H. Roe, J. Lab. Clin. Med. (1952) 40 39.
12. Pozza, G., G. Galarsino, H. Hoffeld, and P.D. Foa, Amer. J. Physiol. (1958) 192, 497.
13. Adelman, R.C., in "Symposium on Clinical and Metabolic Aspects of Fructose", E.A. Nikkila and J.K. Huttunen eds., Acta Medica Scandinavica, Suppl. (1972) 542.
14. Crane, R.K., Physiol. Rev. (1960) 40, 789.
15. Papadopoulos, N.M. and J.H. Roe, Amer. J. Physiol. (1957) 189 301.
16. Bar-On, H., and Y. Stein, J. Nutr. (1968) 94, 95.
17. Nikkila, E.A., Scand. J. Clin. Lab. Invest., 18, Suppl. (1966) 92, 76.
18. Selye, H., "Stress of Life", McGraw Hill, New York (1956).
19. Selye, H., "Hormones and Resistance", Springer-Verlag, Heidelberg, (1971).
20. Axelrod, J., Recent Prog. Horm. Res., (1965) 21, 597.
21. von Euler, U.S., and F. Lishajko, Acta Physiol. Scand. (1961) 51, 348.
22. Weil-Malherbe, H., and E.R.B. Smith, Pharmacol. Rev. (1966) 18, 331.
23. Cooper, J.R., F.E. Bloom and R.H. Roth, "The Biochemical Basis of Neuropharmacology", p. 80, Oxford Univ. Press, London (1970)
24. Blum, J.J., ed., "Biogenic Amines as Physiological Regulators", Prentice-Hall Inc., Englewood Cliffs, N.J. (1970).
25. Szara, J. Axelrod, and S. Perlin, Amer. J. Psychiat. (1958) 15, 162.
26. Palm, J.D., Schizophrenia (1969) 1, 161.
27. Palm, J.D., Schizophrenia (1970) 2, 198.

Literature Cited continued

28. Pisano, J.J., J.R. Crout, and D. Abraham, Clin. Chim. Acta.
    (1962) 7, 285.
29. Gitlow, S.E., L.M. Bertani, A. Rausen, D. Gribetz, and S.W.
    Dziedzic, Cancer (1970) 25, 1377.

The Metabolism of Infused Maltose and Other Sugars

ELEANOR A. YOUNG and ELLIOT WESER

Division of Gastroenterology, Department of Medicine, The University of Texas Health Science Center, San Antonio, Tex. 78284

Introduction

Provision of adequate nutrition when oral feeding or tube-feeding is difficult or impossible, can be achieved if essential nutrients and calories are introduced directly into the vein. For over three hundred years, man has searched for ways to provide life-dependent nutrients intravenously. As early as 1656 Sir Christopher Wren had already utilized a goose quill attached to a pig's bladder to introduce ale, wine and opium into dog veins (1). Richard Lower of Oxford, in 1662 reported intravenous injections into animals, and Jean B. Davis, a French physician in Paris, transfused lamb blood into man in 1667 (1). In 1843, almost two centuries later, Claude Bernard first infused sugars into animal veins (2), and in 1896, Biedl and Kraus reported the intravenous infusion of dextrose solutions in man (3).

Perhaps one of the most exciting and challenging developments in modern medicine, has been the achievement of providing total parenteral nutrition to man. This has been possible largely as a result of advances in the knowledge of the nutritional requirements of man, availability of essential nutrients, and means of parenteral delivery over extended periods of time. Several reviews (4,5,6) and national and international symposia (7,8,9,10, 11,12) attest to the distinguished achievements made within the past decade, largely as a result of numerous clinical trials in which calories and all essential nutrients...amino acids, carbohydrates, fats, vitamins and minerals...have been effectively delivered intravenously to man.

Numerous clinical situations arise in which parenteral nutrition may not only be therapeutic, but essential to life. Some of these are summarized in Table 1. Notwithstanding the recent progress made in parenteral alimentation, current problems focus on superior vena cava catherization via the subclavian vein; infection and sepsis involving catheter entry site, contamination of the catheter and solution; and hyperglycemic, hyperosmolar dehydration (13).

TABLE I

INDICATIONS FOR INTRAVENOUS FEEDING

Malnutrition
Chronic diarrhea
Chronic vomiting
G.I. obstruction
Bowel resection
Inflammatory bowel disease
G.I. fistulas and anomalies
Malignant disease
Anorexia nervosa
Coma
Preoperative preparation
Postsurgical support

The Search For Calorie Sources

From a nutritional point of view, the search for suitable calorie sources has been of fundamental importance. As seen in Table II, a variety of compounds have been explored.

TABLE II

CALORIE SOURCES
FOR INTRAVENOUS FEEDING

Glucose
Fructose
Xylitol
Sorbitol
Ethanol
Maltose
Fat emulsions
Amino Acids

It is the purpose of this paper to review briefly the carbohydrate calorie sources studied to date, and finally to summarize the possibilities of the disaccharide, maltose, as a carbohydrate substrate in intravenous feeding.

Glucose. Since glucose is the carbohydrate normally found in the blood, it would seem to be the obvious and ideal choice of calories. Glucose is an economic and readily available carbohydrate, is efficiently utilized physiologically and also has the highest utilization rate in normal man. Notwithstanding the advantages of glucose as an intravenous source of calories, it

nevertheless has several serious limitations. If a 5% glucose
solution is used as the sole source of calories, 10 liters of
solution would be required to provide the caloric needs of the
average adult male. Infusion of hypertonic solutions of glucose
into peripheral veins may lead to complications such as thrombophlebitis, and high urinary losses of the sugar with a consequent
osmotic diuresis (14,15,16). Furthermore, glucose, being dependent on insulin for its utilization, may be contraindicated in
conditions in which insulin availability and/or activity may be
diminished or absent, such as surgical stress associated with elevated catecholamines and glucocorticoids (17,18,19), as well as in
diabetes (20,21,22,23), hypothermia (17), pancreatitis (20,22),
and sometimes in uremia (20,24). The problems of significantly
impaired glucose tolerance in patients with latent or overt diabetes mellitus, pancreatitis, stress, sepsis or shock, can often be
controlled if the parenteral administration of hypertonic glucose
solutions is initiated at a slow rate to excite increased endogenous insulin response, or, if exogenous insulin is provided (25,
26). Still another limitation of glucose as an intravenous source
of calories is the Maillard reaction that takes place during ster-
ilization and storage of combined glucose-amino acid solutions,
inactivating essential amino acids, especially lysine (27). For
these reasons, other carbohydrates that might overcome some of
the limitations of glucose, have been studied.

   Fructose. Comparative studies of glucose and fructose suggest
that fructose may be more rapidly metabolized than glucose (28,29,
30), infused veins may have a higher tolerance for fructose (31),
and the urinary excretion of fructose is less than that of glucose
(32,33,34). The initial uptake of fructose and its subsequent
phosphorylation to fructose-1-phosphate catalyzed by fructokinase
in the liver and adipose tissue is independent of insulin (16,20,
31,34). Some studies have shown that fructose infusion stimulates
insulin release (36,37), while other studies do not confirm this
(20). Nevertheless, some infused fructose is converted to glucose
(38,39) and consequently requires insulin for its further metabolism (17,32). Thus, while overall utilization of glucose and
fructose are similar in normal man, fructose may have certain advantages over glucose, especially for patients in the immediate
postoperative state when there is a known insulin antagonism (20,
30,40,41), diabetes mellitus (22,23,29), certain liver diseases
(20) and in pancreatectomy (20,22). In spite of the advantages of
fructose as a calorie source for intravenous infusion, a number of
serious limitations have been reported, including an increase in
lactic acid levels in the liver (42,43), increased blood lactate
levels following rapid infusion (44,47), depletion of high-energy-
phosphate as well as inorganic phosphate in the liver (48,49), reduction of inorganic phosphate in the serum (23), and hyperurice-
mia (44,50). The use of intravenous fructose can thus have serious and profound metabolic effects under certain circumstances,

raising serious questions and caution concerning its use as a
calorie substrate in parenteral alimentation (51,53).

Sorbitol. Sorbitol, a hexahydric alcohol with the same caloric value as glucose and fructose (4.1 kcal/g), is not directly
oxidized for energy production, but is converted to fructose via
sorbitol dehydrogenase, and metabolized as is this sugar (54). A
second and quantitatively less important metabolic pathway is the
conversion of sorbitol to glucose via aldose reductase (55). One
advantage of sorbitol is that it does not interact with amino
acids in the Maillard reaction (56). Sorbitol is not reabsorbed by
the renal tubules, and if administered rapidly, can provoke a diuresis (57,58). Thus, from a nutritional point of view, if the
rate of utilization and tolerance is less than that of glucose or
fructose, sorbitol does not offer any important advantage over
these sugars, and shares the limitations of these two sugars as a
calorie source in intravenous feeding (31,56).

Xylitol. The pentiol, xylitol, is a natural intermediate in
carbohydrate metabolism, and is rapidly oxidized to L-xylulose by
sorbitol dehydrogenase, and is then shunted into the pentose
phosphate cycle. Xylitol stimulates insulin release only when
infused at high dosage (20,59), and shares with fructose and sorbitol, its partial insulin-independence characteristics (20,59),
Xylitol can then be readily converted to glucose (27). Infusion
rates are limited (36), and in addition, xylitol raises serum uric
acid and bilirubin (60,62), and has adverse effects with regard to
a wide spectrum of metabolic abnormalities, including metabolic
acidosis, renal tubular epithelial-cell damage, intraluminal de-
posits of calcium oxalate crystals in the renal tubules, altered
cerebral function and hepatocellular injury (60,62). Nevertheless,
Spitz et al (59) have reported successful utilization of xylitol
in healthy subjects and patients with renal disease, and suggest
the use of this calorie source in uremia and in other conditions
characterized by carbohydrate intolerance and insulin resistance.

Ethanol. Ethanol contains 7.1 kcal/g, and thus potentially
is a higher calorie source than other intravenous compounds with
the exception of lipids. Alcohol is oxidized by alcohol dehydrogenase to acetaldehyde, which is then converted to acetyl CoA and
shunted into the tricarboxylic acid cycle for complete oxidation.
It is thought that insulin is not essential for oxidation of alcohol (63). Ethanol has some vasodilator action at the site of fluid
entry and may thus reduce the incidence of thrombophlebitis when
it is used in hyperosmotic carbohydrate solutions (64). In addition ethanol provides calories without an accompanying osmotic
load, and has minimal urinary excretion rates (64). However, the
concentration of ethanol in the body fluids must be kept within
tolerable limits to avoid pronounced pharmacological effects (64).
Direct toxic effects of ethanol on the liver (65) makes the use

of ethanol questionable.

Combination of Calorie Sources. Because no single calorie
source seems to be ideal, several investigators are currently
searching for appropriate combinations of carbohydrate and poly-
alcohol that can be used intravenously. It is postulated that
capitalizing on the most desirable characteristics of each individual source, some ratio of combined sources may prove to be a
more suitable means of providing energy substrate (66). It is
also of importance to note that different carbohydrates have varying insulinogenic potential. The stimulation of insulin is a major key to anabolism and may thus influence the choice of carbohydrate substrate in parenteral feeding.

Utilization of Intravenous Disaccharides as a Source of Calories

After oral ingestion of lactose, sucrose or maltose, only
small amounts of these disaccharides are absorbed intact. Thus,
under normal circumstances circulating levels as well as urinary
excretion of these sugars is minimal. For these reasons, the infusion of the double sugars has received limited consideration as
a possible source of calories in intravenous nutrition. Within the
past decade a variety of animal and human studies suggest that infused maltose, unlike the other disaccharides, may be suitable as
a carbohydrate substrate in intravenous nutrition.

Animal Studies. When radiolabeled lactose or sucrose are administered intravenously in the rat, only small amounts of isotope
appear in the expired CO_2 over a 24-hr period, while 62-68% is excreted in the urine (Table III) (67). This confirms previous
studies which showed that when these two disaccharides are administered parenterally in the rat, they are rapidly and almost quantitatively excreted in the urine (68,69). In contrast, 55-59% of
intravenously administered labeled maltose appears as $^{14}CO_2$, with
minimal urinary excretion of ^{14}C. The recovery of labeled ^{14}C
from maltose was comparable to that from injection of labeled glucose or other monosaccharide mixtures (67).

The extensive metabolism of injected maltose to $^{14}CO_2$ suggested a possible recirculation through the intestinal mucosa with
subsequent oxidation of maltose by intestinal maltases, or, the
possibility that tissues other than small bowel mucosa might possess maltase activity. As seen in Table IV, the hydrolysis and
subsequent metabolism of intravenously administered maltose was
not significantly influenced by selective removal of the small
bowel, kidneys, or 70% of the liver (67). Analysis of maltase activity in selected rat organs (Table V) indicates the presence of
maltase in a variety of tissues (67). Other estimates of rat tissue maltase activity are comparable (70,71,72). It therefore
seems unlikely that circulation of injected maltose to small bowel
mucosa plays a significant role in its over-all metabolism, or

TABLE III

Metabolism of ^{14}C-labeled disaccharides after
*iv administration in the rat**

Sugar	No. animals	$^{14}CO_2$	Urine ^{14}C
		% dose/24 hours	
Glucose-1-^{14}C	5	62.0 ± 11.6	5.3 ± 4.7
Glucose-U-^{14}C	5	64.0 ± 12.0	14.8 ± 10.3
Glucose-1-^{14}C + galactose**	4	52.0 ± 9.7	9.8 ± 6.6
Glucose-U-^{14}C + fructose-U-^{14}C†	5	50.7 ± 7.9	19.3 ± 4.6
Maltose-1-^{14}C	5	54.6 ± 7.0	4.8 ± 3.9
Maltose-U-^{14}C	5	58.6 ± 5.8	3.2 ± 3.0
Lactose-1-^{14}C	6	6.2 ± 2.7	62.1 ± 13.5
Sucrose-U-^{14}C	5	7.6 ± 2.4	68.4 ± 10.8

*Animals received 5 mg of suger in 0.5 ml (1 μc per ml).
**Mixture contained 2.5 mg of each sugar and 0.5 μc glucose-1-^{14}C.
†Mixture contained 2.5 mg and 0.25 μc of each sugar.

Journal of Clinical Investigation (67)

TABLE IV

Oxidation of ^{14}C-labeled sugars to $^{14}CO_2$ after iv injection in partially eviscerated rats

Organ removed	$^{14}CO_2$		
	Maltose-1-^{14}C	Glucose-1-^{14}C	Lactose-1-^{14}C
	% dose/24 hours		
Sham	48.3 ± 7.7 (4)*	55.3 ± 19.5 (3)	2.9 ± 0.9 (3)
Kidneys	46.2 ± 11.3 (4)	45.5 ± 17.6 (3)	16.9 ± 5.9 (3)
Liver (70%)	50.1 ± 9.2 (5)	43.9 ± 4.7 (3)	2.4 (1)
Small bowel	45.0 ± 2.7 (3)		

* Number of rats is given in parenthesis.

Journal of Clinical Investigation (67)

TABLE V

Maltase activity in homogenates of rat organs

Organ	Maltase		
	1	2	3
	U*	U	U
Intestinal mucosa	485	390	205
Kidney	17	61	73
Brain	14		4.0
Liver	2	1.6	1.7
Pancreas		4	5.6
Spleen	1	0.1	0.2
Muscle	0.1	0.3	0.3
Serum	9.1	12.5	8.9
Human serum	0.3	0.1	0.2

*One U equals 1 μmole maltose hydrolyzed per minute per g protein.

Journal of Clinical Investigation (67)

that a single tissue maltase was responsible for maltose oxidation. It is more probable that circulating maltose, unlike lactose or sucrose, may be hydrolyzed by extraintestinal maltases in several tissues and subsequently metabolized.

To explore whether maltosyloligosaccharides were also metabolized in vivo, the oxidation of a tracer dose of uniformly labeled ^{14}C-maltotriose to $^{14}CO_2$ after intravenous injection in the rat was measured (73). As seen in Figure 1, tracer doses of uniformly labeled ^{14}C-maltotriose, as well as uniformly labeled ^{14}C-maltose may be oxidized to $^{14}CO_2$ after intravenous injection in the rat as efficiently as U-^{14}C-glucose, with 64.2 $\pm$ 4.2%, 65.5 $\pm$ 8.3% and 60.5 $\pm$ 4.8% of the infused dose recovered as $^{14}CO_2$, respectively (73).

When insulin is simultaneously administered with glucose-1-^{14} or maltose-1-^{14}C to rats, the percentage of injected ^{14}C expired as $^{14}CO_2$ was the same as the recovery of $^{14}CO_2$ from administration of the sugar without insulin (74). After intravenous injection of glucose-1-^{14}C, 49.3 $\pm$ 8.2% of the isotope appeared in the expired CO_2 over a 6-hr period. When insulin was added to the injection solution, 47.5 $\pm$ 6.6% of the labeled glucose was expired as $^{14}CO_2$. The fraction of injected ^{14}C recovered as $^{14}CO_2$ following maltose-1-^{14}C injection, with and without insulin was also the same, these values being 59.7 $\pm$ 4.9 and 59.7 $\pm$ 5.0%, respectively. Likewise, when the two sugars are compared, there was no significant difference in the amount of glucose or maltose oxidized to CO_2 with or without insulin. As seen in Figures 2 and 3, insulin did cause a more rapid oxidation of both sugars to $^{14}CO_2$. Specific activity curves showed significantly earlier peaks when insulin was given with either glucose or maltose, than when these sugars were administered alone. When the peak excretion curves after maltose and glucose administration are compared, it is consistently observed that the peak oxidation time after maltose is delayed, suggesting a "precursor-product" relationship which requires time for maltose to be hydrolyzed to glucose.

Insulin also enhances the incorporation of intravenously injected glucose and maltose into rat epididymal lipids (Figure 4). The specific activity of extracted lipids of rat epididymal lipids following intravenous infusion of glucose plus insulin was 37% greater than when glucose was infused alone. Of particular interest is the similar response noted when insulin was injected with maltose, representing a 29% increase over incorporation observed when maltose was given alone. Rat epididymal tissue was equally insulin-sensitive when either glucose or maltose was the sugar donating its labeled carbon to the synthesis of lipids (74). These studies indicate that glucose and maltose respond similarly to insulin stimulation.

The oxidation of intravenously administered trehalose has also been studied (75). This double sugar was selected for study because it closely resembles maltose, consisting of two glucose molecules joined in an α -1, 1 linkage. Figure 5 plots the

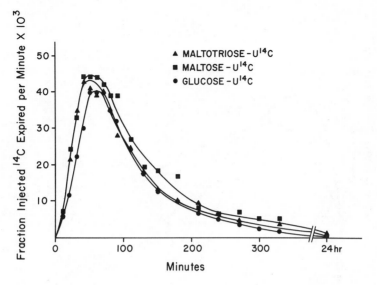

Biochimica et Biophysica Acta

Figure 1.   Oxidation of uniformly labeled [¹⁴C] maltotriose, [¹⁴C] maltose, and [¹⁴C] glucose to ¹⁴CO₂ after intravenous injection in the rat. Each point represents the mean value of five animals (73).

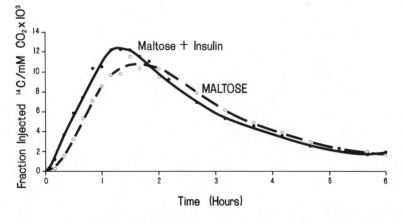

Endocrinology

Figure 2.   Effect of insulin on the oxidation of circulating maltose-1-¹⁴C to ¹⁴CO₂. Specific activity curve following maltose (50 mg) iv (○); maltose (50 mg) plus insulin (0.2 U) iv (●) (74).

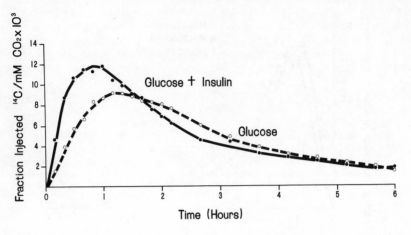

Figure 3.   Effect of insulin on the oxidation of circulating glucose-1-^{14}C to $^{14}CO_2$I.
Specific activity curve following glucose (50 mg) iv (○); glucose (50 mg) plus
insulin (0.2) iv (●) (74).

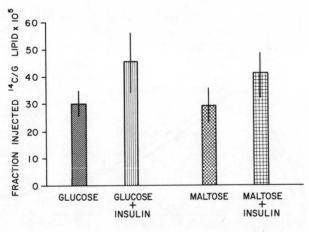

Figure 4.   Effect of insulin on the incorporation of ^{14}C-
labeled glucose, glucose plus insulin, maltose and maltose
plus insulin into rat epididymal tissue. Bars represent the
means and S.D. for 6, 7, 6 and 6 animals, respectively (74).

oxidation of uniformly labeled glucose, maltose, sucrose and trehalose following intravenous administration in the rat. After the
injection of trehalose-U-^{14}C and sucrose-U-^{14}C only 5.26 $\pm$ 0.88%
and 8.11 $\pm$ 1.25% of the isotope appeared in the expired CO_2, respectively. In contrast, after maltose or glucose injection,
59.60 $\pm$ 2.30% and 49.30 $\pm$ 3.50% respectively, was excreted as
$^{14}CO_2$. Only 3 to 5% of the infused maltose and glucose was excreted in the urine, while 40 to 47% of the trehalose and sucrose was
excreted (75). The results of this study indicate that while trehalose and maltose both consist of two glucose molecules, their
metabolic fate is quite different. Unlike maltose, trehalose is
minimally oxidized to CO_2 and largely excreted in the urine. It
has been suggested that the absence of trehalase and sucrase in
rat serum and kidney (71,72,76,77) probably accounts for the minimal oxidation of these sugars. In contrast, maltase is relatively
high in rat kidney (67,77,78) and serum (67,77) which would explain the difference in the metabolism of these disaccharides when
given parenterally. It is postulated that trehalase and maltase
activity in mammalian kidney may play a role in tubular reabsorption of trehalose and maltose, as well as glucose (79). Rat kidney slices have been shown to oxidize ^{14}C-maltose and ^{14}C-malto-
triose to $^{14}CO_2$ more than other tissues, with the exception of
small bowel mucosa (78). After the intravenous administration of
uniformly labeled trehalose and sucrose, the kidney tissue accumulates the highest cpm/g tissue when compared to recovery of the
label in other tissues (75). These studies lend further support
to the suggestion that the presence of the disaccharidase in the
renal tubular tissue may be a major determinant of the efficiency
of disaccharide metabolism subsequent to intravenous infusion. In
an animal such as the rabbit with high trehalase activity in the
kidney (72,78), 64% of intravenously administered trehalose-U-^{14}C
was oxidized to $^{14}CO_2$, while less than 2% was excreted in the
urine (75). The recovery of ^{14}C as $^{14}CO_2$ after infusion of trehalose in the rabbit is seen in Figure 6.

   The efficient oxidation of intravenously administered maltose
poses a question concerning the entry of this sugar into the cell
prior to its metabolism. A comparative study of the uptake of
maltose and other sugars into rat diaphragm cells indicated that
at equilibrium all sugars entered cells by diffusion (80). At all
equimolar concentrations, disaccharide transport into intracellular water was equal, but only 50% that of monosaccharides. When
intracellular sugar was calculated on a weight basis (mg/ml)
transport of all disaccharides and monosaccharides was equal (80).
In cells that possess intracellular disaccharidase activity,
hydrolysis of disaccharides and monosaccharides would account for
their subsequent metabolism.

   The slow 24-hr infusions of nutrient solution containing 25%
maltose hydrate, amino acids, vitamins and electrolytes in rats
over a 14 day period resulted in severe weight losses and up to
52% urinary excretion of the infused maltose. Similar infusions

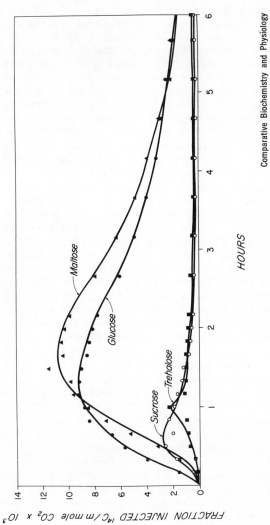

Comparative Biochemistry and Physiology

Figure 5. Oxidation of intravenously administered glucose–U–^{14}*C, maltose–U–*^{14}*C, sucrose–U–*^{14}*C, and trehalose–U–*^{14}*C to *$^{14}CO_2$* in rats over a 6-hour period. Each point represents the mean value for 6, 6, 4 and 7 animals respectively (75).*

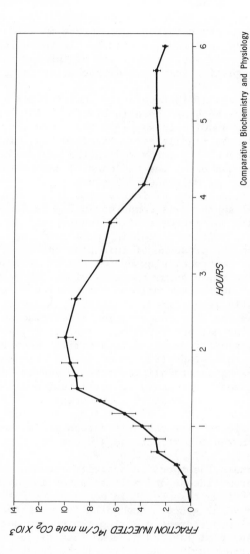

Figure 6.   Oxidation of circulating trehalose to $^{14}CO_2$ in the rabbit. Points represent mean $\pm$ S.D. for one animal (75).

Comparative Biochemistry and Physiology

of glucose solutions resulted in weight maintenance and little or no urinary excretion (81). While this study concludes that long-term parenteral maltose cannot serve as a total caloric substitute for glucose in complete parenteral nutrition, results are limited to observations in only two animals. Additional long-term parenteral studies are needed.

Human Studies. After lactose or sucrose infusion in man, these disaccharides are largely excreted in the urine (67,82). As seen in Table VI, only small quantities of infused maltose appear in the urine, suggesting that this disaccharide is metabolized (67).

Oxidation curves of intravenously administered maltose to healthy, normal subjects are seen in Figure 7 (83). When 10 g maltose containing 5 uCi maltose-U-^{14}C was given intravenously, this disaccharide was readily metabolized to CO_2, with 60% of the administered radioactivity recovered in the expired air over a 6 hr period. Less than 8% of the radioactive carbon was recovered in the urine either as maltose or as glucose (83).

The metabolic response of intravenous infusion of maltose and glucose to normal subjects is compared in Figure 8. Blood glucose concentrations did not increase significantly after maltose infusion, although a significant rise in total reducing substances was noted, indicating the presence of this disaccharide in the blood. This suggests that extracellular hydrolysis of maltose to glucose is minimal. Since human serum contains almost no maltase activity (67,72), it is probable that maltose enters tissue cells intact and is subsequently metabolized. Initially, there was a fourfold increase in serum insulin concentration after glucose and a threefold increase after maltose infusion. Thereafter, serum insulin concentrations gradually declined in a similar manner for both sugars. Data from this study (83) demonstrates that maltose is readily available as a metabolic substrate, and may provide the required metabolite(s) necessary to initiate insulin secretion. The plasma free fatty acids at 15 min decreased 371 uEq/liter after glucose and 338 uEq/liter after maltose infusion. The results of this study indicate that the utilization of infused maltose elicits similar metabolic effects as glucose in the normal subject.

Table VII shows the specific activity (counts/minute per milligram) of serum glucose and maltose after intravenous administration of 55 uCi maltose-U-^{14}C in one subject. Although there was no change in serum glucose concentration, the specific activit of glucose slowly increased during the 60 min period, likely representing reentry of labeled glucose from tissue sources. On the other hand, the specific activity of the injected maltose remained relatively constant (83).

The metabolism of maltose and glucose after intravenous injection was compared in normal and mildly diabetic subjects (84). The recovery of ^{14}C as [14]CO_2 in normal subjects was similar after

TABLE VI

*Disaccharide recovered in 24-hour urine sample after iv
administration of 10 g in adult humans*

| | Disaccharide infused | | |
Subject	Lactose	Sucrose	Maltose
	g	*g*	*g*
J.S.	10.5	7.2	0.09
I.R.	7.1		0.08
B.B.	8.6	4.8	0.12
B.G.		6.8	0.15
Mean ± SD	8.7 ± 1.8	6.3 ± 1.3	0.11 ± 0.03

Journal of Clinical Investigation (67)

TABLE VII

*Specific Activity of Serum Glucose and Maltose after
Intravenous Administration of 10 g Maltose-U-^{14}C* *

| | | | Specific activity | |
Minutes	Serum glucose	Estimated maltose	Glucose	Maltose
	mg/100 ml	*mg/100 ml*	*cpm/mg*	
0	87	0	0	0
15	92	61	209	5773
30	90	50	487	6153
45	90	34	878	5933
60	94	31	1000	6975

*55 μCi Maltose-U-^{14}C.

Journal of Clinical Investigation (83)

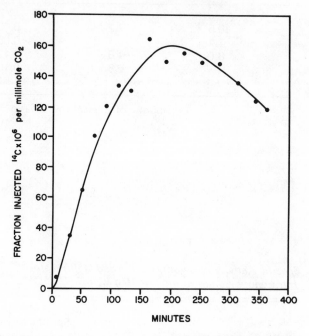

Journal of Clinical Investigation

Figure 7. Fraction of injected ^{14}C recovered as expired $^{14}CO_2$ per millimole CO_2 over a 6-hr period after the intravenous administration of 10 g ^{14}C-labeled maltose. Points are mean values for five subjects (83).

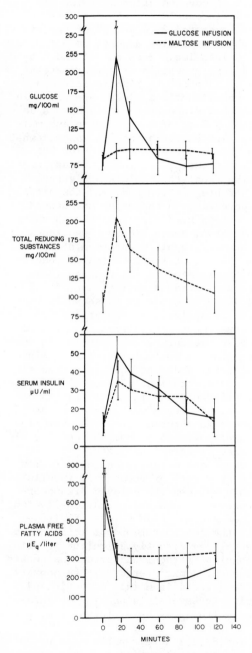

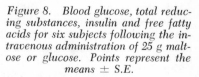

Figure 8. Blood glucose, total reducing substances, insulin and free fatty acids for six subjects following the intravenous administration of 25 g maltose or glucose. Points represent the means ± S.E.

the administration of labeled glucose and maltose, with $33.3 \pm$ 1.6%, $37.7 \pm 3.4\%$ and $36.5 \pm 1.9\%$ recovered after infusion of maltose-U-^{14}C, glucose-U-^{14}C and glucose-1-^{14}C, respectively (Table VIII). Diabetic subjects excreted $25.4 \pm 1.3\%$ of administered maltose-U-^{14}C as $^{14}CO_2$, while a similar amount, $28.3 \pm 0.7\%$ was excreted after glucose-1-^{14}C infusion. Both normal and diabetic subjects showed a delayed peak excretion of approximately 100 min after maltose infusion as compared to glucose infusion. The $^{14}CO_2$ excretion curves for the diabetic subjects are shown in Figure 9. Our studies indicate that diabetic subjects have a decreased capacity to shunt a loading dose of both glucose and maltose into CO_2 pathways. The urinary excretion of ^{14}C was somewhat greater after maltose infusion than after glucose infusion but this difference was not significant except for lower urinary excretion after glucose-1-^{14}C. The renal threshold and clearance rates for maltose in man have not been determined, and the actual amount of glucose and maltose appearing in the urine may depend upon the concentration and rate of infused sugar. Although there is no maltase activity in human serum, human kidney tissue does have maltase activity (85). Chromatographic separation of the urinary ^{14}C indicates that some 50-55% of the excreted radioactivity following maltose infusion is excreted as ^{14}C glucose (84).

The metabolic response to the intravenous infusion of maltose and glucose to normal and diabetic subjects is shown in Figures 10 and 11 and the statistical analysis is summarized in Table IX. Serum glucose concentration after maltose infusion remained less than 95 mg/100 ml over the entire 2-hr period, in contrast to the elevation of serum glucose following glucose administration. The increase in total serum reducing substances was similar after maltose and glucose administration. In normal and diabetic subjects, there was a significant rise in serum insulin after maltose injection, however this increase was greater after glucose. Diabetic subjects showed an abnormal i.v. glucose tolerance test and higher serum insulin levels at 60, 90, and 120 min after glucose infusion as compared to normal subjects. Insulin disappearance curves in both normal and diabetic subjects following maltose infusion indicate a slow rate of removal of insulin from the serum. The relationship between the delayed disappearance of serum insulin and the serum glucose concentrations (which remain below 95 mg/100 ml) is not known. High levels of circulating maltose (as reflected in the concentrations of total serum sugars) at this same time interval may directly stimulate insulin release. It is not known if insulin is required for maltose entry into mammalian cells. Intravenously administered maltose appears to be as efficiently utilized as glucose in mildly diabetic and normal subjects. Further studies in severely diabetic patients are needed to determine whether maltose may be efficiently metabolized despite a reduced insulin response (84).

Several studies in Japan (86,87,88) have reported the use of maltose solutions in a variety of surgical patients. In a study

TABLE VIII

Recovery of ^{14}C after the intravenous administration of 25 g ^{14}C-labeled maltose or glucose to normal and diabetic subjects

Subjects	Carbohydrate	$^{14}CO_2$	Peak^{14}C	Urinary^{14}C
		% Dose	Minutes	% Dose
Normal	I. Maltose-U-^{14}C (5)*	33.3 ± 1.6†	235 ± 10	11.8 ± 1.9
	II. Glucose-U-^{14}C (5)	37.7 ± 3.4	110 ± 13	6.9 ± 1.2
	III. Glucose-I-^{14}C (4)	36.5 ± 1.9	120 ± 6	5.1 ± 0.6
Diabetic	IV. Maltose-U-^{14}C (5)	25.4 ± 1.3	240 ± 10	11.0 ± 2.4
	V. Glucose-I-^{14}C (5)	28.3 ± 0.7	138 ± 15	7.3 ± 2.0
	I vs II+	NS	$p < 0.001$	NS
	I vs III	NS	$p < 0.001$	$p < 0.05$
	II vs III	NS	NS	NS
	IV vs V	NS	$p < 0.001$	NS
	I vs IV	$p < 0.05$	NS	NS
	II vs V	$p < 0.05$	NS	NS

* Number in parenthesis indicates number of subjects.
† Mean ± SE.
+ Statistical comparisons are between groups as indicated.

Journal of Clinical Endocrinology and Metabolism (84)

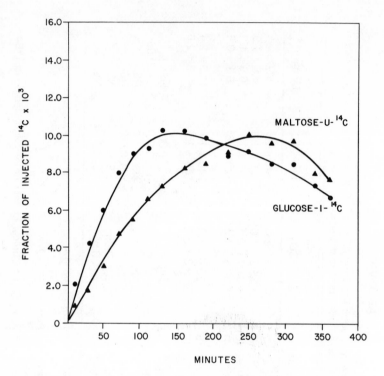

Journal of Clinical Endocrinology and Metabolism

Figure 9. Fraction of injected ^{14}C recovered as expired $^{14}CO_2$ over a 6-hr period after the intravenous administration of 25 g glucose-1-^{14}C or maltose–U–^{14}C to five mildly diabetic subjects (84)

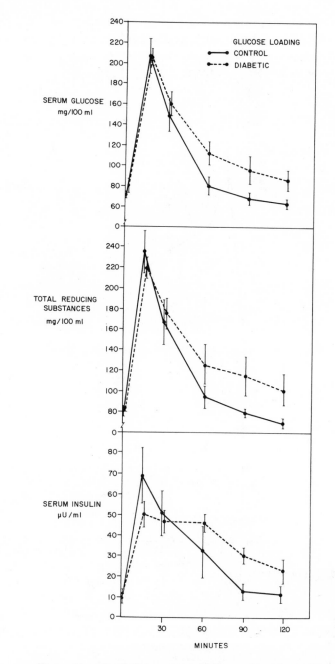

Figure 10.   Metabolic response of 14 control and five mildly diabetic subjects following the intravenous administration of 25 g glucose-1-^{14}C. Each point represents mean value ± S.E.

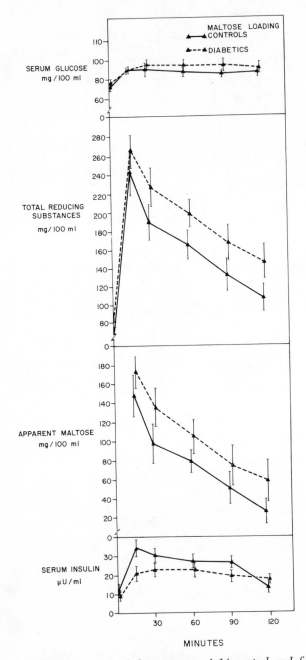

Figure 11. Metabolic response of 14 control and five mildly diabetic subjects to the intravenous administration of 25 g maltose–U–^{14}C. Each point represents mean value ± S.E.

TABLE IX

Statistical comparisons of metabolic response to the intravenous administration of glucose and maltose to normal and diabetic subjects

	Subject groups	Minutes after infusion					
		0	15	30	60	90	120
Serum Glucose mg/100 ml	I vs II	NS*	$p < 0.001$	$p < 0.05$	NS	NS	$p < 0.05$
	III vs IV	NS	$p < 0.001$	$p < 0.001$	NS	NS	NS
	I vs III	NS	NS	NS	NS	NS	NS
	II vs IV	NS	NS	NS	$p < 0.05$	$p < 0.05$	$p < 0.05$
Total Serum Sugars. mg/100 ml	I vs II	NS	NS	NS	$p < 0.01$	$p < 0.01$	$p < 0.01$
	III vs IV	NS	NS	NS	$p < 0.05$	NS	NS
	I vs III	$p < 0.01$	NS	NS	NS	NS	NS
	II vs IV	NS	NS	NS	NS	$p < 0.05$	$p < 0.05$
"Apparent Maltose," mg/100 ml	I vs III	NS	NS	NS	NS	NS	NS
Serum Insulin, μU/ml	I vs II	NS	$p < 0.05$	NS	NS	$p < 0.05$	NS
	III vs IV	NS	$p < 0.01$	$p < 0.01$	$p < 0.01$	NS	NS
	I vs III	NS	$p < 0.05$	NS	NS	NS	NS
	II vs IV	NS	NS	NS	NS	$p < 0.01$	NS

*Statistical comparisons are between subject groups indicated: I. Normal maltose loading. II. Normal glucose loading. III. Diabetic maltose loading. IV. Diabetic glucose loading.

Journal of Clinical Endocrinology and Metabolism (84)

of 67 patients, no secondary effects, clinical abnormalities, or hyperosmolar problems were recognized (84),

Conclusions

To date, there is no ideal carbohydrate source of calories for parenteral alimentation. Studies of intravenously administered disaccharides indicate that maltose and glucose are efficiently and similarly metabolized in man and in the rat. Maltose, because of its caloris density and ability to be metabolized, may be of importance in parenteral nutrition, and warrants further study.

Literature Cited

1. Annan, G. L., Bull. N. Y. Acad. Med. (1939) 15:622.
2. Foster, M. "Claude Bernard". Longmans Green Company, New York. 1899.
3. Biedl, A. and Kraus, R., Wein Klin Wschr. (1896) 9:55.
4. Geyer, Robert P., Physiol. Rev. (1960) 40:150.
5. Law, David H., Adv. Intern. Med. (1972) 18:389.
6. Shils, Maurice E., J. Amer. Med. Assoc. (1972) 220:14.
7. Wretlind, A. (Editor). "Colloquim on intravenous feeding". Colloquim held at The Royal Society of Medicine. London, May 1-2, 1962. Nutr dieta (1963) 5:295.
8. "Parenteral Nutrition Symposium". Symposium held at Kungalv, Sweden, Nov. 9-10, 1962. Acta Chir. Scand. (1964) Suppl. 325: 1.
9. Meng, H.C. and Law, David H. (Editors). "Parenteral Nutrition". International Symposium on Parenteral Nutrition. Vanderbilt University School of Medicine, 1968. Charles C. Thomas, Springfield, 1970.
10. Cowan, G. S. M. and Scheetz, W. L. (Editors). "Intravenous Hyperalimentation". U. S. Army Institute of Surgical Research, San Antonio, Texas. 1970. Lea and Febiger, Philadelphia, 1972.
11. Wilkison, A. W. (Editor). "Parenteral Nutrition". An International Symposium in London, April 20, May 1, 1971. Williams and Wilkins Company, Baltimore, 1972.
12. American Medical Association. "Symposium on Total Parenteral Nutrition". Symposium held at Nashville, Tennessee, Jan. 17-19, 1972. American Medical Association, Council on Food and Nutrition, Chicago, 1974.
13. Dudrick, S. J., Steiger, E., Long, J. M., Ruberg, R. L., Allen, T. R., Vars, H. M. and Rhoads, J. E. In "Intravenous Hyperalimentation". George Cowan, Jr. and Walter Scheetz, (Editors). p. 3. Lea and Febiger, Philadelphia, 1972.
14. Wyrick, W. J., Rea, W. S. and McClelland, R. N., J. Amer. Med. Assoc. (1970) 211:1967.
15. Winters, R. W., Scaglione, P. R., Nahas, G. G. and Verosky, M. J. Clin. Invest. (1964) 43:647.

16. Thoren, L., Nutr. Dieta, (1963) 5:305.
17. Froesch, E. R. and Keller, U. In "Parenteral Nutrition".
    A. W. Wilkinson, (Editor). An International Symposium, London, April 30, May 1, 1971, Williams and Wilkins Company, Baltimore, 1972, p. 105.
18. Hayes, M. A. and Brandt, R. L., Surgery (1952) 32:819.
19. Elman, R. and Weichsclbaum, T. E., Arch. Surg. (1951) 62:683.
20. Mehnert, H., Forster, H., Geser, C. A., Haslbeck, M., Dehmel, K. H., In "Parenteral Nutrition". H. C. Meng and D. H. Law (Editors). International Symposium on Parenteral Nutrition. Vanderbilt University School of Medicine, 1968. Charles C. Thomas, Springfield, 1970, p. 112.
21. Schaefer, H. F., Med. Welt. (1960) 32:1632.
22. Daughaday, W. H. and Weichselbaum. T. E., Metabolism (1953) 2:459.
23. Miller, M., Drucker, W. R., Owens, J. E., Craig, J. W. and Woodward, Jr., H., J. Clin. Invest. (1952) 31:115.
24. Luke, R. G., Dinwoodie, A. J., Linton, A. L. and Kennedy, A. C., J. Lab. Clin. Med. (1964) 64:731.
25. Hinton, P., Littlejohn, S., Allison, S. P. and Lloyd, J., Lancet (1971) 1:767.
26. Dudrick, S. J., MacFadyen, B. V., VanBuren, C. T., Ruberg, R. L., Ann. Surg. (1972) 176:259.
27. Bassler, K. H. In "Parenteral Nutrition". H. C. Meng and D. H. Law (Editors). Proceedings of an International Symposium, Vanderbilt University School of Medicine, Nashville, Tennessee, 1968. Charles C. Thomas, Springfield, 1970, p.96.
28. Weichselbaum, T. E., Elman, R., and Lunc, R. H., Proc. Soc. Explt. Biol. (1950) 75:816.
29. Albanese, A. A., Felch, W. C., Higgons, R. A., Vestal, B. L. and Stephanson, L., Metabolism (1952) 1:20.
30. Elman, R., Amer. J. Clin. Nutr. (1953) 1:287.
31. Thoren, L., Acta. Chir. Scand., (1964). Suppl. 325, p.75.
32. Wretlind, A., Nutr. and Metabol. (1972) 14:Suppl. p.1.
33. Moncrief, J. A., Coldwater, K. B. and Elman, R., Arch. Surg. (1953) 67:57.
34. Miller, M. J., Craig, W., Drucker, W. R. and Woodward, H., Yale J. Biol. and Med. (1956) 29:335.
35. Froesch, E. R., Zapf, J., Keller, U. and Oelz, O., Europ. J. Clin. Invest. (1971) 2:8.
36. Heuckenkamp, P. U. and Zollner, N., Nutr. Metabol. (1972) 14:Suppl. p.58.
37. Aitkin, J. M. and Dunnigan, M. G., Brit. Med. J. (1969) 3:276.
38. Weinstein, J. J. and Roe, J. H., J. Lab. Clin. Med. (1952) 40:47.
39. Pletscher, A., Helv. Med. Acta. (1953) 20:100.
40. Mehnert, H., Mahrhofer, E., and Forster, H., Munchen Med. Wschr. (1964) 106:193.
41. Sunzel, H., Acta Chir. Scand. (1958) 115:235.
42. Berry, M. N., Proc. Roy. Soc. Med. (1967) 60:1260.

43. Woods, H. F., Oliva, P. A., Amer. J. Med. (1970) 48:209.
44. Bergstrom, J., Hultman, E., and Roch-Norlund, A. E., Acta. Med. Scand. (1968) 184:359.
45. Craig, G. M. and Crane, C. W., Brit. Med. J. (1971) 4:211.
46. Sahebjami, H. and Scalettar, R., Lancet (1971) 1:366.
47. Cook, G. C. and Jacobson. J., Brit. J. Nutr. (1971) 26:187.
48. Woods, H. F., Eggleston, L. U. and Krebs, H. A., Biochem. J. (1970) 119:501.
49. Bode, C., Schumacher, H., Goebell, H., Zelder, D., and Pelzel, H., Hormone Metab. Res. (1971) 3:289.
50. Fox, I. H. and Kelley, W. N., Metabolism (1972) 20:713.
51. Pearson, J. F. and Shuttleworth, R., Amer. J. Obstet. Gynec. (1971) 111:259.
52. Woods, H. F. and Alberti, K. G. M. M., Lancet (1972) 2:1354.
53. Harries, J. T. In "Parenteral Nutrition". A. W. Wilkinson (Editor). An International Symposium in London, April 30, May 1, 1971. Williams and Wilkins, Baltimore, 1972, p.266.
54. Blackley, R. L., Biochem. J. (1951) 49:257.
55. Hers, H. G., J. Biol. Chem. (1955) 214:373.
56. Lee, H. A., Morgan, A. G., Waldrom, R., and Bennet, J. In "Parenteral Nutrition". An International Symposium in London, April 30, May 1, 1971. A. W. Wilkinson (Editor). Williams and Wilkins, Baltimore, 1972, p.121.
57. Bye, P. A., Brit. J. Surg. (1969) 56:653.
58. Seeberg, V. P., McQuarrie, E. B., and Secor, C. C., Proc. Soc. Exper. Biol. (1955) 89:303.
59. Spitz, I. M., Rubenstein, A. H., Bersohn, I., and Bassler, K. H., Metabolism (1970) 19:24.
60. Thomas, D. W., Edwards, J. B., and Edwards, R. G., New Eng. J. Med. (1970) 283:437.
61. Schumer, W., Metabolism (1971) 20:345.
62. Forster, H., Meyer, E., and Ziege, M., Klin. Wschr. (1970) 48:878.
63. Mirsky, I. A. and Nelson, N., Amer. J. Physiol. (1939) 127:308.
64. Coats, D. A. In "Parenteral Nutrition". A. W. Wilkinson (Editor). An International Symposium in London, April 30, May 1, 1971. Williams and Wilkins, Baltimore, 1972, p.152.
65. Lieber, C. S., Gastroenterology (1973) 65:821.
66. Bassler, K. H. and Bickel, H. In "Parenteral Nutrition". A. W. Wilkinson (Editor). An International Symposium in London, April 30, May 1, 1971. Williams and Wilkins, Baltimore, 1972, p.99.
67. Weser, Elliot and Sleisenger, Marvin H., J. Clin. Invest. (1967) 46:499.
68. Dahlqvist, A. and Thompson, D. L., Acta. Physiol. Scand. (1964) 61:20.
69. Dahlqvist, A. and Thompson, D. L., J. Physiol. (1963) 167:193.

70. Semenza, G. In "Alimentary Canal". C. F. Code (Editor). Williams and Wilkins, Baltimore, 1968, Vol. 5, Section 6, p.2543.
71. Bittencourt, H., Sleisenger, M. H., and Weser, E. Gastroenterology (1969) 57:410.
72. Van Handel, F., Comp. Biochem. Physiol. (1968) 26:561.
73. Weser, E., Friedman, M., and Sleisenger, M. H., Biochim et Biophys. Acta. (1967) 136:170.
74. Young, J. M. and Weser, E., Endocrinology (1970) 86:426.
75. Flores, M., Weser, E., and Young, E. A., Comp. Biochem. Physiol. (1974) 50B: (In press)
76. Dahlqvist, A. and Brun, A., J. Histochem. Cytochem. (1962) 10:294.
77. Courtois, J. E. and Demelier, J. E., Bull. Soc. Chim. Biol. (1966) 48:277.
78. Sacktor, B., Proc. Nat. Acad. Sci. (1968) 60:1007.
79. Silverman, Melvin., J. Clin. Invest. (1973) 52:2486.
80. Young, E. A. and Weser, E., J. Clin. Invest. (1974) 53:87a.
81. Yoshimura, N. N., Ehrlich, H., Westman, T. L., and Deindoerfer, F. H., J. Nutr. (1973) 103:1256.
82. Deane, N., Schreiner, G. E. and Robertson, J. S., J. Clin. Invest. (1951) 30:1463.
83. Young, J. M. and Weser, E., J. Clin Invest. (1971) 50:986.
84. Young, E. A. and Weser, E., J. Clin. Endocrin. and Metab. (1974) 38:181.
85. Drayfus, J. C. and Alexandre, Y., Biochim. Biophys. Res. Commun. (1972) 48:914.
86. Sunada, Tenitake, et al, Diag. and Treat. (1971) 59:2386. (Japanese)
87. Hayasaka, A., et al, J. New Remedies and Clinics (1972) 21:3   (Japanese)
88. Tanaka, Takaya, et al, J. New Remedies and Clinics (1971) 20:125. (Japanese)

6

The Metabolism of Lactose and Galactose

R. GAURTH HANSEN

Utah State University, Logan, Utah 84322

RICHARD GITZELMANN

Laboratory for Metabolic Research, Children's Hospital, Zurich, Switzerland

Lactose, which is converted to galactose and glucose, is the primary carbohydrate source for developing mammals, and in humans it constitutes 40 percent of the energy consumed during the nursing period. Why lactose evolved as the unique carbohydrate of milk is unclear, especially since most individuals can meet their galactose need by biosynthesis from glucose. Whatever the rationale for lactose in milk, the occurrence of galactose in glyco-proteins, complex polysaccharides, and lipids, particularly in nervous tissue, has suggested specific functions. The organoleptic and physical properties of galactose and, more specifically, the simultaneous occurrence of calcium and lactose in milk, may be significant evolutionary determinants.

Lactose, in contrast to other saccharides, appears to enhance the absorption of calcium, as does vitamin D (1) (2). In man, calcium absorption is associated with the hydrolysis of lactose (3).

The extensive literature concerned with galactose occurrence will not be reviewed, only some relevant examples will be cited. Collagen contains glycosylated hydroxylysine, either as galactose or as glucosyl-galactose (4). Bone collagen mainly contains galactose monosaccharides, which could be important calcium binding centers, since many carbohydrates bind calcium in aqueous solution. In humans an excretion of three oligosaccharides containing galactose is enhanced by lactose ingestion (5). The three oligosaccharides appear to represent nonreducing terminals of the blood's antigenic determinants.

I. Lactose Catabolism

A. **Microorganisms.** The utilization of lactose for energy or structural purposes is preceded by hydrolysis to the hexoses, which can be absorbed. There is considerable potential for improving the properties and acceptability of lactose in foods by hydrolyzing it to the monosaccharides. Toward that end, substantial progress has been made toward isolating and characterizing the relevant enzyme from lactose-fermenting microorganisms (6) (7) (8). In microorganisms, β - galactosidases are induced by galactose and by other sugars that have configurations related to galactose.

B. Mammalian Digestion. In mammals, the rate-limiting step in lactose digestion appears to be the hydrolysis of the disaccharide into absorbable monosaccharides. Most mammalian disaccharidase activity is localized in the brush-border fraction of the mucosal cells of the small intestine (9).

1. Lactase deficiencies. Whether lactase is induced or constitutive in man has not been clearly established. We do know, however, that in populations that traditionally depend on milk as a significant source of energy, throughout life most adults retain an ability to hydrolyze lactose. But when lactose is not a significant component of the adult diet, the capacity to hydrolyze lactose seems to decline over time (10).

By contrast, lactose intolerance is common in many non-milk consuming adult populations. Among these people, the ability to metabolize lactose, obviously present during infancy, disappears between the ages of one and four.

Evidence that lactase levels respond to an altered lactose intake is questionable (11). Neither exposure to extra lactose (12) (13) nor removal of lactose from the diet for periods of 40 to 50 days altered lactase levels in the intestinal tissues of adults. Perhaps of more significance, nine in a group of ten galactosemic children, ages 7 to 17 years, who had carefully avoided lactose-containing materials since early infancy, had normal blood glucose responses to oral lactose loads, suggesting that their lactase levels had not decreased during their long periods of lactose abstinence. The one exception was a 15-year old Negro who was determined by biopsy to be lactase deficient (14).

Any potential for an adaptive response to lactose in humans is insignificant during the life span. A genetic basis for adult lactase deficiency is indicated by the 70 percent of black Americans who are reported to be lactose intolerant, which duplicates the adult intolerance level of black Africans, whose exposure to lactose is probably much less. Although the question has not been conclusively resolved in humans, adult lactase deficiency may be primarily under genetic control.

Intestinal lactase may have occurred initially in adult humans as a consequence of the domestication of milk-producing livestock. This concept is substantiated by the lifelong presence of lactose in most western European adults and in those ethnically derived from Europe. These people can effectively digest the lactose in dairy foods. According to this hypothesis, adaptation to the presence of lactose in the diet required many generations and a period of several thousand years. Adult blacks in the United States have not developed intestinal lactase after exposure to lactose for 300 years.

When milk-producing animals were domesticated it is postulated that some adults with lactase deficiency became lactase producers through gene mutation (15). The specific selective advantage of the lactose-tolerant adult was associated with the lactose-induced enhancement of calcium absorption in an environment that provided a low dietary supply of vitamin D. Milk consumption thus may be advantageous for lactose-tolerant individuals because milk supplies both calcium and a factor promoting its absorption.

The rarely occurring congenital lactose intolerance that is due to a deficiency of lactase was named by Holzel (16) as "Alactasia." A limited number of infants having this defect have been documented, but the mode of inheritance is not clear. Another congenital lactose intolerance is associated with the inability of infants to hydrolyze lactose and the subsequent appearance of lactose in the urine. These phenomena generally seem to be secondary to mucosal damage associated with acute infectious diarrhea, and probably constitute a different and more complex syndrome than alactasia.

A voluminous and important literature is developing describing deficiencies of lysosomal beta- and alpha-galactosidases (17) (18). In Fabry's Disease, there is a deficiency of the α-galactosidase which normally hydrolyzes ceramide trihexoside, resulting in the accumulation of trihexosylceramide in various organs, primarily in kidneys. Three other sphingolipidoses are attributed to the deficiency of an enzyme hydrolyzing β-galactosidic bonds: Krabbe's Disease, Ceramidelactoside Lipidosis, and Generalized Gangliosidosis. Galactosidases obviously play an important role in the regulation of glycolipid levels in tissues.

II. Lactose Biosynthesis

It was early concluded (19) that UDP-galactose was the donor and glucose-1-phosphate the acceptor during the synthesis of lactose. The product of the reaction, the phosphate ester of lactose, was postulated to have a role in its excretion by the glandular tissue. By using C^{14} isotopes in the lactating cow and isolating the postulated intermediates and products, investigators concluded that a major pathway for lactose synthesis had UDP-galactose as the donor, and free glucose (not glucose-1-phosphate) as the acceptor (20). Tissue extracts subsequently were found to catalyze the synthesis of lactose from UDP-galactose and glucose but, contrary to expectations, the yields were

very low (21). This work confirmed the isotope studies in the whole
animal.

A. Lactose Synthetase. Our understanding of lactose synthesis
phenomena was substantially advanced when the lactose synthetase was
resolved into two components: a mixture of "A" protein fractionated
from mammary glands, and of ⍺-lactalbumin, a protein normally
found in milk (22) (23). In the absence of ⍺-lactalbumin, the "A"
protein will catalyze galactosyl transfer to N-acetylglucosamine (24).
Glucose is not a good acceptor, however, having a high apparent
Michaelis constant of 1 M. In the presence of ⍺-lactalbumin, the "A"
protein effectively catalyzes the synthesis of lactose, decreasing the
K_m about 1,000 fold (25). Thus ⍺-lactalbumin is a specifier protein
for the synthesis of lactose. The net effect of ⍺-lactalbumin is to convert a glycosyl transferase enzyme in the biosynthetic pathway of complex polysaccharides to an efficient system for lactose synthesis
(Figure 1).

The mammary gland is unique in that it can produce ⍺-lactal-
bumin, and in so doing it makes glucose an effective substrate for the
galactosyl transferase enzyme. The principal function of the galactosyl
transferases that originate in tissues other than lactating mammary
glands is to transfer galactose to an appropriate carbohydrate side
chain of glycoproteins and lipids. On this basis it is expected that these
transferases are widely distributed. Significantly, bovine ⍺-lactalbu-
min demonstrates a high degree of chemical homology with the amino
acid sequence of hen's egg-white lysozyme (26). Three-dimensional
models of ⍺-lactalbumin and lysozyme also show a high degree of
similarity. Functionally, the biosynthesis of lactose involves the formation of a β (1⟶ 4) glycosidic linkage, and such a linkage is hydrolyzed
in the lysozyme reaction. It has been speculated, therefore, that the
two proteins have related evolutionary origins.

As determined by disc gel electrophoresis, ⍺-lactalbumins
isolated from the milk of pigs, sheep, and goats have two electrophoretically distinct forms, both of which are active in the lactose synthetase reaction and appear to be charged isomers resulting from slight
variations in amino acid composition (27). Genetic variance in bovine
⍺-lactalbumin has been observed in electrophoretic separation, hence
the two forms observed in the pig, goat, and sheep may also represent
genetic variance.

The "A" protein in bovine skim milk has been purified of contaminating proteins. It is a single-chain glycoprotein of molecular weight
of 44,000 (28) (29). In the presence of one of the substrates, the "A"
protein and ⍺-lactalbumin form a stable complex that contains one
molecule of each protein.

III. Galactose Biosynthesis in the Mammary Gland

It is generally assumed that galactose is formed from UDP-glucose in the mammary gland, catalyzed by the C-4 epimerase. In addition to defining a primary pathway of lactose formation, with UDP-galactose and free glucose being the immediate precursors, the previously mentioned isotope studies revealed the interesting possibility of an unusual mode of galactose synthesis (20). When 1, 3^{14}C-labeled glycerol was injected into lactating mammary glands, the patterns of labeling of glucose and galactose differed. The galactose portion of lactose contained more ^{14}C than did glucose. Further, Carbons 4 and 6 of the galactose particularly reflected the injected substrate. UDP-galactose generally contained more label than did UDP-glucose, even though the latter was thought to be the normal biosynthetic precursor.

Alternative explanations have been considered: 1) A cell contains discrete centers of metabolic activity, and glycerol (or glyceraldehyde) is intercepted differentially at these centers. 2) UDP-hexose is labeled by direct incorporation of triose. The earlier but unconfirmed report of UDP-dihydroxyacetone offered one possible intermediate (30). More recently, in the conversion of galactopyranose to galactofuranose at the nucleotide level, an open chain hexose derivative has been postulated that could incorporate triose by a transaldolase-like exchange (31) (Figure 2).

IV. Galactose Metabolism.

Galactose that is consumed in excess of developmental needs is metabolized for energy.

In humans the liver appears to be the primary site for all metabolism of galactose; however, other tissues including the red cell have this capacity and hence can be conveniently used to evaluate the metabolic capability of the individual. Fundamental studies using microorganisms and animals, together with analyses of the metabolic problems in the human genetic disorders, have clarified the pathways of galactose metabolism in man.

The primary metabolic reactions of galactose are illustrated in Figure 3.

A. Reduction of Galactose. A non-specific reduction of the aldehyde at carbon-1 leads to the product galactitol (32) (33). This process is especially significant since the lens of the eye forms galactitol from excess galactose, and, in some genetically defective humans, who have no further capacity to metabolize galactitol, it accumulates and gives rise to cataracts (34).

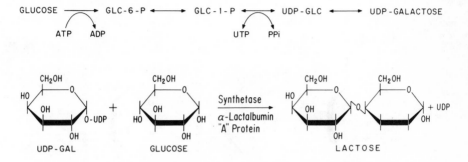

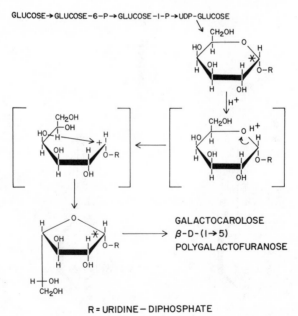

Figure 1. *Biosynthesis of lactose from glucose*

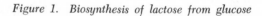

GALACTOCAROLOSE
β-D-(1→5)
POLYGALACTOFURANOSE

R = URIDINE – DIPHOSPHATE

Figure 2. *Galactose furanose formation*

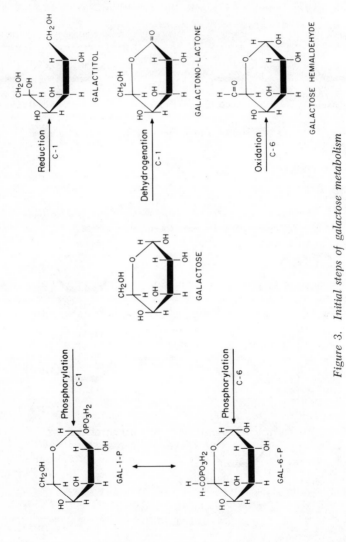

Figure 3. Initial steps of galactose metabolism

B. Dehydrogenation of Galactose. Dehydrogenation at carbon-1, which precedes the formation of galactonic acid, occurs in man and other animals (35). In man, whether galactonic acid arises by the action of a specific enzyme or a general aldehyde dehydrogenase or some phosphorylated intermediates has not been solved, but galactonic acid is excreted in cases of galactosemia and of galactokinase deficiency when galactose is consumed (36) (37). It does serve as a base for quantitative estimation of galactose (38).

C. Oxydation of Galactose. Microorganisms contain an enzyme that catalyzes an oxidation of galactose at carbon-6 to galactose hemialdehyde (39). While this reaction is of no known significance in humans it does provide a basis for quantitative estimates of their levels of galactose and some of its derivatives.

D. Tagatose Pathway. Direct phosphorylation of galactose at carbon-6 is of questionable significance in man. Some evidence for the occurrence of gal-6-P has been presented (40), but as an alternate to direct phosphorylation, the gal-6-P could arise from gal-1-P with a mutase type reaction (41). Indications are that when gal-1-P is present, gal-6-P is not formed (42). In microorganisms, gal-6-P can be metabolized in a manner analogous to the way glc-6-P in glycolysis in a series of reactions (catalyzed by inducible enzymes) that are distinct from those of the glucose pathway (43). The sequential products are gal-6-P, tagatose-6-P, tagatose-1,6-diP, then glyceraldehyde-3-P and dihydroxyacetone-P (two trioses common to the glucose pathway) (Figure 4).

E. Leloir Pathway. Phosphorylation catalyzed by a kinase initiates the Leloir pathway of galactose metabolism in man. The resulting product (gal-1-P) was identified in 1943 in rabbit liver following ingestion of galactose (44). Human liver tissue normally metabolizes most of the ingested galactose through the Leloir pathway, which requires two more enzymes in addition to the kinase, namely, a transferase and an epimerase (45):

a)   kinase
     galactose + ATP $\longrightarrow$ gal-1-P + ADP

b)   transferase
     gal-1-P + UDP-glc $\rightleftharpoons$ UDP-gal + glc-1-P

c)   epimerase
     UDP-gal $\rightleftharpoons$ UDP-glc

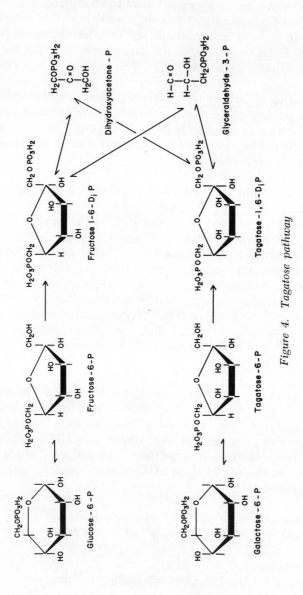

Figure 4. Tagatose pathway

Sum of b + c:

$$\text{gal-1-P} \rightleftharpoons \text{glc-1-P}$$

1. <u>Biosynthesis of uridine diphosphate glucose and uridine diphosphate galactose</u>. In addition to the function of UDP-glc as a co-factor in the Leloir pathway for galactose utilization, it serves broader needs of the cell (46) (47). The synthesis of glycogen requires UDP-glc. Many chemical compounds needed for growth and for differentiation contain a variety of saccharides. UDP-glc is the primary source of glycosyl residues for the biosynthesis of many of these saccharides. It is not surprising, therefore, that the enzyme for catalyzing the synthesis of UDP-glc is ubiquitous and abundant:

d) pyrophosphorylase
$$\text{glc-1-P} + \text{UTP} \rightleftharpoons \text{UDP-glc} + \text{PPi}$$

In aqueous extracts of liver, more than 0.5% of the protein is this synthetase for UDP-glc (48) (49). It is relevant here to note that the reaction is reversible; the equilibrium <u>in vitro</u> favors reactants as written, which fact gives rise to the enzyme being commonly designated as a pyrophosphorylase.

In addition to being abundant, the pyrophosphorylase is not highly specific. It will catalyze the reaction with UDP-gal at about 5% of the rate with UDP-glc (50).

d') $\text{gal-1-P} + \text{UTP} \rightleftharpoons \text{UDP-gal} + \text{PPi}$

F. <u>Pyrophosphorylase Pathway of Galactose Metabolism</u>. Isselbacher (51) has proposed a pyrophosphorylase pathway of galactose utilization which is significant in humans:

d') pyrophosphorylase
$$\text{gal-1-P} + \text{UTP} \rightleftharpoons \text{UDP-gal} + \text{PPi}$$

c) epimerase
$$\text{UDP-gal} \rightleftharpoons \text{UDP-glc}$$

d) pyrophosphorylase
$$\text{UDP-glc} + \text{PPi} \rightleftharpoons \text{UTP} + \text{glc-1-P}$$

Sum d', c and d:
$$\text{gal-1-P} \rightleftharpoons \text{glc-1-P}$$

Due to its low specificity, the UDP-glc pyrophosphorylase will catalyze both reactions d and d' (although claims have been made that a separate enzyme (52) (53) exists in human liver for each of the two reactions).

G. Uridine Diphosphate Galactose C-4-epimerase. The epimerase, which is required together with the pyrophosphorylase, seems to be ubiquitous and occurs early in human development (54). The epimerase-catalyzed reaction is the primary site of glucose formation from galactose when this sugar is being metabolized for energy. Conversely, when galactose is needed for structural purposes, it is derived from glucose at the nucleoside diphosphate hexose level, via the same reaction.

The UDP-gal-C-4 epimerase reaction requires DPN^+ as a cofactor. When the enzyme is fractionated from animal sources, the DPN^+ usually dissociates from the protein. E-coli, and yeast enzymes, however, retain DPN^+ more tenaciously. Reduced pyridine nucleotide strongly inhibits the animal enzymes.

In hemolysates from red cells from newborn infants, two distinct bands of epimerase are distinguishable on electrophoresis, while from adult red cells only one distinctly different band is found (55). When NAD^+ is added to the electrophoresis gel containing epimerase, the two-banded pattern characteristic of infant hemolysate is seen. An NAD^+ dependent structural interchange must be responsible for this observation.

The specific hydrogen atoms involved in the hexose interconversion are removed from one hexose substrate and replaced on the other in the opposite steric mode at Carbon 4. This requires a substantial change in the conformation of the hexoses during the reaction, with the carbon-bound hydrogens being retained. In the epimerase reaction, a keto intermediate at Carbon 4 was established by Nelsestuen (56) and confirmed by an isotope effect on the reaction rate (57) (56) (58) (59) (60).

Ethanol oxidation generates an increase in $NADH_2$, which apparently inhibits the UDP-galactose C-4-epimerase (61). This in turn inhibits the clearance of galactose from the blood (62). Adding NAD^+ to a liver preparation has partially prevented the enhancement effect of ethanol on $NADH_2$.

In pregnant women the capacity of the liver to remove galactose is accelerated and the inhibitory effect of ethanol is greatly reduced (63).

H. Genetic Defects. Galactosemia is an inborn error of metabolism (64) caused by an inherited deficiency of gal-1-P uridyltransferase, which normally catalyzes the second step in the conversion of galactose to glucose. Disease manifestations are cataracts, liver, and kidney dysfunction and disturbed mental development due to organic brain damage. Symptoms are apparent when galactose is ingested and gal-1-P (i.e., the product of the kinase reaction) accumulates.

Defects in catalysis during the other two steps in the Leloir pathway have now been described in humans. Following the discovery of the transferase defect, a number of kinaseless families were reported. In patients with a defect in the kinase (65), galactose and galactitol, but not galactose-1-phosphate, accumulate in the tissues and cataracts develop early in infancy. The other toxic manifestations of transferaseless galactosemia do not occur in persons lacking the kinase. Since cataracts develop in patients with either defect, galactitol must be the causative agent for cataract formation in both the kinase and transferase defects.

Galactokinase deficiency was found in two out of 240 persons who had eye cataracts (66). Both had developed their cataracts during their first year of life.

In humans, an epimerase deficit in blood cells has been reported (67) (54). If the liver and other organs are also epimerase deficient, the function of the epimerase reaction in metabolism would dictate a carefully controlled galactose intake. The dietary problem would be to provide enough galactose to meet the requirements for this sugar and its derivatives, but not so much as to produce toxic quantities of intermediates. In the absence of epimerase, presumably the kinase and pyrophosphorylase reactions would provide a biosynthetic route for UDP-gal.

1. Genetics of transferase deficiency. Since the absence of galactose-1-P-uridyl transferase activity is the basis for diagnosing galactosemia, the development of quantitative methods for measuring the transferase in erythrocytes allowed precise definition of interrelationships in families of patients with the disease (68) (69) (70). Direct measurements of the enzyme in erythrocytes confirmed little or no transferase activity in all tested galactosemics. Further, the parents, some siblings, and some other relatives of the tested patients had, on the average, only half the normal level of enzyme. Both parents, as well as a paternal and a maternal grandparent, must therefore be carriers, or genetic heterozygotes, before the disorder will be expressed in offspring. This finding clearly establishes galactosemia as an autosomal-recessive disease.

In tested galactosemic families, the offspring have demonstrated the expected mendelian ratios of one galactosemic:two heterozygotes: one normal. At least one of the maternal and one of the paternal grandparents of the patient and other relatives have been heterozygotes in the frequency predicted from the hypothesized mode of inheritance.

    2. <u>Genetic variants of transferase deficiency</u>. A so-called
Duarte variant of gal-1-P-uridyl transferase has been defined by a refinement of the chemical assay and by electrophoretic separation of
blood cell proteins having transferase activity. Family relationships
have been defined for the Duarte mutant. The heterozygote has about
three-fourths the normal transferase activity. The homozygote has
one-half the normal value of the transferase. The gal-1-P uridyl
transferase in the Duarte variant appears to be a structural mutation
since starch gel electrophoresis reveals two faster moving proteins
with catalytic activity (71) (72). The importance of having a detailed
structural analysis of the transferase is apparent.

    On the basis of electrophoresis and the uridyl transferase red
cell value, individuals have been identified who have both the classical
and the Duarte structural defects (73). The defective protein of classical galactosemics is revealed by immulogical procedures, but is inactive according to chemical assays (74) (75). Structural alteration is
assumed to prevent the less active Duarte variant and the inactive galactosemia protein from performing its normal catalytic function (76).

    Other transferase variants have been identified. It has been
shown (77) that a so-called Negro variant could have a 10 percent normal transferase activity based on assays of uridyl transferase in liver
and intestinal tissues, even though the red cells showed no activity.
Since this is difficult to explain morphologically, a more rigorous
characterization of this mutant must precede a tenable interpretation.

    The enzyme in the Rennes mutant that was found in two galacto-
semic siblings migrates more slowly than normal transferase on electrophoresis (78). A further variation, which was revealed by an unstable
transferase (Indiana variant), has been found in a galactosemic family
(79).

    A Los Angeles variant of galactosemia displays three transfer-
ase bands during electrophoresis of erythrocyte hemolysates (80). In
contrast to the Duarte variant, the total amount of transferase activity
in the hemolysate is normal or greater.

    I. <u>Galactose-1-phosphate Toxicity</u>. Galactose-1-phosphate is
the toxic agent causing most of the pathology in classical galactosemia.
This can be inferred from the comparison of disease manifestations in
transferase deficiency with those in galactokinase deficiency.

    Cataracts are the only common sign; they are caused by osmotic
swelling and disruption of lens fibers due to the accumulation of galactitol (34). No brain, liver, and kidney pathology is observed in kinase

deficiency and, since gal-1-P cannot be formed in this disorder, one can conclude that it must play the deciding pathogenetic role in transferase deficiency.

Symptoms other than eye cataracts, which are observed in patients with transferase deficiency, may be due to a high concentration of gal-1-P within the cell. The blood glucose levels of some acutely ill infants lacking transferase are subnormal, indicating a disturbed carbohydrate metabolism. Three key reactions involving glucose have been reported to be affected by galactose-1-phosphate: the mutase, dehydrogenase, and pyrophosphorylase reactions shown in Figure 5 (81) (82). In each case the evidence was based on kinetic studies of isolated enzymes, not from human tissues; it is therefore somewhat presumptive. About a 50-fold excess of galactose-1-phosphate over glucose phosphates is required for significant inhibition of the isolated reactions.

Glucose-1-P, uridine mono, di, and tri phosphates, and nucleoside diphosphate-glucose derivatives inhibit the transferase (83). From inhibitor constants and calculated intracellular levels of these compounds it has been deduced that the uridine derivatives and glucose-1-phosphate could have a physiologically regulatory function.

J. Biosynthesis of Galactose-1-phosphate from UDP-galactose. The idea that the pyrophosphorylase pathway is a means of galactose metabolism in the human erythrocyte stems from the following observations: Epimerase and UDP-glc are normal red cell constituents. Hence UDP-gal is also available as a substrate for other reactions. Incubation of hemolysates lacking transferase (84) with UDP-gal produced gal-1-P in a reaction that was absolutely dependent on inorganic pyrophosphate and was stimulated by magnesium; the production of gal-1-P was inhibited by UDP-glc, by UDP and Pi. Under identical conditions, the crystalline enzyme from human liver catalyzes the formation of gal-1-P from UDP-gal (85) (50).

UDP-glucose pyrophosphorylase of both calf and rabbit have also been purified and crystallized (48) (85) (50). The biochemical evidence that one protein catalyzes reactions with both glucose and galactose derivatives is convincing. Throughout purification and crystallization, the ratio of activity of the enzyme towards the various substrates remains constant (86) (85) (50). UDP-gal is bound to the purified enzyme as a function of the number of protomer subunits of pyrophosphorylase (49) (87). This bound UDP-gal may then be stoichiometrically replaced by UDP-glc (87). UDP-glc also limits the synthesis of gal-1-P from UDP-gal by hemolysates (84). It is concluded, therefore, that UDP-gal competes with UDP-glc (although less effectively) for the same site on the enzyme. Immunological evidence supporting this conclusion has also been obtained (88).

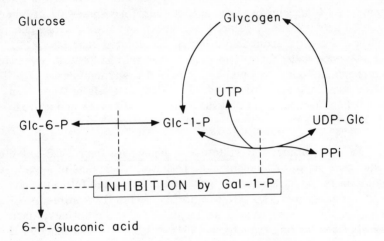

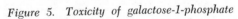

Figure 5. Toxicity of galactose-1-phosphate

The production of gal-1-P from glc-1-P by the pyrophosphory-lase pathway requires the enzymes pyrophosphorylase and epimerase and their substrates, the UDP-hexoses, UTP and PPi. A substantial concentration of UTP is maintained intracellularly for nucleic acid synthesis and for UDP-glc formation. Besides being a precursor of UDP-gal, UDP-glc is a source of glycosyl donors for pentoses, uronic acids, and hexosamines; hence, there is a constant and vital metabolic flux through UDP-glc. Metabolic interconversions of sugars and their derivatives require epimerases, which appear to be generally distributed in nature. Hence, the epimerase-catalyzed formation of UDP-gal from UDP-glc is a common intracellular reaction. Under most circumstances, when nucleotides are extracted from the cell, UDP-gal and UDP-glc are present in a ratio of approximately 1/3 to 2/3, providing ample UDP-gal substrate from which gal-1-P may be enzymatically formed.

Inorganic pyrophosphate is required as the other substrate if gal-1-P is to be produced from UDP-gal. Pyrophosphate is a product of most biosynthetic processes, including the formation of polysaccharides, proteins, and lipids (89). To permit the biosynthesis of gal-1-P from UDP-gal from an equilibrium that favors reactants, PPi is theoretically hydrolyzed by the intracellular pyrophosphatases. Quite aside from the futile energy wastage, if this hydrolysis took place, substantial evidence indicates that not only do the cells realize the potential for productive use of the PPi, but PPi may have a regulatory function as well (90) (91). Furthermore, PPi accumulates in man in sufficient quantity to crystallize with calcium and cause some joint disorders (92). The availability of PPi for gal-1-P synthesis is therefore most probable.

The galactosemic has a special problem since the transferase block promotes an accumulation of gal-1-P from dietary galactose while, at the same time, a substantial need for UDP-gal obviously exists. In galactosemia, the pyrophosphorylase pathway appears to have adequate capacity to form UDP-gal from glc-1-P but cannot readily convert gal-1-P to UDP-gal. Hence, gal-1-P accumulates when galactose is ingested.

The following observation indicates that the pyrophosphorylase pathway is largely responsible for galactose metabolism in red cells from galactosemics. An antibody to crystalline UDP-glucose pyrophosphorylase from human liver has been prepared (88). This antibody, when incubated with extracts of galactosemic red cells, specifically precipitates the enzyme responsible for metabolism of galactose. Hence the galactosemic who lacks the Leloir pathway can convert some galactose to glucose in erythrocytes (and probably other tissues), via the pyrophosphorylase pathway.

K. Uncontrolled Biosynthesis of Galactose-1-phosphate from Glucose. The usual procedure for maintaining patients with galacto-semia is to exclude galactose sources from their diets. When this is carefully done, levels of gal-1-P lower than 4 mg/100 ml are main-tained in most patients. Any galactose ingestion is followed by an immediate rise in red cell gal-1-P. Unfortunately, even when their intake of galactose sources is carefully regulated, uncontrolled biosyn-thesis of gal-1-P from UDP-gal has been observed in some galacto-semics (93).

Much evidence, both clinical and experimental, currently docu-ments biosynthesis of galactose from glucose in man. Mayes and Miller (94) have grown transferase-deficient skin fibroblasts in a medium devoid of galactose and observed the formation of gal-1-P from glucose. The final concentrations (approx. 2 mg/g protein) were simi-lar to those attained by red cells in vitro (approx. 3 mg per g non-Hb protein) (84).

Cultured fibroblasts from galactosemics without transferase activity have converted (1-^{14}C) galactose to $^{14}CO_2$ (95), with an accu-mulation of gal-1-P. Both CO_2 and gal-1-P formation were inhibited by glucose, suggesting a common intermediate. Galactokinase-deficient cells similarly treated did not produce CO_2 from (1-^{14}C) galactose, suggesting the pyrophosphorylase pathway as the alternate route of galactose metabolism in galactosemics.

Galactokinase-deficient children grow and develop normally when maintained on a diet free of galactose. Pregnant women who are heterozygotes for transferase deficiency and have previously had trans-ferase-deficient offspring are routinely subjected to a galactose exclu-sion diet; despite galactose deprivation their fetuses develop normally. One completely transferase-deficient woman who followed a lactose-free regimen throughout pregnancy delivered a healthy infant and, pre-sumably still on the diet, produced lactose (2.8 g/100 ml) in her colos-trum on the second post partum day (96). In galactokinase-deficient twin infants on a suitable diet, small amounts of galactose remained detectable in plasma and urine (97). Both galactokinase- and transfer-ase-deficient infants, though on galactose exclusion diets, excreted some galactitol in the urine (97) (98). High gal-1-P is commonly re-corded in the cord blood of transferase-deficient newborns born of mothers on galactose-restricted diets (99).

The need for galactose-containing polymers to assure functional and structural integrity of cells and tissues is satisfied by the biosyn-thetic reactions that have been detailed. Hence there is a substantial capacity to synthesize galactose and its derivatives at all stages of human development. The gal-1-P of a transferase-deficient newborn (at age 5 hrs) was 17 mg/100 ml of RBC. At the end of his first day, the gal-1-P had actually risen to 26 mg/100 ml, although he had been given intravenous glucose only and had taken no food (88). Clearly his red blood cells had synthesized gal-1-P, either from endogenous galactose stores or (more likely) from glucose.

We have observed what appears to be uncontrolled biosynthesis of gal-1-P in two galactosemic infants. After an initial exposure to milk and following diagnosis, both received a "galactose-free" formula. Very surprisingly, upon initiation of the diet at age 7 and 6 days, respectively, red cell gal-1-P levels dropped rather slowly, and potentially toxic levels were maintained for months. At age 27 days, one infant was fed isocaloric amounts of dextrimaltose in water for 36 hrs; however, the gal-1-P did not drop but rose slightly. The female infant had breast swellings until her 25th day of age. At age 19 days, her breast secretions, collected and compared to those of three other newborns, contained what appeared to be normal concentrations of lactose obviously synthesized from glucose (93).

Such biogenesis of galactose could take place in tissues other than the red cells and the breast glands, e.g., the liver and the central nervous system. It is remarkable in this connection that in the few reported long-term follow-up studies (100) (101), some of the galactosemia patients who had been diagnosed at birth and treated since, showed signs of organic brain damage at school age, evidenced by difficulties in visual perception. Self-intoxication with gal-1-P through a prolonged maintenance of high levels during infant life has been hypothesized as the cause of the damage. Evidently such biosynthesis of gal-1-P has constituted a mechanism of potential self-intoxication in well-treated galactosemic infants (102). Convincing evidence implicates the pyrophosphorylase pathway in such cases (88).

The regulation of this process to limit the amount of UDP-gal formed to that required for biosynthetic reactions and thereby prevent the formation of toxic quantities of gal-1-P is the central problem of some transferase deficient children.

Abbreviations:

glc-1-P:	glucose-1-phosphate
gal-1-P:	galactose-1-phosphate
gal-6-P:	galactose-6-phosphate
UDP-glc:	uridine diphosphate glucose
UDP-gal:	uridine diphosphate galactose
UTP:	uridine triphosphate
ATP:	adenosine triphosphate
ADP:	adenosine diphosphate
Pi:	inorganic phosphate
PPi:	inorganic pyrophosphate

Literature Cited

1. Lengemann, F. W., R. H. Wasserman and C. L. Comar, J. Nutr. (1959) 68:443.
2. Fournier, P., Y. Dupins and A. Fournier, Israel J. Med. Sci. (1971) 7:389.
3. Condon, J. R., J. R. Nassim, F.I.C. Millard, A. Hilbe and E. M. Stainthorpe, Lancet (1970) i :1027.
4. Segrest, J. P. and L. W. Cunningham, J. Clin. Invest. (1970) 49:1497.
5. Lundblad, A., P. Hallgren, A. Rudmark and S. Svensson, Biochem. (1973) 12:3341.
6. Wendorff, W. L., and C. H. Amundson, J. Milk Food Technol. (1971) 34(6):300-306.
7. Strom, Roberto, Domenica Gandini Attardi, Sture Forsén, Paola Turini, Franco Celada and Eraldo Antonini, Eur. J. Biochem. (1971) 23:118-124.
8. Hill, J. A., and R. E. Huber, Biochim. Biophys. Acta. (1971) 250:530-537.
9. Miller, D., and R. K. Crane, Biochim. Biophys. Acta. (1961) 52:293.
10. Simoons, F. J., Amer. J. Dig. Dis. (1970) 15:695-710.
11. Gilat, T., Gastroenterology (1971) 60:346-347.
12. Cuatrecasas, P., D. H. Lockwood and J. R. Caldwell, Lancet (1965) 1(7375):14-18.
13. Keusch, G. T., F. J. Troncale, L. H. Miller, V. Promadhat and P. R. Anderson, Pediatrics (1969) 43:540-545.
14. Kogut, M. D., G. N. Donnell and K. N. Shaw, J. Pediat. (1967) 71:75-81.
15. Flatz, G. and H. W. Rotthauwe, The Lancet (1973) 2:76.
16. Holzel, A., Proc. Roy. Soc. Med. (1968) 61:1095.
17. Brady, R. O., Advances in Enzymology (1973) 38:293-315.
18. Brady, R. O., Angew. Chem. (1973) 85:28-38.
19. Gander, J. E., W. E. Petersen, P. D. Boyer, Arch. Biochem. Biophys. (1957) 69:85-99.
20. Hansen, R. G., Harland G. Wood, Georges J. Peeters, Birgit Jacobson and JoAnne Wilken, J. Biol. Chem. (1962) 237:1034-1039.
21. Watkins, W. M. and W. Z. Hassid, J. Biol. Chem. (1962) 237: 1432-1440.
22. Brodbeck, U. and K. E. Ebner, J. Biol. Chem. (1966) 241:762.
23. Brodbeck, U., W. L. Denton, N. Tanahashi and K. E. Ebner, J. Biol. Chem. (1967) 242:1391-1397.

24. Brew, K., T. C. Vanaman and R. L. Hill, Proc. Nat. Acad. Sci., U. S. (1968) 59:491.

25. Morrison, J. F. and K. E. Ebner, J. Biol. Chem. (1971) 246: 3992-3998.

26. Brew, K., T. C. Vanaman and R. L. Hill, J. Biol. Chem. (1967) 242:3747-3749.

27. Schmidt, D. V. and K. E. Ebner, Biochim. Biophys. Acta (1972) 263:714-720.

28. Clarke, J. T. R., L. S. Wolfe and A. S. Perlin, J. Biol. Chem. (1971) 246(18):5563-5569.

29. Klee, Werner A., and Claude B. Klee, J. Biol. Chem. (1972) 247(8):2336-2344.

30. Smith, E. E. B., B. Galloway and G. T. Mills, Biochem. Biophys. Res. Comm. (1961) 5:148-151.

31. Trejo, A. Garcia, J. W. Haddock, G. J. F. Chittenden and J. Baddiley, Biochem. J. (1971) 122:49-57.

32. Hers, H. G., Biochim. Biophys. Acta (1960) 37:120-126.

33. Hayman, S. and J. H. Kinoshita, J. Biol. Chem. (1965) 240:877-882.

34. Van Heyningen, R., Exp. Eye Res. (1971) 11:415-428.

35. Cuatrecasas, P. and S. Segal, Science (1966) 153:549-551.

36. Bergren, W. R., W. G. Ng, G. N. Donnell and S. P. Markey, Science (1972) 176:683-684.

37. Gitzelmann, R., H. J. Wells and S. Segal, Europ J. Clin. Invest. (1974) 4:79-84.

38. Wallenfels, K. and G. Kurz, "Methods in Enzymology" Vol. IX. p. 112 (W. A. Wood, ed.) Academic Press, New York, 1966.

39. Avigad, G., D. Amaral, C. Asensio and B. L. Horecker, J. Biol. Chem. (1962) 237:2736-2743.

40. Inouye, T., M. Tannenbaum and D. Y.Y. Hsia, Nature (1962) 193:67-68.

41. Posternak, T. and J. P. Rosselet, Helv. Chim. Acta (1954) 37:246-250.

42. Dahlqvist, A. J. Lab. Clin. Med. (1971) 78(6):931-938.

43. Bissett, D. L. and R. L. Anderson, Biochem. Biophys. Res. Comm. (1973) 52:641.

44. Kosterlitz, H. W., Biochem. J. (1943) 37:318-321.

45. Leloir, L. F., Arch. Biochem. Biophys. (1951) 33:186-190.

46. Caputto, R., H. S. Barra and F. A. Cumar, Ann. Rev. Biochem. (1967) 36:211-246.

47. Ginsburg, V. and E. F. Neufeld, Ann. Rev. Biochem. (1969) 38:371-388.

48. Albrecht, G. J., S. T. Bass, L. L. Seifert and R. G. Hansen, J. Biol. Chem. (1966) 241:2968.

49. Levine, S., T. A. Gillett, E. Hageman and R. G. Hansen,
    J. Biol. Chem. (1969) 244:5729-5734.
50. Turnquist, R. L., T. A. Gillett and R. G. Hansen, J. Biol.
    Chem. (1974) in press.
51. Isselbacher, K. J., J. Biol. Chem. (1958) 232:429-444.
52. Abraham, H. D. and R. R. Howell, J. Biol. Chem. (1969)
    244:545-550.
53. Chacko, C. M., L. McCrone and H. L. Nadler, Biochim.
    Biophys. Acta (1972) 268:113-120.
54. Gitzelmann, R. and B. Steinmann, Helv. paed. Acta (1973)
    28:497-510.
55. Bergren, W. R., W. G. Ng and G. Donnell, Biochem. Biophys.
    Acta (1973) 315:464.
56. Nelsestuen, Gary L. and Samuel Kirkwood, J. Biol. Chem.
    (1971) 246(24):7533-7543.
57. Davis, L. and L. Glaser, Biochem. Biophys. Res. Comm.
    (1971) 43:1429-1435.
58. Wee, T. G., J. Davis and P. A. Frey, J. Biol. Chem. (1972)
    247:1339-1342.
59. Wee, T. G. and P. A. Frey, J. Biol. Chem. (1973) 248:33-40.
60. Maitra, U. S., M. A. Gaunt and H. Ankel, J. Biol. Chem.
    (1974) 249:3075-3078.
61. Forsander, Olof A., Biochim. Biophys. Acta (1972) 268:253-256.
62. Isselbacher, K. J. and S. M. Krane, J. Biol. Chem. (1961)
    236:2394.
63. Kesaniemi, Y. A., K. O. Kurppa and K. R. H. Husman, J. Obs.
    and Gyn. (1973) 80:344.
64. Segal, S., "The Metabolic Basis of Inherited Disease" (J. B.
    Stanbury, J. B. Wyngaarden and D. S. Fredrickson, eds),
    pp. 174-195, McGraw Hill, New York, (1972).
65. Gitzelmann, R. Ped. Res. (1967) 1:14.
66. Beutler, E., F. Matsumoto, W. Kuhl, A. Krill, N. Levy,
    R. Sparks and M. Degnan, N. Eng. J. Med. (1973) 288:1203.
67. Gitzelmann, R., Helv. Paediat. Acta (1972) 27:125-130.
68. Donnell, G. N., W. R. Bergren, R. K. Bretthauer and R. G.
    Hansen, Pediatrics (1960) 25:572-581.
69. Schwarz, V., A. R. Wells, A. Holzel, G. M. Komrower,
    Ann. Hum. Gen. (1961) 25:179.
70. Kirkman, H. N. and E. Bynum, Ann. Hum. Gen. (1958-59)
    23:117-126.
71. Mathai, C. K. and E. Beutler, Science (1966) 154:1179-1180.
72. Ng, W. G., W. R. Bergren, M. Fields and G. N. Donnell,
    Biochem. Biophys. Res. Comm. (1969) 37:451.

73. Gitzelmann, R., J. R. Poley and A. Prader, Helv. Paed. Acta (1967) 22:252-257.

74. Hansen, R. G., "Galactosemia" (D. Y. Hsia, ed) p. 55, Charles C. Thomas, Springfield, Ill., (1969).

75. Tedesco, T. A. and W. J. Mellman, Science (1971) 172:727-728.

76. Tedesco, T. A., J. Biol. Chem. (1972) 247:6631-6636.

77. Segal, S., A. Blair and H. Roth, Am. J. Med. (1965) 38:62.

78. Schapira, F. and J. C. Kaplan, Biochem. Biophys. Res. Comm. (1969) 35:451.

79. Chacko, C. M., J. C. Christian, and H. L. Nadler, J. Ped. (1971) 78:454.

80. Ng, W. G., W. R. Bergren and G. N. Donnell. Ann. Hum. Genet. (1973) 37:1.

81. Sidbury, J. B. Jr., "Galactosemia" (D. Y. Hsia, ed) p. 13, Charles C. Thomas, Springfield, Ill., (1969).

82. Oliver, I. T., Biochim. Biophys. Acta (1961) 52:75-81.

83. Segal, S. and S. Rogers, Biochim. Biophys. Acta (1971) 250: 351-360.

84. Gitzelmann, R., Pediat. Res. (1969) 3:279-286.

85. Knop, J. K. and R. G. Hansen, J. Biol. Chem. (1970) 245:2499-2504.

86. Ting, W. K. and R. G. Hansen, Proc. Soc. Exp. Biol. Med. (1968) 127:960-962.

87. Turnquist, R. L., M. M. Turnquist, R. C. Bachmann and R. G. Hansen, Biochim. Biophys. Acta (1974) 364:59-67.

88. Gitzelmann, R. and R. G. Hansen, Biochim. Biophys. Acta (1974) 372:374-378.

89. Lehninger, A. L., "Bioenergetics," p. 183, Benjamin, New York (1965).

90. Schwenn, J. D., R. M. Lilley and D. A. Walker, Biochim. Biophys. Acta (1973) 325:586-595.

91. Levine, G. and J. A. Bassham, Biochim. Biophys. Acta (1974) 333:136-140.

92. Russell, R. G. G., S. Bisaz, H. Fleisch, H. L. F. Currey, H. M. Rubinstein, A. A. Dietz, J. Boussina, A. Micheli and G. Fallet, Lancet (1970) II:899-902.

93. Gitzelmann, R., B. Steinmann, R. G. Hansen, in press (1974).

94. Mayes, J. S. and L. R. Miller, Biochim. Biophys. Acta (1973) 313:9-16.

95. Petricciani, J. C., K. Binder, C. R. Merril and M. R. Geier, Science (1972) 175:1368.

96. Roe, T. F., J. G. Hallatt, G. N. Donnell and W. G. Ng, J. Pediat. (1971) 78:1026-1030.

97. Olambiwonnu, N. O., R. McVie, W. G. Ng, S. D. Frasier and
     G. N. Donnell, Pediatrics (1974) 53:314-318.

98. Roe, T. F., W. G. Ng, W. R. Bergren and G. N. Donnell,
     Biochem. Med. (1973) 7:266-273.

99. Donnell, G. N., R. Koch and W. R. Bergren, "Galactosemia,"
     (D. Y. Y. Hsia, ed) p. 247, Charles C. Thomas, Springfield,
     Ill. (1969).

100. Komrower, G. M. and D. H. Lee, Arch. Dis. Child. (1970)
     45:367-373.

101. Fishler, K., G. N. Donnell, W. R. Bergren and R. Koch,
     Pediatrics (1972) 50:412-419.

102. Gitzelmann, R. and R. G. Hansen, Abstr. Europ. Soc. Ped.
     Res., Ann. Meeting, Sevilla (1973); Pediat. Res. (1974)
     8:137.

Metabolism and Physiological Effects of the Polyols (Alditols)

OSCAR TOUSTER

Department of Molecular Biology, Vanderbilt University, Nashville, Tenn. 37235

I. Introduction

   Polyols, or alditols, are of course not strictly carbohy-drates, but since they are produced chemically and biologically from sugars, we can consider them honorary carbohydrates. They are now established in mammalian metabolism and are of some impor-tance in nutrition and pathology. In this paper I survey the roles of polyols and emphasize some of the most pertinent current uses and problems.

II. Survey of the Occurrence and Enzymology of the Polyols

   The occurrence of polyols in animals is summarized in Table I.

TABLE I.   POLYOLS IN ANIMAL METABOLISM

Occurrence in tissues
      Sorbitol--fetal blood, seminal vesicles and plasma, nerve,
            lens of alloxan-diabetic rats or rats given
            cataractogenic dose of $\underline{D}$-xylose
      Xylitol--lens of rats given cataractogenic dose of $\underline{D}$-xylose
      Dulcitol--various tissues after cataractogenic dose of
            $\underline{D}$-galactose
Occurrence in urine
      Erythritol
      $\underline{D}$-arabitol, $\underline{L}$-arabitol
      Sorbitol
      $\underline{D}$-mannitol
Utilization by mammals in vivo
      High--xylitol, ribitol, sorbitol
      Variable--$\underline{D}$-mannitol (oral dose moderately utilized;
            parenteral--poorly)
      Poor--arabitol ($\underline{D}$ and $\underline{L}$), dulcitol

Sorbitol is most widely distributed, occurring in fetal blood and in seminal vesicles and plasma, where the polyol is undoubtedly a normal metabolic intermediate. Sorbitol accumulates in some tissues of diabetic animals, a matter which is discussed in greater detail below. Xylitol and, to a smaller extent, sorbitol accumulate in the lens of rats given cataractogenic doses of D-xylose (1). Dulcitol, or galactitol, accumulates after cataractogenic doses of D-galactose, and it is also found in the human genetic disease, galactosemia. Several polyols have been isolated from human urine: erythritol (2), arabitol (3), mannitol and sorbitol (4,5).

The utilization of polyols by mammals is also indicated in Table I, with the wide range of utilization indicated. The most appreciably used polyols are xylitol, ribitol, and sorbitol.

The main biochemical reactions of polyols are shown below:

<u>Enzymatic Reactions of Polyols</u>

<u>General</u>

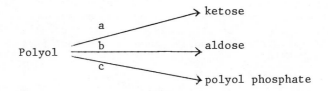

<u>Mammals</u>

$$\text{L-Xylulose} \xrightleftharpoons{a} \text{xylitol} \xrightleftharpoons{a} \text{D-xylulose}$$

$$\text{D-Glucose} \xrightleftharpoons{b} \text{sorbitol} \xrightleftharpoons{a} \text{D-fructose}$$

Polyols undergo oxidation to the corresponding ketose (a) or to the corresponding aldose (b), or phosphorylation to the polyol 1-phosphate (c). Many examples of reactions (a) and (b) are found in mammals. The L-xylulose-xylitol-D-xylulose interconversion occurs in the glucuronate-xylulose cycle. The glucose-sorbitol-fructose interconversion occurs in male accessory organs and undoubtedly in other tissues as well. However, the phosphorylation of polyols occurs in microorganisms but not in mammals. A review on polyols will supply the reader with additional information in this biochemical area (6).

III. Xylitol in Metabolism and Nutrition

Many years ago, when we were investigating the metabolism of
L̲-xylulose, the sugar excreted in gram quantities by humans with
the genetic metabolic abnormality known as essential pentosuria,
we discovered that L̲-xylulose is normally utilized as shown in the
following equations:

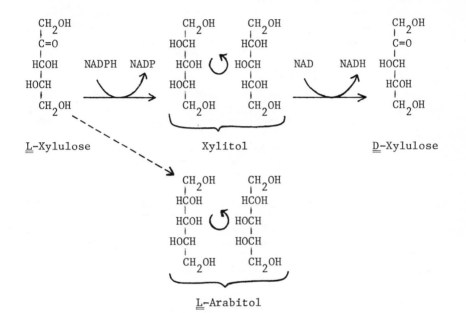

L̲-Xylulose   Xylitol   D̲-Xylulose

L̲-Arabitol

The L̲-xylulose is reduced to xylitol by an unusually specific
NADPH-linked polyol dehydrogenase (7,8). The xylitol is then re-
oxidized to D̲-xylulose by an NAD-linked enzyme of rather broad but
definite specificity. This enzyme is most commonly known as sorbitol dehydrogenase. Pentosuric individuals excrete smaller
amounts of L̲-arabitol, probably as a "detoxication" product of the
accumulated L̲-xylulose.

The substrate specificity of sorbitol dehydrogenase, which is
better expressed by the name, L̲-iditol dehydrogenase, is shown
below:

Sorbitol dehydrogenase is specific for
erythro-1,2,4-polyol configuration.

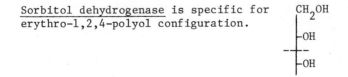

As can be seen from the formula on the right, sorbitol, xylitol, and ribitol are good substrates. The low level of oxidation of L-arabitol by this enzyme even when highly purified has not been explained.

The work on L-xylulose metabolism in our laboratory and of King, Burns and others on L-ascorbic acid biosynthesis led to the formulation of the glucuronate-xylulose cycle (9,10), which is shown in Figure 1. This cycle occurs in all mammals in which it has been studied, the reactions generally occurring in the liver and in the kidney. The function of the cycle is not completely understood. Since an inability to carry out the reduction of L-xylulose to xylitol is apparently not deleterious, pentosuria is an inherited metabolic disorder (11,12), not a metabolic disease. The early reactions in the cycle are obviously important. It appears that most higher animals biosynthesize L-ascorbic acid, although primates, the guinea pig, flying mammals, and insects (13) do not. It has been demonstrated that man, the monkey, and the guinea pig lack the liver microsomal oxidase that converts L-gulonolactone to the keto derivative. I would also point out the numerous oxidation-reductions using pyridine nucleotide-linked coenzymes which effectively move hydrogen from NADPH to NAD, thereby possibly serving a transhydrogenase function. I should also mention that although it is accepted that UDP-glucose and UDP-glucuronate are early members of the cycle, and obviously serve as precursors of sugar moieties in glyco-polymers, there is some uncertainty as to how the free glucuronate is produced.

Since, in the conversion of glucuronate to L-xylulose via L-gulonate, there occurs a decarboxylation of the C_6 carbon of glucuronate, this carbon being the same as C_6 of glucose, this cycle can be considered a C_6 oxidation pathway for glucose. It may then be asked whether much glucose is oxidized normally through this pathway. Specific studies indicate that only a small amount of glucose is handled via this route. From the fact that pentosuric individuals normally excrete several grams of L-xylulose each day and from experiments on the extent of augmentation of this excretion on feeding the precursor D-glucuronolactone, it can be estimated that the carbohydrate flux through the cycle is between 5 and 15 grams per day (14).

It was therefore of some interest that Winegrad and his associates reported several years ago that the C_6 oxidation of glucose is enhanced in alloxan-diabetic rats (15) and that L-xylulose levels in the serum of diabetic humans are several times higher than normal (16). These findings are not well understood. It does appear, however, that in diabetes the so-called insulin dependent pathways are more prominently employed and that more glucose appears to be oxidized via glucuronate and via sorbitol, as will be discussed in more detail below.

The utilization of polyols became of special interest when the metabolic importance of sorbitol and xylitol was discovered. The high conversion of an administered polyol to liver glycogen

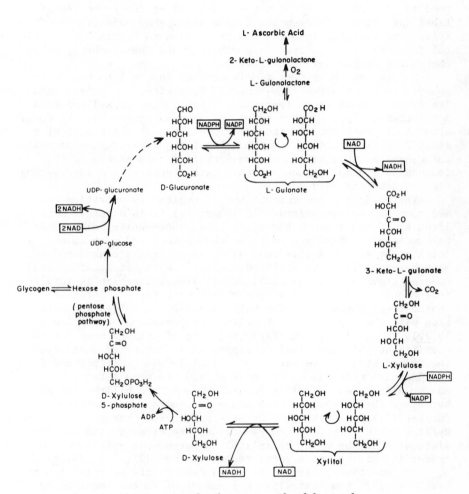

Figure 1.   The glucuronic acid–xylulose cycle

and its considerable oxidation to CO_2 are of course indications
of efficient utilization. The data in Table II show that xylitol
and ribitol are well metabolized to CO_2 and glycogen, whereas D-
arabitol is not. L-Arabitol is poorly utilized and shows a
peculiar discrepancy between the low level of incorporation of
label into liver glycogen and a moderately good oxidation to CO_2.
Xylitol utilization involves its conversion to D-xylulose. Ribitol is similarly converted to D-ribulose and then probably phosphorylated to D-ribulose 5-phosphate.

Xylitol has been very widely studied in the last decade as a
substitute for glucose in parenteral nutrition. In animal studies it was demonstrated that the administration of xylitol does
not increase blood glucose nearly as much as glucose itself does,
a point of importance in the use of xylitol for the treatment of
diabetics. It was also observed that the administration of xylitol causes an increase in plasma insulin far in excess of that
induced by glucose. However, this rather general and interesting
finding does not hold for the human.

The basis for the current use of xylitol in nutrition and
medicine may be summarized as follows: a) It is a normal metabo-
lite, b) it has a sweet taste, c) it is inexpensive, d) it does
not undergo the Maillard reaction when autoclaved with amino
acids or protein hydrolysates, e) it is generally considered to
be non-toxic, f) it is utilized in large doses (at least several
hundred grams per day by man), and g) its utilization is insulin-
independent. Some of these advantages were first pointed out by
Konrad Lang; three symposium volumes may be consulted in connection with the development of xylitol in parenteral nutrition (18,
19,20). These desirable characteristics of xylitol have led to
significant pharmaceutical developments in countries other than
the United States. Intravenous xylitol is well utilized and is
an important clinical agent in Japan and, to some extent, in Ger-
many. High doses of xylitol cause uricemia and bilirubinemia,
but since this effect is also shown by fructose and sorbitol,
Förster (21) does not consider it a particular characteristic of
xylitol administration. For additional references, and further
discussion of the value of xylitol in parenteral nutrition, the
reader is referred to several recent reviews (21,22,23,24,25).

An important influence of the acceptability of xylitol has
been a report from Australia on a number of deaths incurred by
patients who had been given xylitol (24,26). It has been pointed
out, however, that the dosage levels exceeded those generally
employed, that a contaminant may have been present, and that the
histopathological observations were due to the types of patients
involved (27). Until this matter is resolved, the use of xylitol
in America is likely to continue to be severely restricted.

Oral xylitol has been studied in animals and man, with some
evidence resulting to suggest that it reduces dental caries (27,
28,29).

TABLE II.   UTILIZATION OF FREE PENTITOLS BY THE RAT AND GUINEA PIG

Pentitol	Species	% of Administered Tracer Dose			Time (Hrs.)	Ref.
		Oxid. to CO_2	In urine	Liver glycogen		
Xylitol	Rat	–	–	11.8	2	a
	Guinea pig	–	–	23.8	2	a
	Guinea pig	10	25	–	24	a
Ribitol	Guinea pig	–	–	19.75	2	b
	Rat	31.4	29.9	–	24	b
D-Arabitol	Rat or guinea pig	–	–	0.28	2	b
L-Arabitol	Guinea pig	–	–	3.1	2	b
	Rat	–	–	0.95	2	b
	Rat	13.3	37.1	–	24	b

a   McCormick and Touster (9)

b   McCormick and Touster (17)

I should mention that although xylitol absorption from the intestinal tract is slow and in large amounts causes osmotic diarrhea, there is a rapid adaptation by humans which might minimize this problem with oral xylitol (27,30).

IV. Sorbitol and Other Hexitols

From the work of Hers (31,32), the major route of utilization of administered sorbitol is known:

Route of Utilization of Sorbitol and Fructose

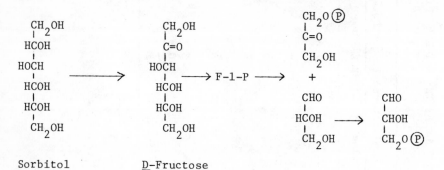

Sorbitol   D-Fructose

Sorbitol is oxidized to fructose, which is then phosphorylated to fructose-1-phosphate followed by cleavage to dihydroxyacetone phosphate and glyceraldehyde. The latter is then phosphorylated to the 3-phosphate. Both triose phosphates are members of the Embden-Meyerhof glycolytic pathway.

Gabbay (33) has recently observed another metabolic interrelationship between fructose and hexitols. Dietary fructose is converted, in about 3% yield, to urinary D-mannitol. He has presented evidence that the enzyme aldose reductase surprisingly has the capacity to catalyze this reduction of fructose to mannitol.

Sorbitol is in fact an important metabolic intermediate as shown below:

$$\text{D-Glucose} \xrightleftharpoons{\text{NADPH}} \text{Sorbitol} \xrightleftharpoons{\text{NAD}} \text{D-Fructose}$$

        (aldose   (sorbitol
        reductase)   dehydrogenase)

The sorbitol pathway (34,35) involves the conversion of glucose to sorbitol through the mediation of the enzyme aldose reductase,

with NADPH as coenzyme. Sorbitol is oxidized to $\underline{D}$-fructose by
sorbitol dehydrogenase. There is some evidence that this pathway
of glucose utilization, as well as the glucuronic-xylulose cycle,
are somewhat more extensively utilized during insulin deficiency
(35). Should glucose enter cells in higher amount than usual and
be converted to sorbitol and fructose, which are poorly permeable,
osmotic changes may occur which are undesirable. The evidence is
strong that this sequence of events is involved in the production
of dulcitol from galactose in the lens and the formation of cataract in individuals with galactosemia (1,36).

Gabbay (37) has emphasized that polyol accumulation in nerve
may be related to the occurrence of diabetic neuropathy. For
example, galactosemia causes increases in nerve dulcitol and
water content, and decreases the motor nerve conduction velocity.
If the animals are then placed on a normal diet, the dulcitol and
water content decrease, and the nerve conduction velocity is
restored to normal. Moreover, artificially-induced diabetes in
the rat causes an increase in sorbitol and fructose as well as in
glucose in peripheral nerve. A decrease in the nerve conduction
velocity occurs concurrently. In an attempt to modify these
events, Gabbay, Dvornik, and their associates have been studying
synthetic inhibitors of aldose reductase as possible agents for
blocking polyol formation in animals. A recent report demonstrates that the inhibitor AY22284 reduces the accumulation of
galactitol in both the lens and sciatic nerve of galactosemic
rats, greatly reduces and delays the formation of detectable
cataracts in galactose-fed rats, and reduces the accumulation of
sorbitol and of fructose, but not of glucose, in the sciatic
nerve of artificially-diabetic rats (38). Of course, little work
has been done on the human in this area, and there will be continued difficulties in doing such investigations on human diabetics. A cause and effect relationship between polyol accumulation
in nerve and decrease in function has not been definitely established even in experimental animals, and even if this were to be
accomplished, it would still remain to be determined whether diabetic neuropathy in the human has the same cause.

The moderate, and dose dependent, utilization of orally
administered mannitol, and the effects of this hexitol on intestinal function, have been extensively studied (39). The use of
mannitol as a diuretic agent has recently been reviewed (40).

V. Maltitol and Isomaltitol

Maltitol has been studied recently at Charles Pfizer and
Company because of reports that this polyol is low caloric and
therefore might be a superior sweetening agent (41,42). Dr. H.
H. Rennard of Pfizer has informed me of his work, some of which
was done in collaboration with Dr. J. R. Bianchine of Johns
Hopkins. The low recovery of administered labeled maltitol in
the urine and feces of the rat indicated that it was efficiently

utilized, and similarly encouraging results were obtained in the human, including high recovery of ^{14}C in expired CO_2. However, the fact that the expired $C^{14}O_2$ peak in rats occurred at 4 to 5 hours after feeding suggested that the label might have been absorbed in the lower gut. It was indeed found that the maltitol was being utilized by intestinal microflora, which apparently were converting the labeled polyol into volatile fatty acids. In addition, intestinal mucosal preparations of rats have a low capacity to hydrolyze maltitol. Therefore, although the utilization of the maltitol is indirect, involving its preliminary conversion to fatty acids, this polyol is considered by Rennard to be a well utilized substance.

The utilization of isomaltitol has also been investigated. From studies on rats it was suggested that it could be a useful ingredient in calorie-reduced foods and beverages (43).

VI. Concluding Remarks

At the present time sorbitol and xylitol are the most important alditols in that they are key metabolic intermediates and are being fed or administered to humans in considerable amounts.

As far as the future is concerned, it appears to me that the problems which will most actively concern investigators are related to the more general use of xylitol, further investigation of the possible role of sorbitol in diabetes, and the possible advantages of polyols in decreasing dental caries.

Literature Cited

1. van Heyningen, R., in "Proceedings of the International Symposium on Metabolism, Physiology, and Clinical Use of Pentoses and Pentitols," Hakone, Japan, August 27-29, 1967 (B. L. Horecker, K. Lang, and Y. Takagi, eds.), pp. 109-123, Springer-Verlag, Berlin, Heidelberg, New York (1969).
2. Touster, O., Fed. Proc. (1960) 19, 977-983.
3. Touster, O. and Harwell, S., J. Biol. Chem. (1958) 230, 1031-1041.
4. Pitkänen, E. and Pitkänen, A., Ann. Med. Exp. Fenn. (1964) 42, 113-116.
5. Ingram, P., Applegarth, D. A., Sturrock, S., and Whyte, J. N. C., Clin. Chim. Acta (1971) 35, 523-524.
6. Touster, O. and Shaw, D. R. D., Physiol. Rev. (1962) 42, 181-225.
7. Hollmann, S. and Touster, O., J. Biol. Chem. (1957) 225, 87-102.
8. Arsenis, C. and Touster, O., J. Biol. Chem. (1969) 244, 3895-3899.
9. McCormick, D. B. and Touster, O., J. Biol. Chem. (1957) 229, 451-461.

10. Burns, J. J. and Kanfer, J., J. Am. Chem. Soc. (1957) 79, 3604-3605.
11. Touster, O., Fed. Proc. (1960) 19, 977-983.
12. Hiatt, H. H., in "The Metabolic Basis of Inherited Disease" (J. B. Stanbury, J. B. Wyngaarden, and D. S. Fredrickson, eds.), third ed., pp. 119-130, McGraw-Hill, New York (1972).
13. Gupta, S. D., Chaudhuri, C. R., and Chatterjee, I. B., Arch. Biochem. Biophys. (1972) 152, 889-890.
14. Hollmann, S. and Touster, O., "Non-glycolytic Pathways of the Metabolism of Glucose," p. 107, Academic Press, New York (1964).
15. Winegrad, A. I. and Shaw, W. N., Am. J. Physiol. (1964) 206, 165-168.
16. Winegrad, A. I. and Burden, C. L., New Engl. J. Med. (1966) 274, 298-305.
17. McCormick, D. B. and Touster, O., Biochim. Biophys. Acta (1961) 54, 598-600.
18. Horecker, B. L., Lang, K., and Takagi, Y., eds., "Proceedings of the International Symposium on Metabolism, Physiology, and Clinical Use of Pentoses and Pentitols," Hakone, Japan, August 27-29, 1967, Springer-Verlag, Berlin, Heidelberg, New York (1969).
19. Lang, K. and Fekl, W., Z. Ernährungswissenschaft (1971) Suppl. 11.
20. Sipple, H. L. and McNutt, K. W., eds., "Sugars in Nutrition," Academic Press, New York, San Francisco, London (1974).
21. Förster, H., in "Sugars in Nutrition" (H. L. Sipple and K. W. McNutt, eds.), pp. 259-280, Academic Press, New York, San Francisco, London (1974).
22. Froesch, E. R. and Jakob, A., in "Sugars in Nutrition" (H. L. Sipple and K. W. McNutt, eds.), pp. 241-258, Academic Press, New York, San Francisco, London (1974).
23. Meng, H. C., in "Sugars in Nutrition" (H. L. Sipple and K. W. McNutt, eds.), pp. 527-566, Academic Press, New York, San Francisco, London (1974).
24. Thomas, D. W., Edwards, J. B., and Edwards, R. G., in "Sugars in Nutrition" (H. L. Sipple and K. W. McNutt, eds.), pp. 567-590, Academic Press, New York, San Francisco, London (1974).
25. van Eys, J., Wang, Y. M., Chan, S., Tanphaichitr, V. S., and King, S. M., in "Sugars in Nutrition" (H. L. Sipple and K. W. McNutt, eds.), pp. 613-631, Academic Press, New York, San Francisco, London (1974).
26. Thomas, D. W., Edwards, J. B., Gilligan, J. E., Lawrence, J. R., and Edwards, R. G., Med. J. Australia (1972) 1, 1238-1246.
27. Brin, M. and Miller, O. N., in "Sugars in Nutrition" (H. L. Sipple and K. W. McNutt, eds.), pp. 591-606, Academic Press, New York, San Francisco, London (1974).

28. Grunberg, E., Beskid, G., and Brin, M., Int. J. Vitamin and
    Nutrition Res. (1973) 43, 227-232.
29. Mäkinen, K. K., in "Sugars in Nutrition" (H. L. Sipple and
    K. W. McNutt, eds.), pp. 645-687, Academic Press, New
    York, San Francisco, London (1974).
30. Bässler, K. H., in "Proceedings of the International Sympo-
    sium on Metabolism, Physiology, and Clinical Use of
    Pentoses and Pentitols," Hakone, Japan, August 27-29,
    1967 (B. L. Horecker, K. Lang, and Y. Takagi, eds.), pp.
    190-196, Springer-Verlag, Berlin, Heidelberg, New York
    (1969).
31. Hers, H. G., Biochim. Biophys. Acta (1960) 37, 127-138.
32. Hue, L. and Hers, H.-G., Eur. J. Biochem. (1972) 29, 268-
    275.
33. Gabbay, K. H., Clin. Research (1974) XXII (3), 468A.
34. Hers, H. G., Biochim. Biophys. Acta (1956) 22, 202-203.
35. Winegrad, A. I., Clements, R. S., and Morrison, A. D., in
    "Handbook of Physiology," (Amer. Physiol. Soc., J. Field,
    ed.), Sect. 7, Vol. I, pp. 457-471, Williams & Wilkins,
    Baltimore, Maryland (1972).
36. Kinoshita, J. H., Invest. Ophthalmol. (1965) 4, 786-799.
37. Gabbay, K. H., New Engl. J. Med. (1973) 288, 831-836.
38. Dvornik, D., Simard-Duquesne, N., Krami, M., Sestanj, K.,
    Gabbay, K. H., Kinoshita, J. H., Varma, S. D., and
    Merola, L. O., Science (1973) 182, 1146-1147.
39. Nasrallah, S. M. and Iber, F. L., Am. J. Med. Sci. (1969)
    258, 80-88.
40. Ginn, H. E., in "Sugars in Nutrition" (H. L. Sipple and K.
    W. McNutt, eds.), pp. 607-612, Academic Press, New York,
    San Francisco, London (1974).
41. Naito, F., New Food Industry (1971) 13, 1.
42. Hosoya, N., Ninth Internat. Congr. Nutrition (1972) Mexico.
43. Musch, K., Siebert, G., Schiweck, H., and Steinle, G., Z.
    Ernährungswissenschaft (1973), Suppl. 15, pp. 3-16.

Metabolism and Physiological Effects of the Pentoses and Uronic Acids

OSCAR TOUSTER

Department of Molecular Biology, Vanderbilt University, Nashville, Tenn. 37235

I. Introduction

The importance of the pentoses needs little comment, since they are so well known to be components of DNA, RNA, coenzymes, ATP, and proteoglycans. Moreover, pentose phosphates are important metabolic intermediates in such processes as CO_2 fixation in photosynthesis. Similarly, uronic acids are components of proteoglycans, or mucopolysaccharides, and of metabolic pathways, including those leading to the pentoses. These structural and metabolic aspects will be briefly reviewed, as well as the utilization of these substances and relevant pathological considerations.

II. The Physiologically Important Pentoses

Table I lists pentoses which are important in mammalian metabolism.

TABLE I.   PHYSIOLOGICALLY-IMPORTANT PENTOSES

D-Ribose - in nucleotides, pentose phosphate pathway

D-2-Deoxyribose - in deoxyribonucleotides

D-Ribulose - in pentose phosphate pathway; Ru-1,5-DP is CO_2 acceptor in photosynthesis

D-Xylulose - in pentose phosphate pathway, in glucuronic acid-xylulose cycle

L-Xylulose - in glucuronic acid-xylulose cycle, excreted in gram quantities by humans with essential pentosuria

D-Xylose - in gal-gal-xyl linkage of mucopolysaccharide to protein

D-Ribose of course is a key component of RNA and other ribo-
nucleotides, and D-ribose 5-phosphate is a member of the pentose
phosphate pathway of carbohydrate metabolism. D-2-Deoxyribose is
a component of the nucleotides in DNA. D-Ribulose, as the 5-
phosphate, is an intermediate in the pentose phosphate pathway
and, as the 1,5-diphosphate, is the CO_2 acceptor in photosynthesis. D-Xylulose as the 5-phosphate derivative is an intermediate
in the pentose phosphate pathway and occurs as the free sugar in
the glucuronate-xylulose cycle, as described in the preceding
paper in this symposium. L-Xylulose is also a member of the
cycle and is noteworthy because of its rather large excretion by
humans with the genetic metabolic disorder known as essential
pentosuria. In proteoglycans (mucopolysaccharides) D-xylose is
the sugar residue attached to serine in the bridge linking the
polymeric carbohydrate to the protein core. The structure of the
galactose-galactose-xylose bridge was mainly worked out through
the work of Lennart Rodén (1). Of course many other pentoses
occur in nature and are ingested in foodstuffs, but those listed
in Table I are of the greatest importance to mammals in their
normal metabolism.

III. Utilization of Pentoses

     Table II summarizes some experiments in which ^{14}C-labeled
pentoses were administered to animals and man and their utilization estimated. Examination of the liver glycogen column shows
that ribose is utilized as effectively as glucose. It should be
borne in mind, however, that since these are tracer quantities of
pentose, it need not be true that equivalent but large amounts of
pentose would be utilized as well as glucose. In man D-xylose,
D-ribose and D-lyxose are oxidized to CO_2 to a moderate extent, a
finding consistent with the fact that most of the label which
appears in the urine occurs in a form that is not the administered sugar. In these experiments the sugars were infused in
human subjects over a 15-minute period. The CO_2 and liver glycogen experiments indicate that L-arabinose is utilized only to a
negligible extent.

     Although D-xylose may be isomerized to D-xylulose by plant
and bacterial enzymes, in mammals this aldopentose is either
reduced to xylitol, an intermediate in the glucuronate-xylulose
cycle (7), or oxidized to D-xylonic acid by an NAD-linked D-
xylose dehydrogenase detected in calf lens by Van Heyningen (8).
D-Ribose is converted to ribose 5-phosphate, an intermediate in
the pentose phosphate pathway. The route of utilization of
D-lyxose has not been established; perhaps it is isomerized to
D-xylulose.

TABLE II. UTILIZATION OF FREE PENTOSES BY MAMMALS

Pentitose	Species	% of Administered Tracer Dose			Time (Hrs.)	Ref
		Oxid. to CO_2	In urine	Liver glycogen		
D-Glucose	Mouse	—	—	8.3	3	a
D-Ribose	Mouse	—	—	10.0	3	a
	Man	48	10	—	6-24	b
	Rat	—	—	7.1	2	c
D-Xylose	Mouse	—	—	1.0	3	a
	Man	16	35	—	6-24	b
	Guinea pig	15	75	—	24	d
D-Arabinose	Mouse	—	—	0.03	3	a
	Man	19	57	—	24	b
L-Arabinose	Mouse	—	—	0	3	a
	Man	0.8	85	—	6-24	b
D-Lyxose	Man	14	72	—	6-24	b

a Hiatt (2)
b Segal and Foley (3)
c McCormick and Touster (4)
d McCormick and Touster (5)

(Table adapted from Hollmann and Reinauer (6))

IV. Pentoses and D-Glucuronic Acid as Metabolic Intermediates

The pentose phosphate pathway for glucose utilization is shown in Figure 1. The main feature of this pathway for glucose oxidation is that 3 molecules of glucose phosphate are oxidized, in NADP-linked steps, to form 3 molecules of pentose phosphate. A series of isomerizations and group transfers occur which have the overall effect of converting 3 molecules of hexose to 3 molecules of fructose phosphate and 1 molecule of glyceraldehyde phosphate plus 3 molecules of CO_2. This is therefore the C_1 oxidation pathway of glucose metabolism. It is the main pathway for the production of NADPH, which is the nucleotide coenzyme commonly used in reductive biosynthetic processes, and it is the route by which ribose is made for the production of nucleotides and for deoxyribose production as well. It should be emphasized that most of the reactions, although not the decarboxylations, are reversible. Most of the ribose 5-phosphate appears to be derived from this pathway reading from right to left, rather than left to right, in other words, from the non-oxidative portion of the pathway. The phosphorylation of ribulose 5-phosphate to ribulose 1,5-diphosphate provides the CO_2 acceptor in plants. We would also point out that all pentoses in this pathway are phosphorylated. From the quantitative point of view, this is a minor pathway for carbohydrate oxidation, in comparison to the Embden-Meyerhof glycolytic route, but a greater amount of glucose is directed through this pathway when there is need for NADPH.

Another route by which pentoses are formed is through the conversion of D-glucuronic acid to the xyluloses in the glucuronic-xylulose pathway, in which the pentose intermediates are not phosphorylated. A pentosuric individual excretes a rather constant amount of L-xylulose. The feeding of D-glucuronolactone elevates the urinary L-xylulose in an amount indicating that the conversion occurs in rather high yield (9). That this is a direct conversion has been demonstrated with labeled lactone. It is relevant to mention that D-glucuronate is poorly converted to L-xylulose in an experiment of this type because, unlike the lactone, the free acid or salt is poorly absorbed or impermeable to cells.

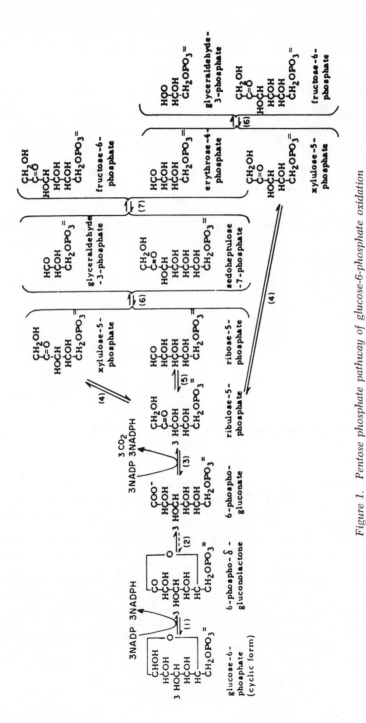

Figure 1.   Pentose phosphate pathway of glucose-6-phosphate oxidation

Related to the D-glucuronic acid-L-xylulose conversion is the production of L-ascorbic acid from D-glucose, a process in which D-glucuronate is an intermediate (10).

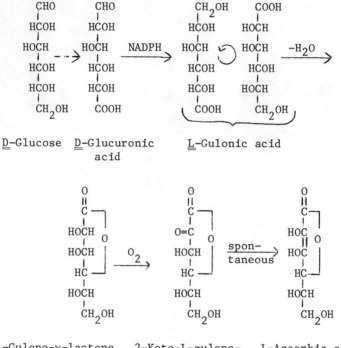

D-Glucose   D-Glucuronic   L-Gulonic acid
                  acid

L-Gulono-γ-lactone   2-Keto-L-gulono-   L-Ascorbic acid
                          γ-lactone

This pathway, largely based on the work of King and Burns in the rat, shows that the D-glucose chain is inverted during its transformation into L-ascorbic acid. The same holds for D-glucuronic acid, but not for the L-gulonic acid derivatives. These and other studies on the biosynthesis of L-ascorbic acid and of L-xylulose led to the formulation of the glucuronate-xylulose pathway (Figure 2) (7,11,12,13).

The functions of the glucuronate-xylulose cycle, which occurs in all mammals studied, are discussed in the previous paper in this volume and will not be further described at this point. However, we should like to mention that there is still uncertainty about the specific reaction(s) by which free glucuronate is formed. We can accept that D-glucuronate is the precursor of L-gulonate, and we know a good deal about the biosynthesis of

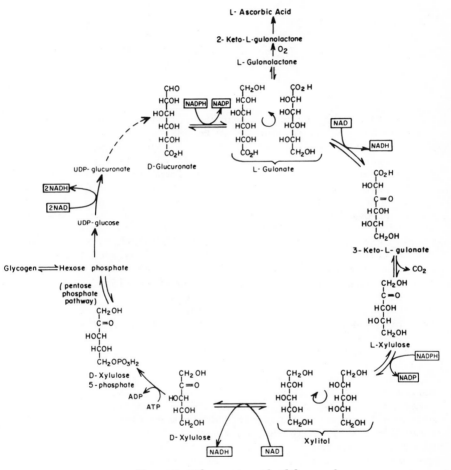

Figure 2.   *Glucuronic acid-xylulose cycle*

UDP-glucuronic acid. There have been two suggestions as to how
D-glucuronate might be formed from UDP-glucuronic acid:

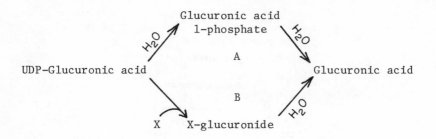

In pathway A, the enzyme UDP-glucuronic acid pyrophosphatase
would cleave the nucleotide sugar to UMP plus glucuronic acid-1-
phosphate, which would then be hydrolyzed by a phosphatase to
free glucuronate. An objection to this route is that the pyrophosphatase has been localized in our laboratory as a constituent
of the plasma membrane of liver cells (14). This relatively non-
specific enzyme, nucleotide pyrophosphatase, is the same enzyme
as phosphodiesterase I. It seems highly unlikely that an enzyme
of such broad specificity and, in particular, one located in the
plasma membrane plays a role in a metabolic pathway such as we
are considering here. A second objection stems from the fact
that the only phosphatases in liver which can hydrolyze glucuronic
acid-1-phosphate are located in the lysosomes (15,16). These
phosphatases also are generally not very specific. A second suggested route (B) has UDPGlcUA donating a glucuronic acid residue
to a hypothetical acceptor, X, to form a glucuronide which either
hydrolyzes spontaneously because of its intrinsic instability to
yield free glucuronic acid or is hydrolyzed by the enzyme β-glucuronidase. Although glucuronide formation is a common reaction
in liver, there is no basis for speculating on the identity of X.
More important, β-glucuronidase is located in the endoplasmic
reticulum and, especially, in the lysosomes. Although β-glucuronidase does produce glucuronic acid from complex glucuronides,
unpublished studies in our laboratory have failed to provide evidence that this enzyme produces the glucuronic acid that is the
precursor of L-ascorbic acid. Whether we are naive about some
aspect of the enzymology or cell biochemistry involved, or
whether there is another route not as yet apparent, is uncertain.
     For some years it was believed that inositol, which occurs
rather commonly in animals and is obviously a food constituent,
might be metabolized through more than one metabolic route. In
addition, a kidney enzyme was discovered which converts inositol
to D-glucuronic acid. Consequently, a joint study by four laboratories was undertaken in which labeled inositol was administered
to normal and pentosuric human beings (17). We found that the

inositol was oxidized to CO_2 to a considerable extent in the normal but was much reduced in pentosuric individuals, a result consistent with the formulation of a pathway from inositol to $\underline{D}$-glucuronic acid, which would then be metabolized through the glucuronate-xylulose cycle. Pentosuric subjects would accumulate labeled $\underline{L}$-xylulose, whereas normal subjects would not have a block at this point. The labeling patterns in isolated metabolites conformed to the postulated metabolic pathways. Myo-inositol labeled at position 2 did in fact yield C_1-labeled urinary $\underline{L}$-xylulose in the pentosuric individuals. There was also a preponderance of radioactivity in C_6 of blood glucose, a finding consistent with the metabolism of the inositol through the xylulose pathway and then on through the pentose phosphate pathway to glucose.

V. Pathological Aspects of the Pentoses

Although essential pentosuria is an inherited metabolic disorder (9,18), not a metabolic disease, because the poor ability to effect the reduction of $\underline{L}$-xylulose to xylitol appears not to be deleterious in any way, the underlying basis of this disorder will be described at this point. For some time this enzymatic localization of the defect (at $\underline{L}$-xylulose reduction) in pentosuria was rather indirect, pentosuric individuals being understandably reluctant to donate a piece of liver for enzymatic analyses. Not long ago Asakura in Japan reported that the two xylitol dehydrogenases are present in red blood cells, a finding which made possible investigation of the normal and mutant enzymes in human red cells. When Wang and van Eys (19) carried out such a study, it was at first surprising to find in pentosuric erythrocytes a moderate amount of activity of the NADP-linked xylitol dehydrogenase catalyzing the reduction of $\underline{L}$-xylulose. However, further study showed that the enzyme was abnormal. Its K_m for NADP is 10 to 20 times higher than that of the normal enzyme, that is, it has a much lower affinity for this substrate than does the normal enzyme. In other words, there is a mutant enzyme present, and it is not very effective. That the block in pentosuria is not total has in fact been apparent from *in vivo* studies.

The feeding of xylose in high amounts to rats causes xylitol cataract (20), but I should emphasize that xylitol administration does not. The xylose is transported into the lens, where it is reduced to xylitol and upsets the osmotic balance. In regard to the medical aspects of xylose, I should mention that oral xylose doses are given to patients in tests of intestinal absorption. Since the xylose is poorly metabolized and is therefore excreted to a considerable extent in the urine, the amount of urinary xylose is a rough measure of the absorptive capacity of the patients.

VI. Physiologically Important Uronic Acids

By far the most important uronic acid in mammals is D-glucuronic acid. As shown in Table III, it is important because it is a constituent of many mucopolysaccharides or proteoglycans and is a constituent of glucuronide derivatives of drugs and hormones. As already indicated above, it is a precursor of L-ascorbic acid and the xyluloses and is the direct product of the metabolic oxidation of inositol in man. Karl Meyer originally discovered that some of the uronic acid in mucopolysaccharides is L-iduronic acid, the 5'-epimer of D-glucuronic acid. Figure 3 shows a portion of the heparan sulfate molecule containing α-linked sulfated N-acetylglucosamine residues interspersed with sulfated L-iduronic acid and D-glucuronic acid. Some time ago the epimerization of UDP-L-iduronic acid by rabbit tissue extracts was reported. However, this work has not been confirmed in any other laboratory, and there is now evidence that the formation of L-iduronic acid occurs at the macromolecular level, i.e., it seems to be formed concurrently with sulfation of the polymer (21).

VII. Utilization and Production of the Uronic Acids

The routes for the utilization of D-glucuronate in various organisms are summarized below (7):

Microorganisms

D-Glucuronate————→D-fructuronate————→D-mannonate

————→2-keto-3-deoxygluconate (KDG)————→KDG 6-phosphate

————→pyruvate + triose phosphate

Plants

D-Glucuronate⟨ glucuronic acid 1-P ——UTP——→UDPGlcUA————→pectins and hemicelluloses
⟩D-glucaric acid

Animals

D-Glucuronate⟨ L-gulonate ⟨ → xylulose pathway
→ →L-ascorbic acid
⟩D-glucaric acid

TABLE III. PHYSIOLOGICALLY IMPORTANT URONIC ACIDS

```
CHO
 |
HCOH        D-Glucuronic acid  - in heparin, hyaluronic acid,
 |                                chondroitin sulfates, etc., and
HOCH                              glucuronides (of drugs and hor-
 |                                mones); involved in metabolism
HCOH                              of inositol, L-ascorbic acid,
 |                                and the xyluloses
HCOH
 |
COOH
```

```
CHO
 |
HCOH
 |
HOCH        L-Iduronic acid  - in heparin and heparan sulfate,
 |                              dermatan sulfate
HCOH
 |
HOCH
 |
COOH
```

Figure 3. Portion of heparin and heparin sulfates

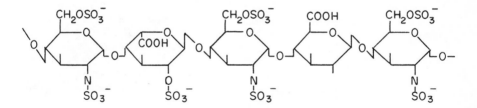

Biosynthesis:

1. Polymerization of GlcNAc and glucuronic acid

2. N-deacetylated

3. N- and O-sulfated with epimerization of some D-glucuronic
    acid to L-iduronic acid.

The metabolism of glucuronate in microorganisms is quite special, as shown by Ashwell and his collaborators several years ago, the first step being epimerization to D-fructuronate. In plants, D-glucuronate can be directly phosphorylated, a reaction that does not occur in animals. UDP-glucuronic acid is a precursor of plant polysaccharides. Glucuronate can also be oxidized to the corresponding dicarboxylic acid, glucaric acid. In animals the conversion to glucaric acid and the presence of the latter in urine have been demonstrated. We have already discussed the reduction of glucuronate to L-gulonate and its conversion to L-ascorbate or its metabolism through the xyluloses.

The utilization and production of glucuronic acid in vivo are summarized below (7):

A. Utilization

    Utilization in vivo is extensive only if administered as the lactone because the acid probably does not enter cells. High extent of utilization is indicated by

    1) high yield of $^{14}CO_2$ from labeled lactone

    2) high yield of urinary L-xylulose in the pentosuric human

B. Production

    Glucuronic acid production is increased by

    1) substances excreted as glucuronides

    2) inducers of the microsomal P-450 system (e.g. steroids, barbiturates). These substances also increase the production of

        a) L-ascorbic acid

        b) glucaric acid

The production of glucuronic acid, that is, of UDP-glucuronate, is responsive to some inducing agents which increase the production of conjugated glucuronides, of L-ascorbic acid, and of glucaric acid and, I might add, of L-xylulose in the pentosuric human. The mechanism of this induction has been studied for many years and is probably still not very clearly understood. Various steroids and barbiturates and other drugs which induce the microsomal P_{450} system are stimulators of the production of glucuronic acid derivatives.

Figure 4 shows that UDP-glucuronic acid is somewhat of a key intermediate in metabolism:

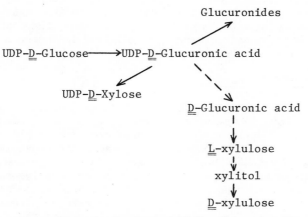

Figure 4. *Reactions of UDP–D-glucuronic acid*

UDP–Glucuronic acid is used in the biosynthesis of glucuronides and proteoglycans; it is the precursor of glucuronic acid which goes to the xyluloses and to ascorbic acid, and it is the precursor of the xylose found in the gal-gal-xyl bridge between mucopolysaccharide chains and polypeptide chains in proteoglycans by virtue of its decarboxylation to UDP-xylose.

VIII. Pathological Aspects of D–Glucuronic and L–Iduronic Acids

There are now two hereditary lysosomal diseases specifically attributable to deficiencies in lysosomal uronidases. Gargoylism, or Hurler's disease, associated with the accumulation of dermatan and heparan sulfates and with mental deficiency and a variety of morphological changes, has recently been shown to be due to an L–iduronidase deficiency in lysosomes (22). In the last few years another type of mucopolysaccharidosis has been found that has some similarity to Hurler's disease. As a result of the work of Sly et al. (23) and of Neufeld and her associates (24), this disease, atypical mucopolysaccharidosis, can be attributed to β–glucuronidose deficiency in the lysosomes. In connection with lysosomal disorders, it is relevant to mention at a symposium such as the present one that severe lysosomal storage abnormalities have been caused by the administration of undegradable polymers, including dextrans and polyvinylpyrrolidone. Great caution should be used in injecting such materials into humans.

Also known are abnormalities in glucuronyl transferase, the enzyme system(s) catalyzing the transfer of glucuronic acid from UDPGlcUA to suitable acceptors. In Crigler-Najjar disease a deficiency of glucuronyl transferase is responsible for insufficient conversion of the heme degradation product bilirubin to bilirubin glucuronide, the rapidly excretable, more water-soluble acidic form. In this disease the unreacted bilirubin accumulates in the nervous system, with deleterious consequences to the infant (25). There seems to be an animal model of this disease, the Gunn rat, in which similar abnormal bilirubin metabolism is observed as well as low transferase levels.

IX. Summary and Prospects

In summary, it is evident that pentoses and uronic acids are extremely important to mammalian biology. I have not commented on certain aspects of utilization of complex uronic acid and pentose-containing polymers, such as pectins, by mammals because in general these seem to be poorly utilized. One area that will certainly witness an interesting future concerns the lysosomal storage disease because so many of the accumulated proteoglycans are rich in uronic acids. Indeed, since pinocytosed chemotherapeutic agents are destined to enter lysosomes, where the metabolic abnormalities are found, these diseases are prime targets for enzyme therapy attempts. Currently, β-glucuronidase is in fact being studied as a chemotherapeutic agent in atypical mucopolysaccharidosis.

Literature Cited

1. Rodén, L., in "Metabolic Conjugation and Metabolic Hydrolysis" (W. H. Fishman, ed.), Vol. II, pp. 345-442, Academic Press, New York (1970).
2. Hiatt, H. H., J. Biol. Chem. (1957) 224, 851-859.
3. Segal, S. and Foley, J. B., J. Clin. Invest. (1959) 38, 407-413.
4. McCormick, D. B. and Touster, O., Biochim. Biophys. Acta (1961) 54, 598-600.
5. McCormick, D. B. and Touster, O., J. Biol. Chem. (1957) 229, 451-461.
6. Hollmann, S. and Reinauer, H., Z. Ernährungswissenschaft (1971) Suppl. 11, pp. 1-7.
7. Touster, O., in "Comprehensive Biochemistry" (M. Florkin and E. H. Stotz, eds.), Vol. 17, pp. 219-240, Elsevier Publishing Company, Amsterdam-London-New York (1969).
8. van Heyningen, R., Biochem. J. (1958) 69, 481-491.
9. Touster, O., Fed. Proc. (1960) 19, 977-983.

10. Burns, J. J., in "Metabolic Pathways" (D. M. Greenberg, ed.), Vol. 1, pp. 341-356, Academic Press, New York (1960).
11. Burns, J. J. and Kanfer, J., J. Am. Chem. Soc. (1957) 79, 3604-3605.
12. Hollmann, S. and Touster, O., J. Am. Chem. Soc. (1956) 78, 3544-3545.
13. Hollmann, S. and Touster, O., J. Biol. Chem. (1957) 225, 87-102.
14. Touster, O., Aronson, N. N., Jr., Dulaney, J. T., and Hendrickson, H., J. Cell Biol. (1970) 47, 604-618.
15. Arsenis, C., Hollmann, S., and Touster, O., Abstracts of the American Chemical Society Meeting, New York, September 1966, C-286.
16. Arsenis, C. and Touster, O., J. Biol. Chem. (1967) 242, 3400-3401.
17. Hankes, L. V., Politzer, W. M., Touster, O., and Anderson, L., Ann. N. Y. Acad. Sci. (1969) 165, 564-576.
18. Hiatt, H., in "The Metabolic Basis of Inherited Disease" (J. B. Stanbury, J. B. Wyngaarden, and D. S. Fredrickson, eds.), 3rd ed., pp. 119-130, McGraw Hill, New York, Toronto, London (1972).
19. Wang, Y. M. and van Eys, J., New Eng. J. Med. (1970) 282, 892-896.
20. van Heyningen, R., in "Proceedings of the International Symposium on Metabolism, Physiology, and Clinical Use of Pentoses and Pentitols," Hakone, Japan, August 27-29, 1967 (B. L. Horecker, K. Lang, and Y. Takagi, eds.), pp. 109-123, Springer-Verlag, Berlin, Heidelberg, New York (1969).
21. Höök, M., Lindahl, U., Bäckström, G., Malmström, A., and Fransson, L.-Å., J. Biol. Chem. (1974) 249, 3908-3915.
22. Matalon, R. and Dorfman, A., Biochem. Biophys. Res. Commun. (1972) 47, 959-964.
23. Sly, W. S., Quinton, B. A., McAlister, W. H., and Rimoin, D. L., J. Pediat. (1973) 82, 249-257.
24. Hall, C. W., Cantz, M., and Neufeld, E. F., Arch. Biochem. Biophys. (1973) 155, 32-38.
25. Schmid, R. in "The Metabolic Basis of Inherited Disease" (J. B. Stanbury, J. B. Wyngaarden, and D. S. Fredrickson, eds.), 3rd ed., pp. 1141-1178, McGraw-Hill, New York, Toronto, London (1972).

9

Role of Carbohydrates in Dental Caries

WILLIAM H. BOWEN

Caries Prevention and Research Branch, National Caries Program, National Institute of
Dental Research, National Institutes of Health, Bethesda, Md. 20014

Dental caries results from the action of specific bacteria
which colonize the tooth surface and metabolize particular components of the diet. The action results in the rapid and sometimes
prolonged production of acid on the tooth surface resulting in
the dissolution of the enamel.

Since the time of Aristotle it has been considered that carbohydrates played an essential role in the pathogenesis of dental
caries. There is now an abundance of evidence accumulated from
epidemiological surveys (1) and animal experimentation (2) which
clearly indicates that dental caries does not develop in the
absence of dietary carbohydrate. In an elegant clinical study
Gustafsson, et.al. (3) showed that the incidence of caries is
related to the frequency of intake of carbohydrate and not to the
total amount consumed. For example, patients who in 1 year consumed 94 kg. of sugar with meals had fewer new carious lesions
than patients who consumed 85 kg., 15 of which was taken between
meals.

The restriction in carbohydrate intake which occurred during
World War II was followed by a dramatic fall in the prevalence in
dental caries in many European countries. (4)(5)(6)

Carbohydrates and sugar in particular apparently can also
affect the maturation of enamel, a process which leads to increased mineral uptake in enamel post-eruptively. It was
observed (7) that the teeth of rats exposed to high sugar diets
showed delayed maturation and were therefore presumably more
susceptible to decay. Rats bred on a diet (8) conducive to the
formation of severe protein-calorie imbalance have been shown to
have enhanced susceptibility to caries. The effect was ascribed
to altered tooth size (9) and to alterations in salivary composition.

The physical form in which sugar is ingested will also influence its cariogenicity. Powdered sugar is more cariogenic than
similar sugars given in an aqueous solution. (10) The size of
particles and the adhesiveness of the diet also influence the
cariogenicity of the diet. (11) In general the longer a poten-

tially cariogenic substance is retained in the mouth the greater
is the likelihood that caries will develop.

The formation of dental plaque is the earliest evidence that
microorganisms and components of the diet are interacting. Dental
plaque is the soft white tenacious material which occurs on tooth
surfaces and is composed of microorganisms enmeshed in a matrix
of carbohydrate and protein.

Specific microorganisms are associated with the early formation of dental plaque and sucrose plays an important role in
their establishment on the tooth surface. (12) Streptococcus
mutans is a prime microbial agent in the pathogenesis of dental
caries. (13)(14) It has several interesting properties; it is
found predominantly on the tooth surface and it forms polyglucan
and polyfructan from sucrose. (15)(16) Strep. mutans can become
reversibly bound to the tooth surface in the absence of sucrose
but following ingestion of this sugar extracellular polysaccharide
is formed. (17) This substance enhances the ability of the micro-
organism to adhere to the tooth surface and also leads to the
aggregation of other microorganisms. (18) The available evidence
indicates that the predominant polyglucan in plaque is composed
of material possessing mainly 1-3 linkages; substantial material
possessing 1-6 linkages is also present. (19) Up to 40% of the
polyglucan formed in plaque is readily metabolizable by plaque
microorganisms. (20) Although polyfructan is also found it is
metabolized very rapidly(21) by substantial numbers of the microorganisms in plaque. (22)

Apart from the contribution that extracellular polysaccharides make to the adherence of microorganisms their precise role
in the pathogenesis of dental caries is unclear. Recent evidence
has shown that phosphorus is tightly bound to the polysaccharide
and that the carbohydrate is charged. (23) This indicates that
the polysaccharide could limit the diffusion of charged substances
into and out of plaque. Acid formed within plaque could not,
therefore, be readily neutralized by the diffusion of such substances as bicarbonate. It is also likely that the extracellular
polysaccharide protects the microorganisms from inimical influences. Whatever the precise role they have in the pathogeneses
of caries there is little doubt that the integrity of the tooth
would be enhanced by either preventing their formation or their
rapid removal.

There is also clear evidence which indicates that microorganisms in plaque can synthesize an intracellular polysaccharide
(IPS) of the amylo pectin type from a wide variety of carbohydrates. (24)(25) This material can be catabolized by plaque
microorganisms during periods when extraneous sources of carbohydrate are lacking. This catabolism is probably responsible for
the comparatively low pH values observed in plaque around carious
lesions even in patients who have been fasting. (26) There is
some evidence to indicate that the number of intracellular polysaccharide forming organisms in plaque is positively correlated

with the number of carious lesions.(27)
    The results of research carried out by Kanap and Hamilton(28)
indicate that both the synthesis and catabolism of IPS is influenced by the presence of fluoride. They have shown that the low
concentrations of fluoride inhibit enolase and glucose-6-p formation without penetrating the cell significantly indicating that
fluoride may affect the transport of sugar into the bacterial
cell. This is probably one of several mechanisms through which
fluoride exercises its cariostatic effect.
    Dental plaque also forms in the absence of dietary carbohy-
drate, (29)(30) e.g., in patients or animals who receive their
complete diet by gastric intubation, but it lacks several properties found in plaque formed under conventional circumstances.
Animals fed in this manner do not develop caries. In addition
the plaque so formed lacks the ability to lower the pH value of
topically applied sugar solutions in contrast to that formed
normally, which may lower the pH value of a sugar solution to 4.5
or less in a matter of minutes. (32) It is generally considered
that rapid demineralization of the tooth surface occurs below pH
5.5.
    The types and proportions of acids formed in dental plaque
are attracting an increasing amount of attention because it is
conceivable that the difference in the cariogenicity of plaques
may reside in some measure in the different types or proportions
of acids present. Gilmour and Poole (33) found that a constant
relationship between the concentration of lactic acid in plaque
and pH decrease was lacking. In some plaques it was found that
the concentration of lactic, propionic and acetic acids accounted
for less than 50% of the titratable acidity. In a study carried
out by Geddes (34) it was observed that 'fasting' plaque contained
3×10^{-5} m moles of acid/mg wet weight and that five minutes after
exposure to sugar the concentration had increased to 5×10^{-5} m
moles. The major change was to a five-fold increase in D (-)
lactate and an eight-fold increase in D (+) lactate.
    There is a positive correlation between the frequency of
sugar intake and the incidence of caries. (35) Each ingestion of
sugar is followed by a rapid fall in pH value on the tooth surface. The pH returns to neutrality over a 20-30 minute period.
The duration for which the plaque has been allowed to accumulate
will influence both the magnitude of the fall in pH and the time
required for its recovery. (36) In general the older the plaque
the greater its pathogenic potential. An extreme example of the
effects of prolonged exposure to sucrose can be seen in infants
who have comforters dipped in a sucrose syrup or similar solution. (37) These children develop rampant caries on the palatal
surfaces of the upper molars and incisors.
    It is occasionally argued that much caries could be elimina-
ted if other sugars were substituted for sucrose in the diet.
Some support for this concept can be found in patients who suffer
from fructose intolerance. These patients must avoid sucrose and

fructose. Fructose intolerant patients have substantially less
caries than normal persons but they are not caries-free. (38)
Clearly such patients must alter their dietary intake considerably, other than merely avoiding sucrose.

Sucrose has probably been blamed as the main dietary culprit
in caries causation simply because it is the sugar which is most
frequently ingested. There is no evidence that its substitution
by glucose or fructose would lead to a significant reduction in
dental decay in humans. Results of many experiments carried in
animals clearly indicate that glucose and fructose can induce
significant levels of decay. (39)(40)(41) Primates which received their complete diet by gastric intubation with the exception of glucose or fructose (i.e. plaque was formed in the presence of these sugars) formed plaque which contained significant
levels of extracellular polysaccharide and in addition this
plaque could lower the pH of sugar solutions rapidly. (42)

The effects of polyols such as sorbitol, mannitol and xylitol
on plaque formation and the development of caries have been investigated in animals and to a lesser extent in man. (43) It was
observed in primates that the ingestion of sorbitol was followed
initially by the formation of plaque which had a syrupy consist-
ency. It was also noted that the numbers of Strep. mutans in
plaque declined markedly when sorbitol was substituted for sucrose even though Strep. mutans ferments sorbitol. Prolonged
ingestion in man (44) or primates did not lead to the development
of a plaque flora with an enhanced ability to metabolize sorbitol.
All the available evidence indicates that sorbitol is substantially less cariogenic in animals than sugars. Xylitol was shown by
Muhlemann, et. al. (45) to be even less cariogenic than sorbitol.

A possible explanation for the lower cariogenicity of sorbitol may be found in the manner in which it is metabolized by
microorganisms. The breakdown of sorbitol produces mainly formic
acid and ethanol; in contrast, the metabolism of glucose results
in the formation of primarily lactic acid. (46)

It is possible that the extensive use of polyols would not
be acceptable by the general public as in some persons even moderate doses have a cathartic effect.

There is little doubt that the incidence of caries would
decline dramatically if the general population would reduce the
frequency of intake of fermentable carbohydrates. However the
ingestion of candy is rarely associated in peoples minds with the
formation of a carious lesion at some future time. Any disease
which affects 95% of the population is unlikely to be controlled
to a significant extent by individual effort. Effective control
calls for public health measures and of these water fluoridation
is the most effective.

Literature Cited

1. Read, T. and Knowles, E. Brit. Dent. J. (1938),64:185.
2. Frostell, G. and Baer, P.N. Acta Odont. Scand. (1971) 29:253.
3. Gustafson, B.E.; Quensel, C.E.; Swenander, L.; Lundquist, C.;
    Grahnen, H.; Bonow, B.; and Krasse, B. Acta Odont. Scand.
    (1954), 11: 232.
4. Toverud, K.V., Kjosnes, E., and Toverud, G. Odont. Tid.
    (1942), 50:529.
5. Sognnaes, R. and White, R. Amer. J. Dis. Child. (1940), 60:
    283.
6. Parfitt, G. J. Brit. Dent. J. (1954), 97:235.
7. Nikiforuk, G. J. Dent. Res. (1970), 49:1252.
8. Menaker, L. and Navia, J. J. Dent. Res. (1973), 52:680.
9. Holloway, P.J., Shaw, J.H. and Sweeney, E.A. Arch. oral Biol.
    (1961), 3:185.
10. Sognnaes, R.F. J. Nutr. (1949), 36:1.
11. Caldwell, R.C. J. Dent. Res. (1970), 49:1295.
12. Krasse, B. Arch. oral Biol. (1966), 11:429.
13. de Stoppelaar, J.D., van Houte, J.V. and de Moor, C.E. Arch.
    oral Biol. (1967),12:1199.
14. Gibbons, R.J., De Paola, P.F., Spinell, D.M., and Skobe, Z.
    Infection and Immunity (1974), 9:481.
15. Gibbons, R.J. and Nygaard, M. Arch. oral Biol. (1968), 13:
    1249.
16. Wood, J.M. and Critchley, P. Arch. oral Biol. (1966) 11:1039.
17. Gibbons, R.J. and van Houte, J. Infection and Immunity.
    (1971), 3:567.
18. Gibbons, R.J. and Fitzgerald, R.J. J. Bacteriol. (1969), 98:
    341.
19. Baird, J.K., Longyear, V.M. and Ellwood, D.C. Microbios.
    (1973), 8:143.
20. Wood, J.M. Arch. oral Biol. (1969), 14:161.
21. van Houte, J. and Jansen, H.M. Arch. oral Biol. (1968), 13:
    827.
22. da Costa, T. and Gibbons, R.J. Arch. oral Biol. (1968), 13:
    609.
23. Melvaer, K.L., Helgeland, K. and Rolla, G. Arch. oral Biol.
    (1974), 19:589.
24. van Houte, J., Winkler, K.C. and Jansen, H.M. Arch. oral
    Biol. (1969), 14:45.
25. Gibbons, R.J. and Socransky, S.S. Arch. oral Biol. (1962),
    7:73.
26. Stephan, R.M. J. Dent. Res. (1944), 23:257.
27. Loesche, W.J. and Henry, C.A. Arch. oral Biol. (1967), 12:
    189.
28. Kanapka, J.A. and Hamilton, I.R. Arch. Biochem. and Biophys.
    (1971), 146:167.
29. Littleton, N.W., Carter, C.H. and Kelley, R.T. J. Amer. Dent.
    Assoc. (1967), 74:119.

30. Bowen, W.H. and Cornick, D.E.R.   Int. Dent. J. (1970),20:382.
31. Kite, O.W., Shaw, J.H. and Sognnaes, R.F.   J. Nutr. (1950),
     42:89.
32. Stephan, R.M. and Miller, B.F.   J. Dent. Res. (1943), 22:45.
33. Gilmour, M.N. and Poole, A.E.   Caries Res. (1967), 1:247.
34. Geddes, D.   ORCA Abstracts (1973), Zurich.
35. Zita, A., McDonald, R.E. and Andrews, A.L.   J. Dent. Res.
     (1959), 38:860.
36. Kleinberg, I.   J. Dent. Res. (1970), 49:1300.
37. Winter, G.B., Hamilton, M.C. and James, P.M.C.   Arch. Dis.
     Child. (1966) 41:216.
38. Marthaler, T.M. and Froesch, E.R.   Brit. Dent. J. (1967),
     124:597.
39. Stephan, R.M.   J. Dent. Res. (1966), 45:1551.
40. Campbell, R. and Zinner, D.D.   J. Nutr. (1970), 100:11.
41. Green, R. and Harltes, R.   Arch. oral Biol. (1969), 14:235.
42. Bowen, W.H.   Arch. oral Biol. (1974), 19:231.
43. Shaw, J.H. and Griffths, D.   J. Dent. Res. (1960), 39:377.
44. Cornick, D. and Bowen, W.H.   Arch. oral Biol. (1972), 17:1637
45. Muhlemann, H., Regolati, B. and Marthaler, T.M.   Helv. Odont.
     Acta (1970), 14:48.
46. Dallmeier, E., Bestmann, H.J. and Kroncke, A.   Deutsch.
     Zahnaerztl. Z. (1970), 25:887.

10

The Role of Trace Elements in Human Nutrition and Metabolism

R. W. TUMAN and R. J. DOISY

Department of Biochemistry, State University of New York,
Upstate Medical Center, Syracuse, N. Y. 13210

Introduction

The ultimate goal of nutritionists, food chemists, and
food technologists is to answer the question: What is adequate
nutrition?

The answer to this most important question requires knowledge of the nutrients required for good health, the amounts
needed, and food sources which can supply the necessary nutrients.

In the past, efforts to define human requirements have been
preoccupied with discussions of the major essential nutrients,
including: clarification of amino acid, vitamin and macro-
element requirements, recommending a proper balance of carbohydrate, fat and protein, and defining appropritate energy requirements (1). Very little attention has been given to the so-called
trace elements.

Only recently, however, have scientists begun to appreciate
the full extent of the biochemical role of trace elements and
their interactions with human health and nutrition.

At the present time, the 14 trace elements listed in Table 1
have been identified as being essential for either human or
animal nutrition (2). These include iron, iodine, copper, manganese, zinc, cobalt, molybdenum, selenium, chromium, tin, vanadium, fluorine, silicon, and nickel.

It is interesting to note (Table 1) that during the first
100 plus years since iron was found to be essential, only five
additional trace elements were discovered to be required for
good health, including iodine, copper, manganese, zinc, and cobalt.

In contrast with this rather slow early recognition of the
importance of trace elements, during the 20 year period from
1953-1973, a total of eight additional trace elements have been
found to be essential, including molybdenum, selenium, chromium,
tin, vanadium, fluorine, silicon, and nickel. Furthermore, no
less than 5 of these 8, namely, nickel, tin, silicon, fluorine,
and vanadium, have emerged as essential nutrients only in the

156

TABLE 1

DISCOVERY OF ESSENTIAL TRACE ELEMENTS REQUIREMENTS

1. Iron . . . . . 17th Century
2. Iodine . . . . 1850 Chatin, A.
3. Copper . . . . 1928 Hart, E. B., H. Steenbock, J. Waddell, and C. A. Elvehjem
4. Manganese. . . 1931 Kemmerer, A. R. and W. R. Todd
5. Zinc . . . . . 1934 Todd, W. R., C. A. Elvehjem, and E. B. Hart
6. Cobalt . . . . 1935 Underwood, E. J. and J. F. Filmer; Marston, H. R.; Lines, E. W.
7. Molybdenum . . 1953 DeRenzo, E. C., E. Kaleita, P. Heytler, J. J. Oleson, B. L. Hutchings and J. H. Williams; Richert, D. A. and W. W. Westerfeld
8. Selenium . . . 1957 Schwarz, K. and C. M. Foltz
9. Chromium . . . 1959 Schwarz, K. and W. Mertz
10. Tin. . . . . . 1970 Schwarz, K., D. B. Milne, and E. Vinyard
11. Vanadium . . . 1971 Schwarz, K., D. B. Milne; Hopkins, L. L. and H. E. Mohr
12. Fluorine . . . 1972 Schwarz, K. and D. B. Milne
13. Silicon. . . . 1972 Schwarz, K. and D. B. Milne; Carlisle, E. M.
14. Nickel . . . . 1973 Nielsen, F. H.

Adapted from: Schwarz, K., Federation Proceedings, (2).

last 3-4 years. Indicative of the increased recognition trace
elements are receiving in human, as well as animal nutrition,
is the rapidity with which the list of essential trace elements
is growing.

Table 2 describes the periodic distribution of those
elements generally considered to be micro-nutrient elements.
Examination of Table 2 reveals several interesting points: 1)
With the recent addition of vanadium and nickel to the list of
essential trace elements, a continuous set of 8 essential elements is created in the first transition series, from vanadium
(atomic number 23) through zinc (atomic number 30). Furthermore,
when one includes molybdenum (atomic number 42), 9 of the 14
essential trace elements are transition elements. Therefore, the
transition series elements, in general, constitute a region of
the periodic table with special interest and importance (2).

2) With the exception of fluorine (atomic number 9) and
silicon (atomic number 14), all of the essential trace elements
are located above calcium (atomic number 20) and none of the 39
elements beyond iodine (atomic number 53) have ever been shown
to be essential for animals or man (2).

3) More than 20 other trace elements shown in Table 2 are
potentially important and are currently under special consideration with respect to essentiality (2). Progress in discovering
new essential trace elements has relied on improved research
techniques. In this respect, establishing the essentiality of
the newer trace elements (tin, vanadium, fluorine, silicon, and
nickel) has relied on the development and introduction of the
ultra-clean environment and plastic isolator techniques, as
well as the use of pure crystalline amino acids and vitamins in
preparing the diets of laboratory animals.

Recent developments in trace element analysis, particularly
sensitive methods involving atomic absorption spectroscopy and
neutron activation, have further advanced the state of trace
element nutrition. At the present time, the list is composed of
14 essential trace elements, however, the absolute number of
required trace elements is still not known. It is probable that
some or all of the elements listed in Table 2 as potentially
important will be found to participate in vital processes as
still newer experimental techniques are refined and applied.

Several trace elements and their derivatives, for example,
cadmium, mercury, arsenic, and lead have been shown to be toxic.
The detrimental effects of lead and methyl-mercury on the central
nervous system are well known. Beryllium and arsenic are highly
carcinogenic in laboratory animals, and nickel carbonyls and
chromates have been implicated as a cause of lung cancer (3).

However, it is obvious from past results, that toxicity cannot be used as a valid argument against potential essentiality.
Most essential elements become toxic at sufficiently high levels
and the margin between toxic and beneficial doses may be small.
For example, the toxicity of selenium was demonstrated well

Table 2

PERIODIC TABLE

DISTRIBUTION OF TRACE ELEMENTS OF KNOWN AND POTENTIAL
IMPORTANCE FOR HUMAN AND ANIMAL NUTRITION

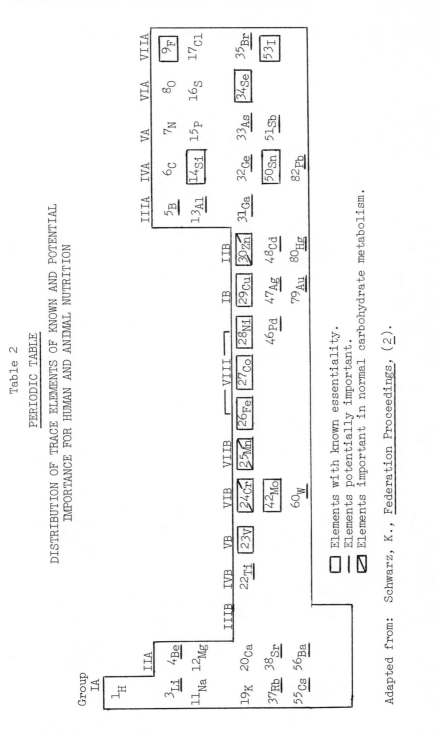

Adapted from: Schwarz, K., *Federation Proceedings*, (2).

before its essentiality, and it is now known that selenium possesses both toxic and beneficial properties, depending on the dose and chemical form (4). A more recent example of this concept is the report by Schwarz (5) of a growth-promoting effect of very low doses of lead in rats maintained in an isolator environment. Thus, it would not be surprising if other trace elements, usually regarded as toxic, will also be found to be beneficial or essential.

The biological properties of the 14 trace elements now recognized to be essential are very diverse (Table 3).

Individual Trace Elements

Iron. It is well recognized that iron is essential as an integral component of hemoglobin and as a component of some flavoproteins and the oxidative respiratory chain. Suboptimal dietary iron intake results in iron-deficiency anemia. The wide-spread incidence of marginal iron deficiencies in segments of the United States' population was recently documented in the Ten-State Nutrition Survey (6). The RDA for iron in the 8th edition of Recommended Dietary Allowances published by the Food and Nutrition Board of the National Research Council has remained at 10 mg/day for adult males and post-menopausal females and 18 mg/day for women of childbearing age (7). This latter amount is difficult to obtain by dietary means since it has been estimated that a balanced, average American diet provides only about 6 mg iron per 1,000 kcal (8). Therefore, women of childbearing age would be required to eat a 3,000 kcal diet to meet the recommendation of 18 mg iron, an undesirable caloric intake for most women. Thus, the major change in the 1974 RDA for iron is a recommendation for supplemental iron intake (30-60 mg) for childbearing women (7). The use of iron enriched foods has been suggested as a means to meet the RDA for iron.

Iodine. The only known function of iodine in human and animal physiology is its essential role in formation of the thyroid hormones, thyroxin, and triiodothyronine. Iodine deficiency results in goiter. The dietary allowance for iodine reported in the latest RDA's has not changed. For the prevention of goiter, an iodine intake of 1 ug/kg body weight is recommended with additional iodine intake recommended for growing children and pregnant women (7). The adequacy of an individual's iodine intake is difficult to assess and intakes vary widely. Thus, it is still suggested that to prevent deficiencies only iodized salt be used.

Zinc. Zinc plays an essential role in a number of important processes including: 1) enzymatic function, 2) protein synthesis and 3) carbohydrate metabolism (9). There are at least 18 known zinc-containing enzymes, including lactate dehydrogenase, carbon-

Table 3

TRACE ELEMENTS WITH BENEFICIAL EFFECTS IN MAN AND ANIMALS

Element [*]	Adult RDA	Biological Function
Iron (Fe)	10-18 mg	integral component of Hb, cytochrome and enzymes.
Iodine (I)	100-150 μg	essential for thyroxine formation and prevention of goiter.
[*]Copper (Cu)	Estimated 80 μg/kg	component of several enzymes, eg. cytochrome oxidase c; role in tissue Fe mobilization and Hb synthesis.
[*]Manganese (Mn)	Estimated 2-3 mg	required by several enzymes, eg. glucokinase, phosphoglucomutase, acetyl CoA synthetase, arginase.
Zinc (Zn)	15 mg	component of several Zn dependent enzymes, eg. lactate dehydrogenase, carbonic anhydrase, peptidases
[*]Cobalt (Co)	3 μg as Vit. B_{12}	integral component of Vit. B_{12} and RBC formation.
[*]Molybdenum (Mo)	Estimated 2 μg/kg	integral component of several en-enzymes, eg. xanthine oxidase, alde-hyde oxidase.
[*]Selenium (Se)	Not es-tablished	integral component of glutathione peroxidase.
Chromium (Cr)	Not es-tablished	integral part of Glucose Tolerance Factor; required for normal insulin response and CHO metabolism.
[*]Tin (Sn)	Not es-tablished	required for optimal growth by rats (1-2 ppm of diet).
[*]Vanadium (V)	Not es-tablished	required for optimal growth by rats and chickens.
[*]Fluorine (F)	Not es-tablished	prevention of dental caries and maintenance of normal skeleton; required for optimal growth by rats.
[*]Silicon (Si)	Not es-tablished	required for optimal growth by rats and chickens; important role in normal bone calcification and struc-tural connective tissue.
[*]Nickel (Ni)	Not es-tablished	required for normal liver function by rats and chickens.

[*]Clinical evidence of deficiency in ADULT man unknown.

ic anhydrase, and several peptidases (10). Zinc deficiency in
animals has resulted in decreased synthesis of both DNA and RNA,
and reduced protein synthesis has been observed in zinc-deficient
rats. The role of zinc in carbohydrate metabolism is still controversial; however, impaired glucose tolerance has been reported
in zinc-deficient rats (11).

More recently, pathological conditions that appear to be a
consequence of inadequate zinc nutriture have been identified in
man. Dietary deficiency of zinc in man is associated with
anorexia, hypogeusia (impaired taste) and hyposmia (impaired
smell), retarded growth, delayed sexual maturation, and impaired
wound healing (12, 13, 14). Zinc deficiency was recently reported in 8 percent of 150 children from middle-income families in
Denver, with another 36 percent of these children probably
marginal in their zinc intake. These deficient children showed
poor growth (below 10th percentile), poor appetite, impaired
taste acuity, and low hair zinc levels. Dietary histories revealed that the diets of these children were low in zinc and all
symptoms improved with zinc supplementation (15). In the Middle
East, zinc deficiency, associated with hypogonadism and dwarfism,
has been demonstrated in man (16). These studies suggest that
marginal zinc deficiency may be more widespread than previously
thought and that dietary intake of zinc in the United States cannot be assumed to be optimal.

It is estimated that a typical American diet supplies between 10 and 15 mg zinc per day to meet an estimated daily
requirement of 10 mg/day (12). Thus, the average daily intake is
only slightly more than the estimated daily requirement, and does
not provide a sufficient safety margin. Therefore, people who
consume foods which are lower than average in available zinc,
such as meat analogs made from vegetable protein, may suffer
from marginal zinc intakes (12). In view of the above, the 1974
RDA's for the first time include a recommendation for zinc, with
15 mg being suggested for adult men and women, and 20 to 25 mg
during pregnancy and lactation (7).

Chromium. Chromium is essential for the maintenance of
normal carbohydrate metabolism in at least three species of
experimental animals. Trivalent chromium is an integral part of
Glucose Tolerance Factor (GTF), and functions as a cofactor for
the peripheral action of insulin. In the rat, the first observed
consequence of mild chromium deficiency is an impairment of
glucose tolerance, caused by a reduced sensitivity of peripheral
tissues to insulin. A more severe degree of chromium deficiency
leads to fasting hyperglycemia, glycosuria, and mild growth
retardation (17, 18).

There is considerable evidence that chromium is also essential for man. Impaired glucose tolerance is the hallmark of
chromium deficiency in man. There has been speculation that
chromium deficiency may contribute to the development of

atherosclerosis (19), and it is of interest that serum cholesterol levels increase with age as tissue chromium levels decrease with age (19). Evidence for the occurrence of chromium deficiency in man and the effect of dietary chromium supplementation will be discussed subsequently in this paper.

Cobalt. Cobalt is essential to man only through its function as an integral part of Vitamin B_{12} and no other functions for cobalt in human nutrition are known. Cobalt deficiency has never been produced in a nonruminant animal and the role of cobalt in human nutrition is only a question of adequate dietary intake of Vitamin B_{12}, rather than of cobalt itself (13). The RDA for Vitamin B_{12} is 3 ug per day (7).

Copper. The nutritional essentiality of copper derives from its role in the structure and function of several cuproenzymes including cytochrome oxidase, ceruloplasmin, amine oxidase and ascorbic acid oxidase. Copper-containing enzymes and copper-containing proteins are required for cellular respiration, normal hemoglobin synthesis, and normal bone formation. The copper-containing protein ceruloplasmin is reported to be intimately involved in tissue iron mobilization (1, 13).

Absolute copper deficiency has never been observed in human adults; however, copper deficiency has been described in patients suffering from general malnutrition and in infants inadvertantly fed formulated diets low in copper (1).

The normal dietary copper intake of between 2-5 mg per day is sufficient to meet the recommended dietary allowance of 2 mg per day. Thus, copper deficiency does not appear to be a problem in this country (20).

Manganese. Manganese functions as a cofactor for several metallo-enzymes including: glucokinase, phosphoglucomutase, acetyl CoA synthetase and arginase. The existence of manganese deficiency has been demonstrated in pigs, poultry, rats, mice, cattle, and sheep; however, evidence of human deficiency has never been obtained. Manganese deficiency was accidentally induced in man through the feeding of a synthetic ration (21). The manifestations of manganese deficiency in animals include growth retardation, reduced fertility, skeletal abnormalities and disorders of the central nervous system (ataxia of the newborn) (1, 13). In addition, manganese plays an important role in normal carbohydrate metabolism, as suggested by the impaired glucose tolerance and hypoplastic pancreatic islet cells observed in manganese deficient guinea pigs (22).

The daily manganese requirements for man are unknown; however, from intake and balance studies, it is estimated that a manganese intake of 2-3 mg/day is adequate for adults (7, 20).

Molybdenum. Molybdenum plays an essential role as an integral component of several enzymes including, xanthine oxidase, aldehyde oxidase and sulfite oxidase. Molybdenum deficiency has been demonstrated in lambs, chicks, and turkey poults using highly purified diets with a low molybdenum content (approximately 20 μg/kg). Feeding this low molybdenum diet resulted in depressed growth (23) and decreased activity of the enzyme xanthine oxidase (24).

Molybdenum deficiency has never been reported in humans. An RDA for molybdenum has not been established; however, balance studies indicate that positive balance in man can be maintained with a molybdenum intake of about 2 μg/kg body weight per day.

Selenium (13, 23). It has recently been demonstrated (29) that selenium is an integral component of the enzyme glutathione peroxidase. Glutathione peroxidase is involved in the reoxidation of reduced glutathione. The enzyme has been isolated from sheep red blood cells; it has a molecular weight of approximately 80,000; and it contains one atom of selenium per protein subunit of approximately 20,000 molecular weight (2).

Selenium deficiency is intimately related to Vitamin E deficiency diseases. For example, the simultaneous deficiency of selenium and Vitamin E causes a variety of pathologies in animals including: fatal exudative diathesis in chicks and turkeys, liver necrosis in the rat and pig, multiple necrotic degeneration of heart, liver, muscle, and kidney in the mouse, and muscular dystrophy in lambs, calves, and chicks (white muscle disease).

Recent studies in chicks have demonstrated that simple selenium deficiency, uncomplicated by inadequate Vitamin E, causes impaired growth, poor feathering, and fibrotic degeneration of the pancreas (25). Selenium deficiency in the rat is manifested by impaired growth, impaired hair coat development, and reproductive failure (26). Furthermore, feeding a selenium-deficient diet containing adequate Vitamin E to subhuman primates results in hepatic necrosis, nephrosis, degenerative changes in cardiac and skeletal muscle, weight loss and death (27).

As stated earlier, selenium possesses both beneficial and toxic properties. Naturally occurring selenium poisoning in animals results in the acute toxicity syndrome, "blind staggers", and the chronic toxicity syndrome of "alkali disease".

In adult man, no evidence of either selenium deficiency or toxicity has been demonstrated, however, selenium deficiency has been reported in children with protein-calorie malnutrition (28). Due to lack of sufficient information, it has not been possible to establish an RDA for selenium in humans.

Tin, Vanadium, Fluorine, Silicon, Nickel

The five trace elements discussed below have recently been found to be essential for laboratory animals (2, 30, 31).

Tin. Tin was recently found to be required for optimal growth in rats. Tin deficiency has been produced in rats by housing in an isolator environment and be feeding highly purified amino acid diets low in tin. Significant growth stimulation was observed when the diets were supplemented with 1-2 mg tin/kg (ppm) of diet (2, 30, 31, 32).

Vanadium. Vanadium is essential in at least two animal species, the chick and the rat. Vanadium deficiency in chickens (diets containing less than 10 µg/kg) results in poor feather growth (33) and retarded bone development (30, 31). In the rat, diets supplying less than 100 ng vanadium/g of diet (100 ppb) showed decreased body growth (34) and recently it was shown that rats respond to 50-100 ng vanadium/g of diet with significant growth stimulation (2).

Fluorine. In addition to the essential role of fluorine, as fluoride, in the prevention of dental caries and in the maintenance of a normal body skeleton (13), recently fluorine has been shown to be essential for optimal growth in the rat. Significant growth effects were produced with 250 µg fluorine/100 g of diet (2.5 ppm) (2).

Silicon. Silicon has been shown to be essential for normal growth in animals. Silicon deficiency in chicks and rats causes depressed growth, and abnormal bone calcification. Silicon also plays an essential role in mucopolysaccharide metabolism and normal connective tissue development. Silicon was recently reported to have a growth-promoting effect in rats (2, 30).

Nickel. Nickel appears to be essential for animals, and pathology consistent with nickel deficiency has been produced in chicks, rats, and swine. Nickel deficiency in these animals causes metabolic abnormalities in the liver, including a decreased oxygen uptake by liver homogenates in the presence of α-glycerophosphate, increased liver lipids, increased phospholipid and cholesterol fraction, and hepatocyte ultrastructural abnormalities (30, 31). Furthermore, in the rat, nickel deficiency resulted in abnormal reproduction as suggested by increased fetal mortality (30).

At the present time, no evidence for human essentiality has been demonstrated for these five newer trace elements. No estimate of man's requirements for these newer essential trace elements can be offered in view of the current insufficient evidence and knowledge of intakes in humans.

Future Considerations

As brought out at a recent symposium (35) little is known about the interactions that occur between essential trace ele-

ments. Knowledge of trace element interactions is of utmost
importance to any valid recommendation of dietary intake. That
is to say, a high dietary intake of a given element may reduce
availability of some other element. Such known relationships as
high calcium intake antagonizing (or reducing) copper availability is but one example of such an interaction. Tungstate is
known to antagonize molybdate, and copper and zinc also interact.
For example, people who are receiving therapeutic doses of zinc
for burns may have an increased copper requirement. Thus, know-
ing the daily intake of any given element is only part of the
problem. The intake of other (interfering) elements and their
balance is of utmost importance. These interrelations are only
beginning to unfold and much more work is needed on this aspect
of trace elements in nutrition.

Role of Chromium in Human and Animal Nutrition

Schwarz and Mertz identified trivalent chromium as an integral component of the biologically active Glucose Tolerance
Factor (GTF) in 1959 (36). Since that time a large body of
convincing experimental evidence has accumulated suggesting that
GTF is required for the maintenance of normal carbohydrate metabolism by both animals and man (18). Chromium nutrition in man
has recently been reviewed by Hambidge (18) and Doisy, et al.
(37) and will not be dealt with in detail in this paper.
The characteristics of GTF as known at this time are
summarized below (17):
GTF is a naturally occurring, dialyzable, heat and acid
stable, organic compound of low molecular weight (400-600 dal-
tons). It can be extracted and concentrated from brewers yeast,
while liver and kidney are also recognized as potentially rich
sources. The precise structure of GTF is not yet known; however,
Mertz (39) recently suggested that the complex contains two
nicotinic acid molecules per chromium atom. Furthermore, glycine,
cysteine, and possibly glutamic acid may be requisite amino acids.
The amino acids may only be required to make the complex water
soluble, and the biological activity may be due to the chromium
and nicotinic acids in a unique coordination complex. Recently,
Mertz has prepared biologically activie synthetic chromium-
nicotinic acid complexes which seem to be similar to, but not
identical with, the naturally occurring GTF complex (39).
GTF contains trivalent chromium as the active metal ion.
The biological effect of chromium "in vitro" and "in vivo", is
solely dependent on the valency state and only trivalent chromium
exhibits biological activity. The biological effects of GTF-
chromium are qualitatively similar, but quantitatively much
greater than simple inorganic chromium complexes. For example,
much smaller quantities of chromium are required "in vivo" to
restore normal glucose tolerance in rats if given in the form of
GTF. Furthermore, the bio-availability of chromium to animals

and man is dependent on the chemical form. Chromium in the
form of GTF, is biologically available and better absorbed than
simple inorganic chromium salts. For example, less than 1 percent of an oral dose of chromium in the form of chromic chloride
is absorbed as compared to 10-25 percent of the chromium in an
oral dose of GTF (38). The chemical form of chromium also de-
termines its distribution in tissues. Only chromium in the form
of GTF is concentrated in the liver and only GTF chromium is
available to the fetus through placental transport.

"In vitro" studies suggest that GTF functions by potentiat-
ing the action of insulin and, as such, it is a required cofactor
for maximal insulin response in all insulin-sensitive tissues
(17). As a result of an uncorrected deficiency of chromium, a
normal insulin response may only be achieved with unphysiologi-
cally high concentrations of insulin.

Evidence for Chromium Deficiency in Man

It is well established that chromium deficiency can be induced (both accidentally and deliverately) in animals by feeding
a diet that is low in available chromium (36, 40, 41, 42).
Evidence has accumulated which suggests that chromium deficiency
also exists in certain segments of the human population. This
evidence is indirect and is based on the following observations:
1) tissue chromium levels decrease with increasing age in the
United States (43, 44); 2) absence of an acute rise of serum
chromium following an insulin or glucose challenge in diabetic
subjects (45), and in pregnant woment with impaired glucose
tolerance (46); 3) diabetes is associated with low chromium
levels in hair (47) and liver (48) compared to nondiabetic controls; 4) insulin-dependent diabetics metabolize chromium in a
manner that is abnormal as compared to non-diabetic subjects
(49) and 5) subjects with impaired glucose tolerance, including
some maturity-onset diabetics (50), middle-aged subjects (51),
children in Jordan suffering with kwashiorkor (52), children in
Turkey suffering from marasmus (53), and some elderly subjects
(37, 49, 54) show improved glucose tolerance after oral chromium
supplementation of the diet. Thus it appears likely that
marginal or overt chromium deficiency occurs in the United States
and elsewhere in the world.

Effects of Chromium and GTF Supplementation of the Diet

The fact that tissue chromium levels decrease with age in
the United States and are exceptionally low in elderly subjects,
is compatible with, but not proof of chromium deficiency. However, these data suggest a role for chromium in explaining the
etiological basis for impaired glucose tolerance which is exhibited by the majority of elderly subjects over 70 years of age.
Hence, a tempting conclusion is that many elderly individuals

have impaired glucose tolerance on the basis of nutritional
chromium deficiency. Therefore, if a deficiency is suspected,
increasing the dietary intake of chromium should relieve the
deficiency and normalize the glucose tolerance. This has been
done with elderly subjects thought to be chromium deficient.

In the original study by Levine, et al. (37, 54), 86 percent
of the elderly population living in the Onondaga County Home
displayed abnormal glucose tolerance tests. Table 4 summarizes
the results obtained when ten elderly subjects, with abnormal
glucose tolerance, were treated with 150 μg daily of supplemental
inorganic chromium for periods up to four months. In addition,
two young subjects originally thought to be normal and one subject with hemochromatosis are included. Shown are the mean two
hour glucose tolerance tests on seven subjects, before and after
dietary chromium supplementation. The criteria used for abnormality in these and subsequent studies are a peak plasma glucose
level above 185 mg/dl and/or a two hour level above 140 mg/dl
(criteria adapted from Conn and Fajans). As shown in Table 4,
the mean plasma glucose levels while on the chromium supplement,
particularly at 60, 90, and 120 minutes, are lowered considerably in all seven subjects compared to the pre-chromium baseline
control tests. In addition, the mean peak plasma glucose level
of the four "responding" elderly subjects as a group was lowered
from 182 to 146 mg/dl and the mean plasma sugar level 2 hours
after a glucose load declined from 156 to 115 mg/dl. Thus,
inorganic chromium supplementation of the diet was effective in
restoring the impaired glucose tolerance to normal in these
seven subjects, and it was concluded that these subjects were,
in fact, chromium deficient. It should be noted that of the ten
elderly subjects treated, only four (40%) responded favorably to
chromium supplementation. However, it should also be pointed
out that there are many etiologies for impaired glucose tolerance,
including infection, emotional stress, etc., and only those
subjects with a pre-existing chromium deficiency would be expected to benefit from chromium supplementation.

On the other hand, a failure to respond to inorganic chromium
does not exclude the possibility of a GTF deficiency. It is possible that the subjects that did not respond to inorganic chromium may have lost the ability to convert inorganic chromium to GTF.
These subjects may have a more favorable response to dietary
supplementation with GTF.

More recently, the effect of dietary GTF supplementation on
abnormal glucose tolerance in elderly subjects was studied (37).
In this case, 45 percent (14/31) of the subjects over the age
of 65 displayed impaired glucose tolerance. Each of twelve
subjects, who volunteered to go on a commercial brewers yeast
extract containing GTF, received a daily supplement (4_xg Yeasta-
min/day) for a period of one to two months. Yeastamin[*] has been

_____
[*]See footnote following Literature Cited.

Table 4

MEAN GLUCOSE TOLERANCE TESTS OF RESPONDERS $\pm$ Cr PLASMA GLUCOSE
CONCENTRATION mg/dl

Elderly Subjects/	Age	Cr	0	30	60	90	120	No. of Tests
GF		−	84	143	149	163	170	2
	79	+	82	138	129	125	106	2
HH		−	67	122	186	197	167	2
	78	+	83	132	139	126	123	2
Ech		−	82	153	180	165	153	2
	88	+	81	136	157	140	131	3
FW		−	98	148	181	152	135	2
	96	+	101	142	152	111	100	3
Young Subjects	Age							
AG		−	90	161	192	151	115	2
	22	+	91	161	126	82	104	3
LS		−	81	146	194	127	120	2
	24	+	81	160	147	132	118	3
Subjects with Hemochromatosis	Age							
		−	111	209	225	166	125	2
	49	+	97	155	170	150	139	2

Supplement: 50 µg of Cr three times daily ($CrCl_3 \cdot 6H_2O$).
*Reprinted by permission of publisher. Doisy, et al., "Effects
and Metabolism of Chromium in Normals, Elderly Subjects, and
Diabetics", In: Trace Substances in Environmental Health-II, D.
D. Hemphill, Ed., University of Missouri, Columbia, pp. 75-82
(37).

shown by Mertz to possess potent GTF activity. It is recognized
that the observed responses may or may not be due to the GTF
content of Yeastamin. That GTF is the active component must
await the availability of pure GTF. The mean effect of supplementation of the diet on glucose tolerance in six "responding"
elderly subjects is shown in Table 5. The subjects display
severely impaired glucose tolerance prior to GTF supplementation,
with a peak plasma glucose level greater than 200 mg/dl and a
two hour glucose value of 178 mg/dl. Following dietary GTF
supplementation, however, six of the elderly subjects show an
improved glucose tolerance to values within normal limits, with
the one and two hour plasma glucose levels being significantly
reduced to 162 and 132 mg/dl respectively.

In addition (Table 5), the serum insulin levels measured
during the tests are decreased while on the supplement, particularly at two hours. Thus, the work load of the pancreas is
decreased and less endogenous insulin, as indicated by lower
serum levels, is needed to maintain normal glucose tolerance
when adequate amounts of GTF are available. This is in agreement
with the role of GTF as a cofactor for normal insulin response.

Furthermore, in addition to the reduction in plasma glucose
and insulin levels, some subjects also respond to GTF supplementation with a significant reduction in fasting serum cholesterol
levels. Cholesterol levels were significantly reduced in these
six subjects from a mean value of 245 to 205 mg/dl, a decrease
of 40 mg/dl. In those subjects with elevated triglyceride levels
there is also a reduction in plasma triglyceride.

Another group of subjects displaying an incidence of impaired glucose tolerance which is clearly greater than that observed
in the general population are the siblings of known diabetics.
The effects of dietary GTF supplementation on the glucose tolerance of a sibling of an insulin-requiring diabetic are described
in Table 6 (37). It is apparent from the two initial screening
GTT's that this subject displays "diabetic-like" glucose tolerance, with elevated plasma glucose levels greater than 200 mg/dl
and serum insulin levels greater than 200 µU/ml, at two time
points during each test. In addition, the subject is hypertriglyceridemic. After approximately eight months of dietary
supplementation with 4-8 grams of Yeastamin/day, glucose tolerance is normalized. In the last test (4/19/74) normal glucose
levels are accompanied by a significant reduction in glucose-
induced plasma insulin levels. Furthermore, plasma triglycerides
have been reduced to within normal limits.

As of this writing, approximately 80 other subjects with
impaired glucose tolerance are on a dietary supplement containing
GTF. Although not all subjects respond with improved glucose
tolerance, the results described here are more or less typical of
the responses obtained in the majority of subjects. One major
difference between subjects is the variation in the length of
time on the supplement before improvement is observed. This is

Table 5

EFFECT OF GTF* SUPPLEMENTATION OF THE DIET ON GLUCOSE TOLERANCE TESTS IN
ELDERLY SUBJECTS WITH IMPAIRED TOLERANCE

Mean Plasma Glucose Levels mg/dl

Time in hours --	0	1	2	Cholesterol mg/dl	Triglyceride mg/dl
Before GTF (11)*	106 ± 4	201 ± 7	178 ± 8	245 ± 9†	121 ± 8
After GTF (9)	99 ± 4	162 ± 11	132 ± 5	205 ± 10	112 ± 12
Significance	NS	0.01	0.001	0.01	NS

Mean Serum Insulin Levels microunits/ml

	0	1	2		
Before GTF	24 ± 6	78 ± 17	118 ± 17		
After GTF	26 ± 12	70 ± 8	83 ± 8		

*Number of tests in parentheses.
 Mean ± SE
†Using paired t test, difference is significant.
Supplement: 4 g of Yeastamin/day.
GTT: 100 g oral load.
Reprinted by permission of publisher: Nutrition Foundation Monograph, Academic Press, NY, (37).

Table 6
EFFECT OF GTF SUPPLEMENT ON GLUCOSE TOLERANCE/SIBLING
OF DIABETIC, AGE 30, MALE

Date	Time	Glucose mg/dl	Insulin μunits/ml	Choles- terol	Triglycer- ides
8/10/73	0'	117	35	194	265
	30'	251	>200		
	60'	267	>200		
	120'	150	95		
	180'	96	27		
8/23/73	0'	108	38	198	256
	15'	176	200		
	30'	220	>200		
	45'	206	183		
	60'	167	163		
	90'	158	138		
	120'	97	39		
GTF 8/24/73					
1/4/74	0'	112	5	150	68
	15'	162	52		
	30'	212	110		
	45'	204	125		
	60'	185	166		
	90'	156	130		
	120'	85	25		
	150'	73	12		
	180'	76	12		
4/19/74	0'	92	10	206	134
	30'	154	57		
	60'	131	52		
	90'	126	44		
	120'	117	35		
	150'	75	22		
	180'	63	10		

Subject gained 8 lbs. between 1/4/74 to 4/19/74.
Supplement: 4 g of Yeastamin per day 8/24/73 - 11/9/73.
             8 g of Yeastamin per day 11/10/73 - 4/19/74.
Reprinted by permission of publisher: Nutrition Foundation Mono-
graph, Academic Press, NY (37).

understandable since the degree of chromium and/or GTF deficiency
might be expected to vary with each subject. For example, the
elderly subjects responded in 1-2 months time, whereas in some
siblings of diabetics 6-8 months are required before normalization occurs.

Thus, evidence is accumulating suggesting that chromium
deficiency does exist in certain segments of our population.
The risk and incidence of chromium deficiency appears to be
greatest in the following population groups: 1) in older age
groups, 2) in children with protein-calorie malnutrition, 3) in
insulin-requiring diabetics, 4) in pregnant women, particularly
multiparae (gestational diabetes), and 5) subjects maintained on
formulated diets for long periods of time may be a high risk for
chromium deficiency. It is proposed that chromium deficiency
may be caused by inadequate dietary intake and/or poor availability of chromium from foodstuffs.

The average American diet supplies only small quantities of
chromium, with intakes in the USA varying from 5 µg/day to over
100 µg/day (1, 18). The average chromium intake for the elderly
subjects (54) was 52 µg daily. The daily urinary loss of
chromium in normal adults ranged from 3-50 µg/day (46, 55) thus,
this is the minimal amount that must be replaced in order to
maintain balance in the adult. As indicated earlier, absorption
of chromium can vary from less than 1 percent to 25 percent of a
given dose, depending on the form in which it is present. Therefore, the dietary intake required to balance the urinary loss
could vary from 50 µg to 500 µg. Diets exceptionally low in
chromium which do not adequately replace losses could lead to
chromium deficiency. The importance of evaluating foodstuffs on
the basis of biologically meaningful chromium rather than total
chromium content was recently discussed (56). Due to inadequate
knowledge of the forms and biological availability of chomium in
foods, an RDA cannot be established. However, it has been
suggested that a daily intake of 10-30 µg of chromium in the
form of GTF would meet our daily requirement (20).

It has also been suggested that inadequate dietary intake
of chromium may occur because of losses of chromium in food refining processes (57, 58). The chromium content of various
wheat and sugar products and the marked loss of chromium that
occurs during the refining of these food staples are described
below.

Whole grain wheat contains 1.75 µg chromium/g Dry Wgt. compared to 0.23 µg/g Dry Wgt. for refined white flour and 0.14 µg/
g Dry Wgt. for white bread. This represents an 87% loss of
chromium in the refinement of whole wheat to white flour and a
92% loss of chromium in going from natural wheat to the consumer
item of white bread. Whole wheat bread retains a little more
of the original chromium, but there is still a greater than 70%
loss of chromium in the refining process.

Similar losses of chromium occur in the refining of sugar.

Refined white table sugars retain very little of the original
chromium contained in the raw sugars. There is a 77-94% loss of
chromium on a dry weight basis in going from unrefined raw sugar
to the resulting consumer item which the American people use
much of (106-120 lbs/person/annum). Raw sugar provides 6-8.8 µg
Cr/100 kcal compared to only 0.5-2.5 µg Cr/100 kcal for refined
sugar. Most of the chromium is removed during the refining
process, i.e., final molasses (47 µg Cr/100 kcal).

Therefore, it is obvious from data of this kind that modern
methods of food processing remove a large percentage of chromium
from two very important food items, wheat and sugar. Thus, diets
high in refined sugar and refined wheat products could contribute
to marginal chromium intakes.

However, chromium is not the only essential trace element
that is significantly decreased during the process of refining
of wheat (59). The losses of six other essential trace elements
that occur during the refining of wheat are described below.
In addition to 76% of the ash content, from 48 to 99% of six
essential trace metals are removed during the milling of wheat
to white flour. The losses in flour include: 76% of the original iron content, 78% of the zinc, 86% of the manganese, 68% of
the copper, 48% of the molybdenum, and 89% of the cobalt. As
with chromium, the highest concentration of these trace elements
is found in the less refined fractions like germ and bran.

Similar losses of essential trace elements occur when other
important food items are divided into their component parts by
either refinement or extraction (58). As a result of partition-
ing rice, significant amounts of five essential trace elements
are lost, including: 75% of the chromium, 46% of the manganese,
75% of the zinc, 27% of the copper, and 38% of the cobalt. In
addition, 83% of the magnesium is removed in the polishing process. In going from corn to corn meal, there is a marked loss
of three essential trace elements including: a 56% loss of
chromium, a 56% loss of manganese, and a 51% loss of zinc. In
addition to the already noted high loss of chromium in refined
sugar, there is a greater than 80% loss of four other essential
trace elements in the production of white table sugar. These
losses include 90% of the manganese, 98% of the zinc, 83% of the
copper, 88% of the cobalt, as well as 98% of the macro-element
magnesium.

From these data, it is apparent that the trace mineral content of many of our major foodstuffs, including refined flour,
cereal products, refined sugar and rice, are markedly reduced
during the refining processes. Increased consumption of highly
refined foods, snack foods, and food analogs could lead to
American diets that may be marginal with respect to adequate
intakes of several trace element essential for good health, and
intentional excessive consumption of these low nutrient foods
might lead to nutritional deficiency diseases through replacement
of conventional food nutrients.

The National Research Council has recently recommended
"enrichment" of foods made from wheat, corn, and rice with ten
vitamins and minerals, including iron, zinc, calcium, and
magnesium.

It can be anticipated that future recommendations may include additional essential trace elements not now included in
this suggested enrichment program. Scientific proof of marginal
or overt deficiency must be obtained before any future additions
would be considered. The evidence for chromium deficiency is
slowly accruing, but further work remains to be done.

Acknowledgement:
    This investigation was supported by part by USPHS Grants
AM 15,100 and RR 229.

Literature Cited

1. WHO Expert Committee on Trace Elements in Human Nutrition,
    (1973), World Health Organization Technical Report Series,
    No. 532, Geneva, 1-65.
2. Schwarz, K., Fed. Proc., (1974), 33 (6), 1748-1757.
3. Maugh, T. H., Science, (1973), 181, 253-4.
4. Allaway, W. H., "Trace Elements in Environmental Health (II)"
    (D. D. Hemphill, ed.) Columbia, Missouri: University of
    Missouri Press, (1969), pp. 181-206.
5. Schwarz, K., "Trace Element Metabolism in Animals - 2",
    University Park Press, Baltimore, (1974), pp. 355-380.
6. Ten-State Nutrition Survey 1968-1970: I. Historical Devel-
    opment, and II. Demographic Data; III. Clinical, Anthropo-
    metry, Dental, IV. Biochemical; V. Dietary and Highlights.
    DHEW Pubs. No. (HMS) 72-8130,-8131,-8132,-8133, and -8134
    (1972).
7. Recommended Dietary Allowances, 1974. Food and Nutriton
    Board, National Academy of Sciences - National Research
    Council, Washington, D.C., 8th edition, Publ. 2216.
8. Mertz, W., Journ. Am. Dietet. Assoc. (1974), 64, 163-167.
9. Halsted, J. A., Smith, J. C., and Irwin, M. I., Jour. of
    Nutr., (1974), 104 (3), 347-378.
10. Parisi, A. F., and Vallee, B. L., Am. J. Clin. Nutr., (1969),
    22, 1222-1239.
11. Quarterman, J., Mills, C. F., and Humphries, W. R., Biochem.
    Biophys. Res. Commun., (1966), 25, 354-358.
12. Sandstead, H. H., Am. J. Clin. Nutr. (1973), 26, 1251.
13. Underwood, E. J., "Trace Elements in Human and Animal Nutri-
    tion", Academic Press, New York, 3rd edition (1971), p. 208.
14. Henkin, R. I., In: "Newer Trace Elements in Nutrition"
    (Mertz, W. and Cornatzer, W. E., ed.) Marcel Dekker, New York,
    (1971), p. 255.
15. Hambidge, K. M., Hambidge, C., Jacobs, M. A., and Baum, J. D.,

Pediat. Res., (1972), 6, 868.

16. Halsted, J. A., Ronaghy, H. A., Abadi, P., Haghshenass, M.,
    Amirhakemi, G. H., Barakat, R. M., and Rheinhold, J. G., Am.
    J. Med. (1972), 53, 277.

17. Mertz, W., Physiol. Rev., (1969), 49, 169-239.

18. Hambidge, K. M., Am. J. Clin. Nutr., (1974), 27, 505-514.

19. Schroeder, H. A., Nason, A. P., and Tipton, I. H., J. Chron.
    Dis., (1970), 23, 123.

20. Mertz, W., Ann. N.Y. Acad. Sci. in Geochemical Environment in
    Relation to Health and Disease, (H. C. Hopps and H. L. Cannon
    Editors), (1971), 199, 191-199.

21. Doisy, E. A., Jr., "Trace Element Metabolism in Animals-2",
    University Park Press, Baltimore, (1974) pp. 668-670.

22. Everson, G. J., and Shrader, R. E., J. Nutr., (1968), 94, 89.

23. Reid, B. L., Kurnick, A. A., Suacha, R. L., and Couch, J. R.,
    Proc. Soc. Exp. Biol., (1956), 93, 245.

24. Higgins, E. S., Richert, D. A., and Westerfeld, W. W., J.
    Nutr., (1956), 59, 539.

25. Thompson, J. M. and Scott, M. L., J. Nutr., (1969), 97, 335.

26. McCoy, K. E. M., and Weswig, P. H., J. Nutr., (1969), 98,
    383.

27. Muth, O. H., Weswig, P. H., Whanger, P. D., and Oldfield, J.
    E., Am. J. Vet. Res., (1971), 32, 1603.

28. Burk, R. F., Jr., Pearson, W. N., Wood, R. P., and Viteri, F.,
    Am. J. Clin. Nutr., (1967), 20, 723.

29. Rotruck, J. T., Pope, A. L., Ganther, H. E., Swanson, A. B.,
    Hafeman, D. G., and Hoekstra, W. G., Science, (1973), 179,
    588.

30. Nielsen, F. H. and Sandstead, H. H., Am. J. Clin. Nutr.,
    (1974), 27, 515-520.

31. Nielsen, F. H., Food Technology, (January, 1974), 38-44.

32. Schwarz, K., Milne, D. B., and Vinyard, E., Biochem. Biophys.
    Res. Commun., (1970), 40, 22.

33. Hopkins, L. L., Jr., and Mohr, H. E., In: "Newer Trace
    Elements in Nutrition", (W. Mertz and W. E. Cornatzer),
    Marcel Dekker, New York, (1971), p. 195.

34. Strasia, C. A., Ph.D. Thesis, Ann Arbor, Michigan, University
    Microfilms, (1971).

35. Hill, C. H., "Interactions of Trace Elements", Symposium:
    Trace Elements and Human Disease, Wayne State University
    School of Medicine, Detroit, Michigan, July 1974, in press.
    Nutrition Foundation Monograph Academic Press, New York, NY.

36. Schwarz, K., and Mertz, W., Arch. Biochem. Biophys., (1959),
    85, 292-295.

37. Doisy, R. J., Streeten, D. H. P., Friberg, J. M., and
    Schneider, A. J., "Chromium Metabolism in Man and Biochemical
    Effects", Symposium: Trace Elements and Hyman Disease, Wayne
    State University School of Medicine, Detroit, Michigan, July
    1974, in press. Nutrition Foundation Monograph, Academic
    Press, New York, NY.

38. Mertz, W. and Roginski, E. E. In: "Newer Trace Elements in Nutrition", (Mertz, W. and Cornatzer, W. E., ed.), Marcel Dekker, New York, (1971), p. 123.
39. Mertz, W., Fed. Proc. (1974), 33 (3), 659 (Abstract).
40. Doisy, R. J., Endocrinology, (1963), 72, 273-278.
41. Schroeder, H. A., Life Sci., (1965), 4, 2057-2062.
42. Davidson, I. W. F., Lang, C. M., and Blackwell, W. L., Diabetes, (1967), 16, 395-401.
43. Schroeder, H. A., Balassa, J. J., and Tipton, I. H., J. Chronic Dis., (1962), 15, 941-964.
44. Hambidge, K. M. and Baum, J. D., Am. J. Clin. Nutr., (1972), 25, 376-379.
45. Glinsmann, W. H., Feldman, F. J., and Mertz, W., Science, (1966), 152, 1243.
46. Hambidge, K. M., In: "Newer Trace Elements in Nutrition", (Mertz, W. and Cornatzer, W. E., editors), Marcel Dekker, New York, (1971), p. 169.
47. Hambidge, K. M. and Rodgerson, D. O., and O'Brien, D., Diabetes, (1968), 17, 517-519.
48. Morgan, J. M., Metabolism, (1972), 21, 313-316.
49. Doisy, R. J., Streeten, D. H. P., Souma, M. L., Kalafer, M. E., Rekant, S. I., and Dalakos, T. G., In: "Newer Trace Elements in Nutrition", (mertz, W. and Cornatzer, W. E., editors), Marcel Dekker, New York, (1971), p. 155.
50. Glinsmann, W. H., and Mertz, W., Metabolism, (1966), 15, 510-520.
51. Hopkins, L. L., Jr., and Price, M. G., In: Western Hemisphere Nutrition Congr., Puerto Rico, (1968), 2, 40-41. (Abstract).
52. Hopkins, L. L., Jr., Ransome-Kuti, O., and Majaj, A. S., Am. J. Clin. Nutr., (1968), 21, 203-211.
53. Gurson, C. T. and Soner, G., Am. J. Clin. Nutr., (1973), 26, 988-991.
54. Levine, R. A., Streeten, D. H. P., and Doisy, R. J., Metabolism, (1968), 17, 114-125.
55. Wolf, W., Greene, F. E., Mitman, F. W., "Determination of Urinary Chromium by Low Temperature Ashing-Flameless Atomic Absorption", (1974), Fed. Proc., 33 (3), 59 (Abstract).
56. Toepfer, W. W., Mertz, W., Roginski, E. E., and Polansky, M. M., Food Chem., (1973), 21, 69.
57. Schroeder, H. A., Am. J. Clin. Nutr., (1968), 21, 230-244.
58. Schroeder, H. A., Am. J. Clin. Nutr., (1971), 24, 562-573.
59. Czerniejewski, C. P., Shank, C. W., Bechtel, W. G., and Bradley, W. B., Cereal Chemistry, (1964), 41, 65-72.

---

*Yeastamin, a brewers yeast extract obtained from A. E. Staley Co., Vico Asmus Division, Chicago, Illinois.

Part B

Carbohydrases (Glycosylases) and Their Roles in Normal and Abnormal Metabolism: Introduction

EDWARD J. HEHRE

Albert Einstein College of Medicine, New York, N.Y. 10461

There is every good reason to examine the physiological effects of food carbohydrates. They form the main dietary component for all segments of the world population and represent about half of our own caloric intake. Furthermore, as a nation, we are considered by some to have a high proportion of overfed and overweight people and, hence, to be inviting too high an incidence of cardiovascular and other diseases. As a physician, I know that a society can moderate the degree of illness resulting from a particular set of causes, provided the causes have been truly defined and a serious effort made to counteract them. Let us by all means learn as much as possible about what the body, through its enzymes, can do with carbohydrates - and what ingested carbohydrates can do for and to the body. These are large and complex questions, however, as the gross effects of food carbohydrates are known to be modulated by the quality and quantity of other dietary components, as well as by age, genetic background, and physical activity of the individual.

A further factor precluding simplistic answers to what the body does with ingested carbohydrates, and how these foods affect the human organism, is the circumstance that man is not a pure biological entity. All of us carry a highly diversified and metabolically active microbial flora on our mucous membranes. Bacteria indigenous to various parts of the alimentary tract form associations as complex as the plant covers on meadows and mountainsides. The combined enzymic equipment of this flora provides for the degradation of a considerably wider range of carbohydrate structures than do the digestive enzymes elaborated by salivary glands, pancreas, and intestinal mucosal cells. The body's utilization of certain unusual food carbohydrates, for example, raises the question of whether bacterial enzymes may play a contributory part by depolymerizing resistant polysaccharides to saccharides which the host enzymes can then deal with. The use of germ-free (gnotobiotic) animals offers an approach to this problem and to learning about the ways in which the microbial flora may contribute to, or detract from, the utilization of carbohydrates for the physiological well being of the host.

Finally, I should like to comment on the term "carbohydrase" used to characterize this session. This term was coined and used long ago for enzymes whose only known activities were to cause the hydrolysis of particular polysaccharides, oligosaccharides, and/or glycosides. Over the past few decades, most of these enzymes have been found to have capacities extending beyond that of hydrolyzing glycosidic linkages. In addition, during this period, a large number of new enzymes have been discovered which act on glycosidic linkages in a way that does not involve water as a reactant. I believe there is increasing evidence that these two until now dissociated groups of so-called Glycoside Hydrolases and Glycosyl Transferases form a great natural class of interrelated Glycosylases [Hehre, E. J., Okada, G., Genghof, D. S., Avan. Chem. Series (1973) 117, 309]. All of their actions are expressions of one of Nature's most versatile biochemical type-reactions: the interchange of a glycosyl group and a proton. It is in this all-inclusive sense of "enzymes of glycosyl mobilization," that the scope of this session may best be construed. At least one speaker, Dr. Segal, will be dealing with enzymes that function in man and higher animals to synthesize or degrade glycogen and maltosaccharides without involving water as a reactant. Most of the papers before us, however, are concerned with enzymes still classed as hydrolases, and whose functioning in mammalian organisms is assumed to be restricted to causing hydrolysis of specific glycosidic linkages. Perhaps this is their complete functional role. But we should not lose sight of the fact that these enzymes have additional catalytic capacities and that, as yet, nothing is known about whether those other capacities have a place in the metabolic scheme.

11

Oligosaccharidases of the Small Intestinal Brush Border

GARY M. GRAY

Division of Gastroenterology, Department of Medicine, Stanford University
School of Medicine, Stanford, Calif. 94305

Carbohydrates represent an important and inexpensive source of calories for man but must be digested to monosaccharides before absorption can occur in the small intestine. Until the last few years, it was commonly believed that all hydrolysis occurred within the intestinal lumen under the influence of secretions from the intestinal wall, the so-called succus entericus. However, the work of Crane and his colleagues (1-3) localizing disaccharidase activities to the brush border membrane of the intestine drew attention to the potential role of the small intestinal cell in carbohydrate digestion.

Table 1 outlines important carbohydrates in the diet of man, the amounts and proportion of each ingested (4), and the site of hydrolysis. Notably only starch and glycogen are partially hydrolyzed within the intestinal lumen. Hydrolysis of the residual oligosaccharide products of starch and of the disaccharides sucrose and lactose occurs under the influence of enzymes integral to the intestinal brush border membrane.

Table 1

DIGESTION OF CARBOHYDRATE

FOOD SOURCE	% OF CHO	LUMINAL HYDROLYSIS	INTESTINAL HYDROLYSIS
STARCH (AMYLOPECTIN AMYLOSE)	60	→MALTOSE, MALTOTRIOSE, α-DEXTRINS	→GLUCOSE
LACTOSE	10	NONE	→GLUCOSE +GALACTOSE
SUCROSE	30	NONE	→GLUCOSE +FRUCTOSE

Intraluminal Digestion of Polysaccharide

Despite the common belief of 15-20 years ago that starches are hydrolyzed completely to glucose, Whelan and his colleagues (5,6) carried out extensive experiments demonstrating that the final products under physiological conditions are the oligosaccharides maltose, maltotriose and the α-limit dextrins

181

containing five to nine glucose molecules and one or more α 1,6 branching links. This presumably reflects a) the poor affinity of α-amylase for α 1,6 branching links and for α 1,4 links adjacent to the 1,6 links (5,6) and b) the preference of the active site of the enzyme for linear oligosaccharides of five or more glucose units by cleavage of the penultimate bond at the reducing end of the molecule (7).

Despite claims that α-amylase secreted from the pancreas may bind to the intestinal surface prior to its action on polysaccharides (8), intestinal fluid contains α-amylase at 10 times the concentration required to explain the in vivo starch hydrolysis in man (9). Hence it appears that digestion of starch and glycogen to oligosaccharides is primarily an intraluminal process.

Oligosaccharidases of the Intestinal Surface

There is only a trace of oligosaccharidase activity in the luminal fluids of the small intestine;   instead, the carbohydrases are concentrated in the brush border surface membrane of the intestine.

Table 2 lists the enzymes from human small intestine that have been identified and characterized. All of these are large glycoproteins. Notably there is only a single β-galactosidase (10) but several α-glucosidases (11,12) in the brush border. There are other carbohydrases within the interior of the intestinal cell that do not appear to have a digestive function and these will not be considered here. All of the α-glucosidases except trehalase are capable of hydrolyzing maltose but it seems preferable to name them according to the substrate for which they are peculiarly specific. The α 1,4 malto-oligosaccharide and α-limit dextrin products of amylase action on starch are hydrolyzed by glucoamylase and the α-dextrinase subunit of sucrase-α-dextrinase respectively. The only intestinal carbohydrase that appears to have little physiological role in digesting carbohydrate in the diet of modern man is trehalase since its appropriate substrate is found only in insects and mushrooms.

At least one of these enzymes, sucrase-α-dextrinase consists of a complex of two proteins, each of which has its own, independently acting enzyme site (12). This particular hybrid enzyme has been cleaved into active, distinct subunits of slightly different molecular size that retain the same biochemical characteristics as found in the native hybrid (12). The α-dextrinase moiety is commonly called "isomaltase" because it is capable of hydrolyzing the 1,6 linkages but the α 1,6 linked disaccharide, isomaltose, is not a saccharide product of amylase action on starch and hence is not a physiological substrate presented to the intestinal surface. The reason for union of sucrase and α-dextrinase moieties to form a hybrid molecule is unknown since these enzymes, whether present in hybrid or monomeric form, hydrolyze the appropriate disaccharide substrate in an identical

TABLE 2

HUMAN BRUSH BORDER OLIGOSACCHARIDASES

Enzyme Type Name	Principal Substrate	% Total Maltase Activity	$\dfrac{Km}{mM}$	Mol. Wt.
β-Galactosidase				
Lactase	Lactose	---	18	280,000
α-Glucosidase				
Glucoamylase	Malto-oligosaccharides ($G_2{}^{\dagger}$ --→ G_9)	25	3.8 --→ 1.1 (G_2) (G_9)	210,000
Sucrase-α-dextrinase*	Sucrose	25	20	280,000
	α-Dextrins	50	4.3 (iso-maltose)	
Trehalase	Trehalose	---	3	---

*Commonly called sucrase-isomaltase although isomaltose is not a physiological substrate in the intestine.

†G indicates glucose and the subscript the number of α 1,4 linked glucose units.

manner. However, experiments using a purified α-limit dextrin as
substrate have not yet been accomplished and it is possible that
the sucrase active site hydrolyzes adjacent α 1,4 linkages while
the α-dextrinase site simultaneously hydrolyzes the α 1,6
branching point of the branched saccharide. Such cooperativity
might greatly facilitate hydrolysis of the oligosaccharide to
free glucose. There is some suggestion that lactase may also
exist as a hybrid with an α-glucosidase (13) and that glucoamylase may be complexed with an oligo 1,6 glucosidase (14) but
sufficiently pure preparations of these enzymes are not yet
available to establish this.

Development of Brush Border Oligosaccharidases

The human intestinal carbohydrases develop at various stages
of uterine life (15) as outlined in Figure 1. The reason for the
differential times for acquisition of these enzymes is unknown.
Small intestinal cells have a remarkably short life span that
appears to be regulated by the rapid maturation and migration of
cells from crypt up along the villus for discharge of senescent
cells from the villus tip.
    The oligosaccharidases, although not present in the immature
cells of the intestinal crypts, are acquired as crypt cells
develop morphologically and migrate onto the villus, as shown
schematically in Figure 2.

Regulation of the Oligosaccharidases

The feeding of sucrose (16), fructose (16) or glucose (17)
produces a doubling in intestinal sucrase activity. Whether
this occurs by virtue of an increase in synthesis of the enzyme
or a decrease in degradation, i.e. stabilization, has not been
clearly defined but it seems likely that feeding of carbohydrates
retards degradation of the enzyme (18,19). Although the synthesis and degradation of other oligosaccharidases have not been
shown to be directly regulated by substrate or products, the monosaccharide products released into the intestinal lumen do compete
for the active hydrolytic site, thereby retarding the rates of
hydrolysis (20).

Role of Surface Oligosaccharidases in Digestion

The final oligosaccharide products from glycogen and starch
digestion and the dietary disaccharides sucrose and lactose are
hydrolyzed very efficiently at the brush border surface of the
intestine so that the released monosaccharides are produced in
great abundance. Hence, neither hydrolysis in the intestinal
luminal contents by α-amylase nor surface hydrolysis by oligosaccharidases integral to the intestine are rate-limiting in the
overall process of hydrolysis and transport in vivo (21,22).

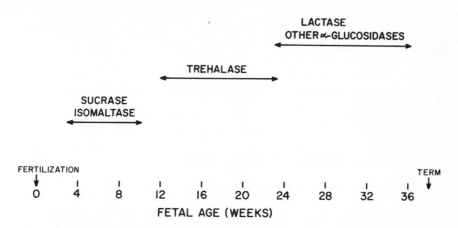

Figure 1. *Development of human brush border oligosaccharidases in the fetus. The lines locate the range of fetal age during which full activity is acquired.*

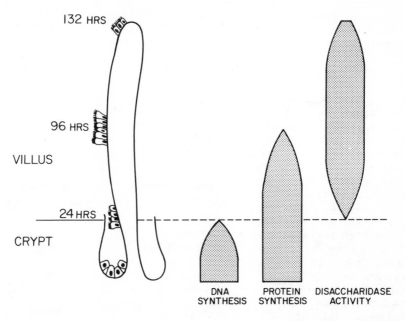

Figure 2. *Functional localization of intestinal cells from the time of their birth at the crypt base until cells migrate up the villus and are shed from the villus tip 132 hours later. Width of shaded vertical bars indicates relative amounts of the particular activity, and vertical position denotes location of the activity in the crypt–villus unit.*

Instead, rate-limiting phenomena appear to be involved princi-
pally in the final transport of the released monosaccharides.
The sole exception to this is the hydrolysis of lactose which is
much slower than hydrolysis of other oligosaccharides, as shown
in Figure 3, so that hydrolysis is even slower than transport of
released monosaccharides (22). Thus normal man is at a relative
disadvantage for the digestion of lactose as compared to other
dietary saccharides, and this appears to become particularly
important when intestinal disease is present.

Deficiency of Intestinal Oligosaccharidase

Since entry into the interior of the intestinal cell is
reserved for monosaccharides, absence or marked reduction of an
oligosaccharidase restricts the offending oligosaccharide to the
intestinal lumen. This can have dire consequences, as outlined
in Figure 4 since the oligosaccharide attracts water by virtue
of its osmotic force. As the saccharide passes down to distal
small intestine and colon, bacteria metabolize it to two and
three carbon fragments that are poorly absorbed in lower bowel.
Hence, the osmotic effect is increased several fold so that ingestion of only 50 grams of a disaccharide may produce diarrhea of
2000-3000 ml of fluid on an osmotic basis alone. Other factors
such as the low pH produced by the metabolized fragments and stimulation of intestinal motion because of distention of the walls
of the hollow gut may also contribute to the diarrhea and may
secondarily produce malabsorption of other nutrients (Figure 4).

Primary Oligosaccharidase Deficiencies

Lactase Deficiency. Lactase is the intestinal saccharidase
that is most commonly deficient, but the enzyme is usually
normally active in children and only becomes reduced in adoles-
cence and adulthood. Interestingly enough, most of the world's
population has adult lactase deficiency (23-36), as shown in
Table 3. Thus, it is com-
monly believed that lac-
tase deficiency is a gen-
etic condition. However,
many of the racial groups
with a high prevalence of
adult lactase deficiency
suffer from poor nutri-
tion and have an appre-
ciable incidence of
small intestinal
disease conditions
which are known to
depress intestinal
lactase out of

Table 3

PREVALENCE OF LACTASE DEFICIENCY

GROUP	% LACTASE DEFICIENT
WHITE	
SCANDINAVIAN	3
NORTH AMERICAN	5-20
BLACK	
AMERICAN	70
AFRICAN	50
OTHER	
CHINESE	80-100
INDIAN	55
FILIPINO	95
ABORIGINE (AUSTRALIAN)	85
ISRAELIS	60

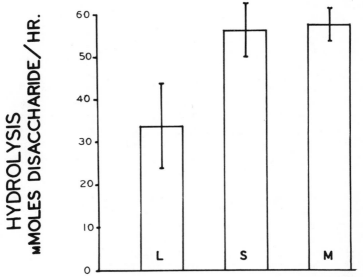

Figure 3. Hydrolysis rates of lactose (L), maltose (M), and sucrose (S) from perfusion of a 30-cm segment of human jejunum in vivo *(22). Brackets indicate ± 2 SE. Lactose is hydrolyzed much more slowly than the other disaccharides (P < 0.01).*

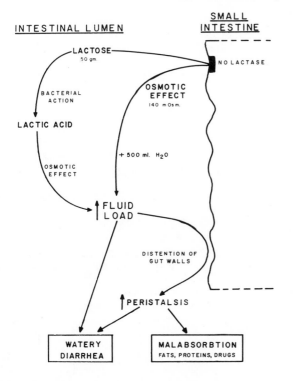

Annual Review of Medicine

Figure 4. Schematic of the effect of disaccharidase deficiency on the fate and action of a dietary disaccharide (see text for elaboration). If intestinal lactase were present in normal concentrations, hydrolysis would occur on the surface of the intestine and the monosaccharide products would be assimilated (41).

proportion to that found for other oligosaccharidases.

Sucrase-α-Dextrinase Deficiency. This hybrid enzyme has
been found to be markedly depressed or absent in about 100 documented cases (37-40). The malady appears to be inherited as an
autosomal recessive. All patients with sucrase deficiency appear
to have markedly depressed levels of α-dextrinase when isomaltose
is used as the substrate, but some dextrinase activity usually
persists. This finding, coupled with the fact that sucrase and
α-dextrinase are distinct proteins (12), suggests that the primary genetic defect constitutes the aleration or absence of the
sucrase subunit with secondary reduction of its α-dextrinase
partner.

Symptoms produced upon ingestion of sucrase are identical
with those discussed above for lactase deficiency. Amylopectin
is usually well tolerated even though appreciable quantities of
α-dextrins are released within the intestine. This may reflect
the relatively large molecular weight of the α-dextrins or the
fact that appropriate bacteria in colon may not be present in
sufficient numbers to metabolize them to small osmotically active
fragments; also, some hydrolysis of these α-dextrins may occur by
action of the residual α-dextrinase subunits or perhaps other
surface α-glucosidases such as glucoamylase.

Treatment of Disaccharidase Deficiencies

Although it appears to be possible to administer enzymes
along with a dietary oligosaccharide to promote digestion, the
expenseusually makes this impractical. By far the simplest form
of therapy is the elimination of the offending carbohydrate since
no single carbohydrate constitutes an obligate source of calories.

References

1. Miller, D. and Crane, R.K. Biochim. Biophys. Acta (1961)
   52:281-293.
2. Eichholz, A. and Crane, R.K. J. Cell Biol. (1965) 26:687-691.
3. Maestracci, D., Schmitz, J., Preiser, H. and Crane, R.K.
   Biochim. Biophys. Acta (1973) 323:113-124.
4. Hollingsworth, D.F. and Greaves, J.P. Am. J. Clin. Nutr.
   (1967)20:65-72.
5. Roberts, P.J.P. and Whelan, W.J. Biochem. J. (1960) 76:
   246-253.
6. Bines, B.J. and Whelan, W.J. Biochem. J. (1960) 76:253-263.
7. Robyt, J.F. and French, D. J. Biol. Chem. (1970) 245:3917-
   3927.
8. Ugolev, A.M. Physiol. Rev. (1965) 45:555-595.
9. Fogel, M.R. and Gray, G.M. J. Appl. Physiol. (1973) 35:
   263-267.

10. Gray, G.M. and Santiago, N.A. J. Clin. Invest. (1969) 48: 716-728.
11. Kelly, J.J. and Alpers, D.H. Biochim. Biophys. Acta (1973) 315:113-120.
12. Conklin, K.A., Yamashiro, K.M. and Gray, G.M. J. Biol. Chem. (1975) in press.
13. Lorenz-Meyer, H., Blum, A.L., Haemmerli, H.P. and Semenza, G. Europ. J. clin. Invest. (1972) 2: 326-331.
14. Eggermont, E. and Hers, H.G. Eur. J. Biochem. (1969) 9:488-496.
15. Dahlqvist, A. and Lindberg, T. Clin. Sci. (1966) 30:517.
16. Rosensweig, N.S. and Herman, R.H. J. Clin. Invest. (1968) 47:2253-2262.
17. Deren, J.J., Broitman, S.A., Zamcheck, N. J. Clin. Invest. (1967) 46:186-195.
18. Das, B.C. and Gray, G.M. Clin. Res. (1970) 18:378.
19. Das, B.C. and Gray, G.M. In preparation.
20. Alpers, D.H. and Cote, M.N. Amer. J. Phys. (1971) 221:865-868.
21. Gray, G.M. and Ingelfinger, F.J. J. Clin. Invest. (1966) 45:388-398.
22. Gray, G.M. and Santiago, N.A. Gastro. (1966) 51-489-498.
23. Bayless, T.M. and Rosensweig, N.S. J. Am. Med. Assoc. (1966) 197:968.
24. Huang, S.-S. and Bayless, T.M. Science (1968) 160:83.
25. Newcomer, A.D. and McGill, D.B. Gastroenterology (1967) 53:881.
26. Littman, A., Cady, A.B., Rhodes, J. Is. J. Med. Sci. (1968) 4:110.
27. Gudmand-Høyer, E., Dahlqvist, A., Jarnum, S. Scand. J. Gastroenterol. (1969) 4:377.
28. Sheehy, T.W. and Anderson, P.R. Lancet (1965) 2:1.
29. Welsh, J.D., Rohrer, V., Knudsen, K.B., Paustian, F.F. Arch. Int. Med. (1967) 120:261.
30. Littman, A., Cady, A.B., Rhodes, J. Is. J. Med. Sci.(1968) 4:110.
31. Cook, G.C., Kajubi, S.K. Lancet (1966) 1:725.
32. Chung, M.H. and McGill, D.B. Gastro. (1968) 54:225.
33. Elliott, R.B., Maxwell, G.M., Vawser, N. Med. J. Aust. (1967) 1:46.
34. Davis, A.E. and Bolin, T. Nature (1967) 216:1244.
35. Desai, H.G., Chitre, A.V., Parekh, D.V., Jeejeebhoy, K.N. Gastro. (1967) 53:375.
36. Gilat, T., Kuhn, R., Gelman, E. and Mizrahy, O. Dig. Dis. (1970) 15:895-904.
37. Burgess, E.A., Levin, B., Mahalanabis, D., Tonge, R.E. Arch. Dis. Childhood (1964) 39:431.
38. Prader, A. and Auricchio, S. Ann. Rev. Med. (1965) 16:345.
39. Sonntag, W.M. et al. Gastro. (1964) 47:18.

40. Auricchio, S. et al. J. Pediat. (1965) 66:555.
41. Gray, G.M. Annual Review Medicine (1971) 22:391-404.

*Research supported by USPHS Grant AM 11270 and Research Career
Development Award AM 47443 from the National Institutes of
Health.

12

Lactose Intolerance and Lactose Hydrolyzed Milk

DAVID M. PAIGE, THEODORE M. BAYLESS, SHI-SHUNG HUANG,
and RICHARD WEXLER

Johns Hopkins Medical Institutions, 615 North Wolfe St., Baltimore, Md. 21205

Prevalence

Low levels of intestinal lactase activity have
been found in many otherwise healthy adults and children in populations of American Negroes (1-5), Asians
(6-10), Bantu tribes (11-12), South American Indians
(13-14), Thais (15-17), and other population groups
(18-20). Current evidence would indicate these low
levels to be the norm for most populations of the world
with notable exceptions being Scandinavians and those
of northern European extraction.

Approximately 70% of the world's adult population
is lactose intolerant (21). It appears that those who
have genetically acquired low lactase levels as adults
are able to drink milk as infants; but gradually become increasingly lactose-intolerant after infancy. The
onset of acquired lactose intolerance depends on the
population studied. In developing countries, as our
data from Peru indicates, 50% of the population is intolerant by 3 years of age (13). In a more technologi-
cally developed country such as the United States, 40%
of the black population is lactose intolerant by the
end of the first decade (Figure I). The difference
between the accelerated loss of enzyme activity in
children in developing areas, contrasted with the slower
decline in blacks in this country, may reflect a relatively better nutritional state influencing and retarding the genetic expression of this event.

Normally, ingested lactose is hydrolyzed by the
enzyme lactase found within the brush border of micro-
villous area of the jejunal mucosa, splitting the lactose into glucose and galactose, which are then absorbed. If enzyme activity is low, the ingested
lactose is not hydrolyzed. Fluid then enters the intestinal lumen to dilute this hypertonic load, causing

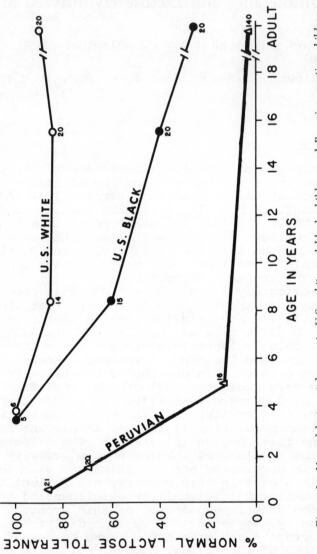
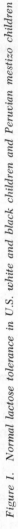

Figure 1. Normal lactose tolerance in U.S. white and black children and Peruvian mestizo children

abdominal distention, cramps and increased peristalsis. In addition, the unabsorbed lactose is fermented to lactic acid which serves as a cathartic. Carbon dioxide and hydrogen is also produced by this fermentation and contributes to the frothy diarrhea.

Milk Drinking

There are variations in how much lactose will cause symptoms in persons with low lactase levels. Some note symptoms of intolerance after one glass of milk, while others are not troubled unless they drink three or four glasses at one time. It should be stressed that not everyone who has low lactase levels and develops symptoms after a lactose tolerance test load (50 g/m^2) will be aware of symptoms after drinking one 8 ounce glass of milk (12 g of lactose).

Data recently reported by Mitchell, Bayless, Paige et al (22), however, indicates that over half of 13 teenagers experiencing a flat tolerance curve and symptoms with a test dose of 50g of lactose will also experience symptoms with 12g of lactose as well as the consumption of 8 ounces of milk (Figure II).

A low level of milk consumption is often implicated as the cause of low lactase levels. Yet, milk drinking does not seem to affect lactase levels. Although some deficient individuals can gradually increase their milk intake, prolonged lactose or milk feeding will not increase lactase activity. Keusch and his workers fed Thai adults lactose for 14 weeks and were unable to effect any change in the levels of intestinal lactase or the individual's lactose tolerance. In another attempt to alter lactase activity, Rosensweig and Herman (23) were unable to bring about any changes after 14 days. Cuatrecasas attempted to alter low lactose levels by lactose feedings for 45 days and was unsuccesful. Newcomer and McGill (24) were unable to alter lactase levels in two subjects after lactose loading for ten days. Gilat et al were unable to induce lactase activity in ten lactose deficient adult Israelis after giving them more than 1 liter of milk per day for 6-14 months (25).

On the other hand, prolonged abstinence from lactose in those individuals destined to have high lactase levels does not appear to inhibit lactase activity. Nine white children with galactosemia, 7 to 17 years, had normal lactose tolerance tests, despite their avoidance of all lactose-containing foods since early infancy (26). In adults, complete lactose deprivation for 42 days was not associated with a significant change

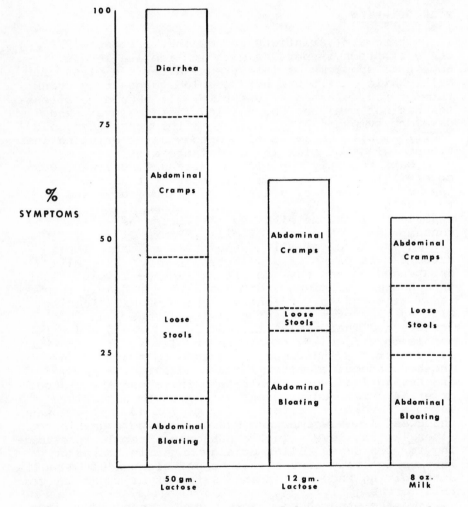

Figure II. Symptoms in lactose-intolerant blacks with the consumption of 50 g and 12 g of lactose as well as 8 ounces of milk (N = 13)

in lactase activity or in lactose tolerance (27).

 As there is a gradient of symptoms with lactose ingestion, the fact that some individuals are intolerant of a lactose load equivalent to 3-4 glasses of milk does not necessarily mean he will experience symptoms with smaller quantities of milk. There is evidence that even though intolerant subjects may not manifest symptoms with this smaller quantity of lactose, it is still not being digested. Individuals experiencing incomplete lactose digestion may, therefore, continue consuming milk despite the fact that they are not realizing its full nutritional value. Milk taken without a meal seems to cause more symptoms than if taken with food. The food may possibly dilute the milk; or it may delay gastric emptying, and permit only small amounts of lactose to enter the small intestine enzyme system at any one time.

Absorption

 We have reported (28) that there appears to be little difference in the ability to physiologically digest a lactose load when smaller amounts are ingested (29). Our data suggests that in lactose intolerant children irrespective of the lactose load; whether it is the test dose of 2 g/kg or the commonly consumed amount of approximately 0.5 g or the intermediate level of 1.0 g/kg of body weight, there is an inadequate blood glucose rise in the lactose intolerant subjects. In the lactose tolerant control, the blood sugar rise is normal and exceeds 26 mg% over the fasting glucose level with all three doses. In addition, all 8 subjects had symptoms with 2.0 g/kg of lactose. When 1.0 and 0.5 g/kg of lactose were given, 5 of the 8 subjects were symptomatic (Figure III).

 Beyond the inadequate rise in glucose, other nutrients appear to be less than adequately absorbed when the results of our short term balance studies of 4 lactose intolerant and 2 lactose tolerant Peruvian children are analyzed (30-31). On a diet of casein, cottonseed oil, and carbohydrate as sucrose or lactose, there is increased loss of water, nitrogen, potassium and sodium in the stool when the lactose intolerant subjects are switched from a nine day period on sucrose to a nine day period on lactose. These values return to control levels when the sucrose replaces lactose in the diet (Figure IV).

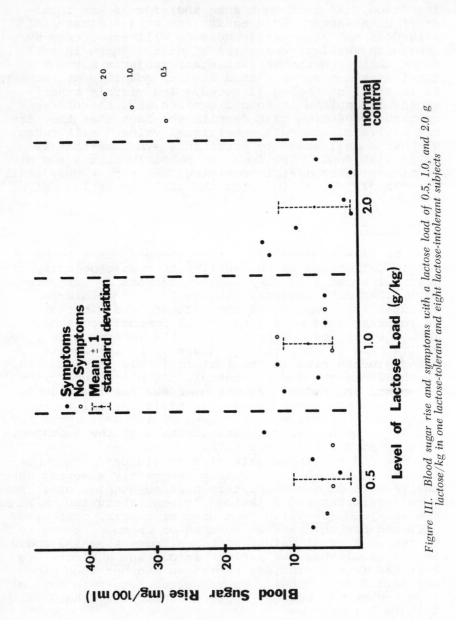

Figure III. Blood sugar rise and symptoms with a lactose load of 0.5, 1.0, and 2.0 g lactose/kg in one lactose-tolerant and eight lactose-intolerant subjects

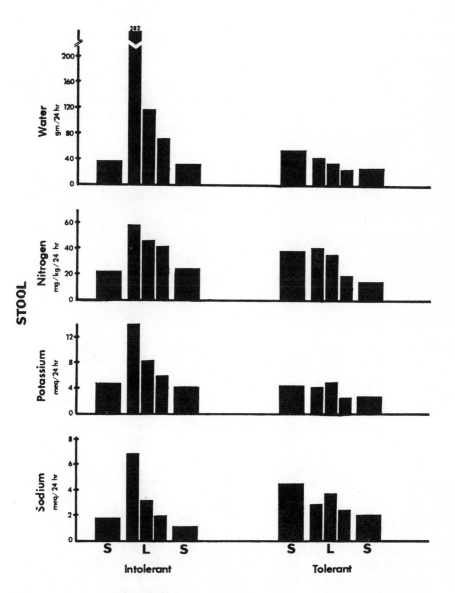

Figure IV.   Stool water, nitrogen, potassium, and sodium of lactose-intolerant and lactose-tolerant children consuming sucrose (S) or lactose (L)

Lactose Intolerance and Milk Rejection

What then is the effect of these physiological differences on the pattern of milk consumption in lactose intolerant groups? Does lactose tolerance play any role in determining milk drinking habits? The data indicates that milk rejection by black elementary school children in an organized school feeding program is significantly higher than in similarly matched white children (5). Overall, the frequency of failure to consume moderate amounts of milk in blacks is 20% as compared to 10% in whites. More important, however, a significant association exists in the black children between nonmilk drinking and lactose intolerance. Seventy-seven percent of this group had an abnormal lactose tolerance test with 85% of these children exhibiting symptoms with the test. (Table I)

Indeed, when one plots the level of milk rejection in black and white children and adults against the level of lactose intolerance in these same groups, a close relationship is noted; milk rejection in both black and white children and adults parallels the prevalence of lactose intolerance in the population studied (32) (Figure V).

This data would suggest that solutions be sought for this situation inasmuch as milk is an important food with a potential for providing nutrients and other much needed protein to disadvantaged populations, domestically and internationally. It is, therefore, important to have lactose intolerant individuals both consume milk without symptoms and utilize its nutrients without interference and loss. While it is apparent that lactose intolerant populations are heterogeneous with respect to their milk drinking habits, with many experiencing little or no symptoms with the consumption of commonly consumed amounts of milk, it is doubtful that all nutrients contained therein are being satisfactorily utilized. Obvious controversy exists as to the precise inferences to be drawn from the experimental data on the clinical consequences of lactose intolerance, yet many agree that viable options should be considered for approaching this prevalent condition.

Suggestions have centered on continued milk consumption despite the presence of known intolerance. Human experimental data has failed, however, to demonstrate induction of lactose activity through continued milk consumption in lactose intolerant individuals. Others have considered the combination of milk and other liquids, such as orange juice, to lower the lactose content to more acceptable levels. Recently, emphasis has

Table I.   Lactose Tolerance Test Results in White and Black Milk Drinking and Non-milk Drinking School Children

| | N | Lactose Tolerance Test ($50g/m^2$) | |
		Abnormal Blood Sugar Rise	Symptoms
White Milk Drinkers	15	20% (3)	(0)
White Non Milk Drinkers	12	17% (2)	(3)
Black Milk Drinkers	14	35.7% (5)	(7)
Black Non Milk Drinkers	17	76.5% (13)	(12)

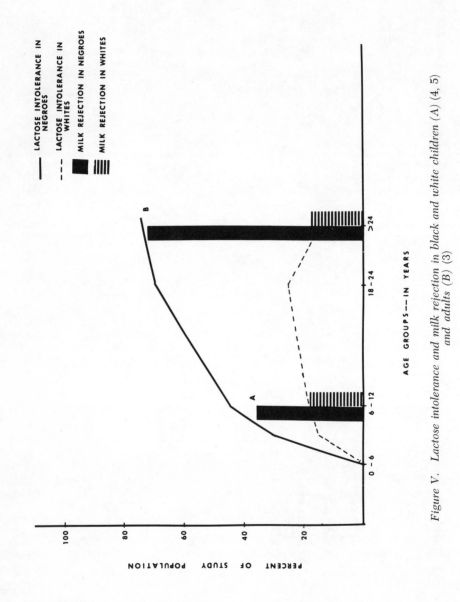

Figure V. Lactose intolerance and milk rejection in black and white children (A) (4, 5) and adults (B) (3)

been given to the prehydrolysis of lactose into its absorbable monosaccharides prior to general distribution.

Lactose Hydrolyzed Milk

A comparison of carbohydrate absorption in lactose tolerant and intolerant adolescents who consumed untreated whole milk and lactose hydrolyzed milk was undertaken by our group (34). The population studied consisted of 32 Baltimore City adolescent volunteers ranging in age from 13-19 years with a mean age of 15.5 years. They were equally divided by sex with all of the subjects being black. The youngsters were drawn from the lower socio-economic census tracts within the city with over 80% coming from the lowest decile census tract. All subjects had a lactose tolerance test performed to categorize their ability to handle a lactose load. They were given 50 g of lactose per meter square of body surface after an overnight fast.

Twenty-two of the 32 subjects (69%) evidenced a flat lactose tolerance curve with a mean peak blood sugar rise in this group of 9.3 mg% and were considered lactose intolerant. The 10 lactose tolerant subjects (31%) had a mean peak blood sugar rise of 36.5 mg%. Twenty of the 22 lactose intolerant subjects experienced symptoms along with the test; 3 of the tolerant subjects experienced symptoms with the lactose load.

Lactose Tolerance Test Results
(N = 32)

	%	Mean Peak Blood Sugar Rise (Mg/100ml)	Standard Deviation
Lactose Intolerant (N=22)	69	9.3	7.2
Lactose Tolerant (N=10)	31	36.5	7.4

After the initial lactose tolerance test, the study population, using a double blind design, was given on alternate days; 8 ounces of untreated whole milk containing approximately 12 g of lactose, 8 ounces of 50% hydrolyzed whole milk containing 6 g of lactose, and 8 ounces of 90% lactose hydrolyzed whole milk containing approximately 1.2 g of lactose.

The test milk was prepared and provided by the
U. S. Department of Agriculture, Dairy Products Laboratory pilot plant in Washington, D.C. Fresh mixed raw
whole milk was treated with the fixed enzyme lactase
isolated from the yeast saccharomyces lactis to hydrolyze up to 90% of the lactose in milk into glucose and
galactose.

The mean maximum blood sugar rise in the 22 lactose intolerant subjects drinking 8 ounces of untreated
whole milk was 4.4 mg%; with 50% hydrolyzed milk, 8.8
mg%; and with 90% lactose hydrolyzed milk, 14.5 mg%.
In the 10 lactose tolerant subjects, the mean peak
blood sugar rise was not appreciably different whether
they consumed untreated whole milk or lactose hydrolyzed milk.

Blood Sugar Rise With Test Milk

	Untreated	50%	90%
Lactose Intolerant (N=22)	4.4	8.8	14.5
Lactose Tolerant (N=10)	12.2	13.3	13.7

The difference between the blood sugar rise in the
lactose intolerant and tolerant subjects with the consumption of 8 ounces of untreated whole milk is significant at the .01 level. No significant differences
are noted when the tolerant youngsters consumed lactose
hydrolyzed milk.

Significant intragroup differences are observed
between the peak blood sugar rise after the consumption
of 8 ounces of the test milks. In the intolerant group
the difference between untreated and 90% hydrolyzed
milk is significant at the .001 level; and between 50%
and 90% hydrolyzed milk at the .02 level. No statistically significant differences are noted between 50%
hydrolyzed and untreated whole milk. In the lactose
tolerant teenagers, no significant intragroup differences are noted irrespective of the test milk studied.

Intra-Group Significance

	Untreated/90%	90%/50%	50%/Untreated
Lactose Intolerant	.001	.02	N.S.
Lactose Tolerant	N.S.	N.S.	N.S.

Due to the presence of glucose and galactose with the hydrolysis of lactose, alteration in the taste of milk were considered important. Eighty-eight percent of the 32 subjects considered the untreated whole milk to be "just like or similar to milk". Twelve percent reported that the untreated milk was "sweeter than milk".

The 50% hydrolyzed milk was described by 81% of the respondents to be "just like or similar to milk". Nineteen percent indicated that it was "sweeter than milk".

The 90% lactose hydrolyzed milk was reported as "sweeter than milk" by the majority of the subjects, 56%. The rest of the subjects described the milk as being "just like other milk".

Taste Response
(N = 32)

	Sweeter Than Milk %	Just Like Milk/Other %
U.W.M. (32)	12	88
50% (27)	19	81
90% (32)	56	44

Facial expressions chosen by the subjects to reflect their opinion of the various test milks paralleled and reinforced the verbal assessment of the test milk.

Discussion

It appears that low lactase activity is the more common situation in populations around the world. Data further suggests that the absence of symptoms with the consumption of 8 ounces of milk does not assure the pre-sence of sufficient lactase activity to hydrolyze lac-tose. Indeed, adolescents with lactose intolerance consuming 8 ounces of untreated whole milk containing 12 g of lactose have a significantly lower peak blood sugar rise than similar youngsters with normal lactose absorption. The differences in carbohydrate absorption are eliminated when lactose malabsorbers are given milk in which 90% of the lactose has been converted by hy-drolysis to glucose and galactose. A more modest im-provement in absorption is noted with hydrolysis of 50% of the lactose in milk. Youths with normal lactose absorption have a comparably high peak blood sugar rise irrespective of the lactose content of the milk.

The decreased blood sugar rise observed occurred even in subjects who did not complain of symptoms with the milk. Diarrhea could not be considered a factor in the significantly lower blood sugar rises inasmuch as none of the adolescents in this study experienced this symptom. The intolerant subjects studied do not, therefore, utilize a significant portion of the carbo-hydrate and caloric content of a glass of whole milk, irrespective of the presence or absence of symptoms. Furthermore, it appears that an appropriate level of lactose hydrolysis should approach 90% inasmuch as sig-nificant differences in blood sugar rise are noted between 50 and 90% hydrolysis.

The prehydrolysis of lactose did result in a re-ported increase in sweetness of the 90% hydrolyzed milk, but did not seem to interfere with the acceptance of the product in this study. The results suggest that 90% lactose hydrolyzed milk should be more broadly evaluated as a more appropriate milk for major popula-tion groups with low lactase levels. The provision of lactose hydrolyzed milk, may provide a more ra-tional answer to providing much needed nutrients to many intolerant groups both domestically and inter-nationally in need of nutritional reinforcement.

Supported in part by grants MC-R-240278-01-0 from the Maternal and Child Health Services and HD-07179-01 from the National Institute of Health.

Literature Cited

1. Bayless, T.M. and Rosensweig, N.S., Journal of the American Medical Association, (1966), 197, 968-972.
2. Paige, D.M., Bayless, T.M. and Graham, G.G., American Journal of Clinical Nutrition, (1973), 26, 238-240.
3. Cuatrecasas, P., Lockwood, D.H. and Caldwell, J.R., Lancet, (1965), 1, 14-18.
4. Huang, S.S. and Bayless, T.M., New England Journal of Medicine, (1967), 276, 1283-1287.
5. Paige, D.M., Bayless, T.M., Ferry, G.D. and Graham, G.G., Johns Hopkins Medical Journal, (1971), 129(3), 163-169.
6. Huang, S.S. and Bayless, T.M., Science, (1968), 160, 83-84.
7. Chung, M.H. and McGill, D.B., Gastroenterology, (1968), 54, 225-226.
8. Bolin, T.D., David A.E., Seah, C.H., et al, Gastroenterology, (1970), 59, 76-84.
9. Bolin, T.D., Crane, G.G. and Davis, A.E., Australian Annals of Medicine, (1968), 17, 300-306.
10. Davis, A.E. and Bolin, T.D., Nature, (1967), 216, 1244-1245.
11. Cook, G.C. and Kajubi, S.K., Lancet, (1966), 1, 725-729.
12. Jersky, K. and Kinsley, R.H., South African Medical Journal, (1967), 41, 1194-1196.
13. Paige, D.M., Leonardo, E., Cordano, A., Nakashima, J., Adrianzen, B. and Graham, G.G., American Journal of Clinical Nutrition, (1972), 25, 297-301.
14. Alzate, H., Gonzales, H. and Guzman, J., American Journal of Clinical Nutrition, (1969), 22, 122-123.
15. Keusch, G.T., Troncale, F.J. and Miller, L.G., Pediatrics, (1969), 43, 540-545.
16. Keusch, G.T., Troncale, F.J., Thavaramara, G., et al., American Journal of Clinical Nutrition, (1969) 22, 638-641.
17. Flatz, G., Saengudom, C. and Sanguanbhokai, T., Nature, (1969), 221, 758-759.
18. Paige, D.M., Bayless, T.M. and Graham, G.G., American Journal of Public Health, (1972), 62(11), 1486-1488.
19. Gudmand-Hoyer, E. and Jarnum, S., Acta Medica Scandia, (1969), 186, 235-237.
20. Gilat, T., Kuhn, R., Gelman, E., et al., American Journal of Digestive Diseases, (1970), 15, 895-904.
21. Bayless, T.M., Paige, D.M. and Ferry, G.D., Gastroenterology, (1971), 60, 605-608.

22. Mitchell, K.J., Bayless, T.M., Paige, D.M., Goodgame, R.W., Huang, S.S., "Intolerance of 8 Ounces of Milk in Healthy Teenagers", Pediatrics, (1974), In Press.
23. Rosensweig, N.S. and Herman, R.H., The Journal of Clinical Investigation, (1968), 47, 2253-2262.
24. Newcomer, A.D. and McGill, D.B., Gastroenterology, (1967), 53, 881-889.
25. Lancet, (1969), 1, 613, "Off Milk", Editorial.
26. Kogut, M.S., Donnell, G.N. and Shaw, K.N.F., Journal of Pediatrics, (1967), 71, 75-81.
27. Knudsen, K.B., Welsh, J.D., Kronenberg, R.S., et al., American Journal of Digestive Diseases, (1968), 13, 593-597.
28. Leichter, J., American Journal of Clinical Nutrition, (1973), 26, 393-396.
29. Paige, D.M., Leonardo, E., Nakashima, J., Adrianzen T., B., and Graham, G.G., American Journal of Clinical Nutrition, (1972), 25, 467-469.
30. Paige, D.M. and Graham, G.G., Pediatric Research, (1972), 6, 329.
31. Graham, G.G., Paige, D.M., Symposia of Swedish Nutrition Foundation XI, (1972), 45-51.
32. Paige, D.M., Graham, G.G., American Journal of School Health, (1974), 44(1).
33. Paige, D.M., Bayless, T.M., Huang, S.S. and Wexler, R., "Lactose Hydrolyzed Milk", American Journal of Clinical Nutrition, (1974), In Press.

Oligosaccharides of Food Legumes: Alpha-Galactosidase Activity and the Flatus Problem

JOSEPH J. RACKIS

Northern Regional Research Laboratory, U.S. Department of Agriculture, Peoria, Ill. 61604

The raffinose family of oligosaccharides--including stachyose and verbascose--occurs in seeds of food legumes at levels that cause flatulence in man and animals. These carbohydrates escape digestion because there is no α-galactosidase activity in mammalian intestinal mucosa and because they are not absorbed into the blood. Consequently, bacteria in the lower intestinal tract metabolize them to form large amounts of carbon dioxide and hydrogen and to lower the pH. The amount and pattern of expelled gases reflect differences in type, location, and abundance of intestinal microorganisms possessing α-galactosidase activity in a favorable nutrient environment.

Water and aqueous alcohol extraction, as well as enzymatic hydrolysis, can be used to process food legumes into products having low flatus activity. According to in vitro and in vivo studies, antibiotics and naturally occurring substances can inhibit bacterial activity in the intestinal tract; however, it is unlikely such additives would be approved for human consumption. Breeding soybeans low in oligosaccharide content holds little promise.

Food legumes, which include oilseeds, peas, and beans, provide important sources of protein and calories. While population is expanding worldwide, and is expected to double in the next 30 years, more and more reliance is being placed on the direct consumption of these sources of protein. The Protein Advisory Group of the United Nations (1) recommends urgent research attention to eight species of food legumes. A challenging scientific problem, flatulence, is one of the priorities in this research and will become important as food legumes are consumed in ever increasing quantities.

There are many causes for the formation in the alimentary canal of gas (2, 3) which may lead to nausea, cramps, diarrhea, abdominable rumbling, and social discomfort with ejection of excessive rectal gas. Here, I shall restrict my discussion of flatulence associated with the consumption of foods to those containing the oligosaccharides--raffinose, stachyose, and verbascose. These oligosaccharides are related by having one or more α-D-galactopyranosyl groups in their structure. Figure 1 illustrates their structural interrelationships, where the α-galactose units are bound to the glucose moiety of sucrose. α-Galactosyl groups are also found in nature joined to other sugars and nonsugars (4), but whether these constituents cause flatulence is unknown.

Oligosaccharides in Food Legumes

The content of the raffinose family of oligosaccharides in various types of food legumes is given in Table I. Soybeans contain the highest levels of raffinose and stachyose, whereas other legumes have the highest levels of verbascose. Dehulled, defatted soybean meal contains 15-18% polysaccharide and 13% oligosaccharide (Table II). There is no starch in mature soybeans, whereas in other food legumes, starch is the predominant carbohydrate. The oligosaccharide content reported by Kawamura (5) represents average values for six U.S. and three Japanese soybean varieties. Oligosaccharide content of varieties and strains of soybeans was determined by Hymowitz et al. (6) in establishing whether these carbohydrates could be eliminated genetically (Table III). Since there is a high degree of stability in the oligosaccharide content of soybeans, elimination of flatulence by breeding holds little promise unless new soybean strains are discovered which contain little or no oligosaccharides.

Oligosaccharides: Metabolism in the Intestinal Mucosa

Gitzelmann and Auricchio (7) found no α-galactosidase (EC 3.2.1.22, α-D-galactoside galactohydrolase) activity in human intestinal mucosa. They demonstrated that a normal child and a galactosemic child were unable to digest raffinose and stachyose since there was no absorption of galactose in the blood. Only trace amounts of raffinose and stachyose were excreted into the urine of the two children. Ruttloff et al. (8) also found no enzymatic hydrolysis of raffinose in the intestinal mucosa of rats, pigs, and humans. Other studies on the absorption and degradation of oligosaccharides containing α-galactosyl groups show that less than 1% of the administered dose was able to pass through the intestinal wall of man and animals (9, 10) (Figure 2). In the absence of α-galactosidase activity in the mucosa, these oligosaccharides remain intact and enter the lower intestine where they can be metabolized by existing microflora.

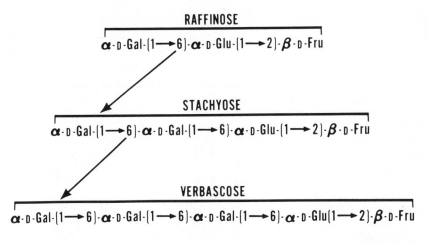

Biochimica et Biophysica Acta

Figure 1.   Structural relationships between the raffinose family of oligosaccharides

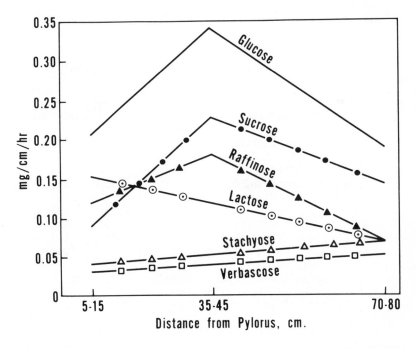

Ernaehrungsforschung

*Figure 2.   Absorption rates of sugars and oligosaccharides in the small intestine
of the rat (10)*

Table I. Oligosaccharides in Leguminous Seeds

Legume	Raffinose a	Raffinose b	Stachyose a	Stachyose b	Verbascose a	Verbascose b
Beans, black mung, dry	0.5	---	1.8	---	3.7	---
Beans, green mung, dry	0.8	---	2.5	---	3.8	---
Chick peas	1.0	1.1	2.5	2.5	4.2	---
Cow peas	0.4	0.4	2.0	4.8	3.1	0.5
Field beans	0.5	0.2	2.1	1.2	3.6	4.0
Horse gram	0.7	---	2.0	---	3.1	---
Lentils	0.6	0.9	2.2	2.7	3.0	1.4
Lima beans, canned	---	---	0.2	---	---	---
Peas, green, dry	---	0.6	---	1.9	---	2.2
Peas, yellow, dry	---	0.3	---	1.7	---	2.2
Pigeon peas	1.1	---	2.7	---	4.1	---
Soybeans, dry	1.9	0.8	5.2	5.4	---	---

[a] Hardinge et al. (30), % of edible portion.

[b] Cristofaro (17), % of dry matter.

Table II. Carbohydrate Constituents of Dehulled, Defatted Soybean Meal

Constituent	% of Meal
Polysaccharide content, total[a]	15-18
Acidic polysaccharides	8-10
Arabinogalactan	5
Cellulosic material	1-2
Oligosaccharide content, total[b]	13.3
Sucrose	6.6
Stachyose	5.3
Raffinose	1.4
Verbascose	Trace

[a] Aspinall et al. (31).

[b] Kawamura (5).

Table III. Strain, Maturity Groups, and Average Weight of
Total Sugar, Sucrose, Raffinose, and Stachyose in Soybean Seed

Strain	Maturity[a] groups	Total sugar	Sucrose	Raffinose	Stachyose
		Weight in g/100 g seed			
Ada	00	9.68	6.33	0.54	2.80
Flambeau	00	9.86	6.43	0.74	2.69
Morsoy	00	10.11	6.38	0.95	2.78
Clay	0	10.04	6.78	0.77	2.49
Merit	0	10.07	6.33	0.69	3.05
M60-92	0	10.22	6.76	0.78	2.68
Chippewa 64	I	9.29	6.15	0.86	2.28
M59-120	I	9.33	5.71	0.60	3.02
Hark	I	9.41	6.11	0 68	2.62
Beeson	II	9.04	5.64	0.72	2.68
Corsoy	II	9.25	5.76	0.59	2.89
Amsoy	II	9.79	6.28	0.65	2.86
SL-9	III	8.57	5.52	0.82	2.23
Wayne	III	9.08	5.71	0.88	2.48
Calland	III	9.44	5.90	0.94	2.60
L66-1359	IV	8.30	5.06	0.80	2.46
Kent	IV	8.37	5.10	0.76	2.48
Cutler	IV	8.65	5.28	0.78	2.59
Mean		9.36	5.96	0.75	2.65
Range of means		8.30-10.11	5.06-6.78	0.54-0.95	2.23-3.05

Hymowitz et al. (6).

[a] For maturity groups 00, 0, I, II, III, and IV average
values are for 10, 12, 23, 33, 27, and 24 locations, respectively.

Flatulence in Humans

When a human experiences flatulence following a meal containing cooked dry beans, there is a sudden increase in passage
of flatus that reaches a maximum in about 4-5 hr, whereas with
a diet containing soy flour, the gas peak occurs in about

8-10 hr. The increase in flatus is due primarily to increased amounts of two gases--carbon dioxide and hydrogen. Appreciable amounts of methane may also be produced. Composition of gases in various segments of the intestinal tract under different dietary and physiological conditions has been compiled (3). Analysis of orally and rectally expelled gases reflects differences in type, location, and abundance of intestinal microorganisms that possess α-galactosidase activity (11).

Four male graduate students volunteered to determine the flatus activity of various commercially manufactured, toasted soy protein products [Table IV, (12)]. The gas-producing factor resides mainly in two products, whey solids and 80% ethanol extractives. These fractions contain about 55% carbohydrate, primarily as sucrose, raffinose, and stachyose. Glucosides of sapogenins, sterols, and isoflavones are also present in small amounts.

Table IV. Effects of Soy Products on Flatus in Man

Product[a]	Carbohydrate content, %	Daily intake, g	Flatus volume, cc/hr Average	Range
Full-fat soy flour	27	146	30	0-75
Defatted soy flour	33	146	71	0-290
Soy protein concentrate	25	146	36	0-98
Soy proteinate	<1	146	2	0-20
Water-insoluble residue[b]	75	146	13[d]	0-30
Whey solids[c]	56	48	300[d]	---
80% Ethanol extractives[c]	55	27	240	220-260
Navy bean meal		146	179	5-465
Basal diet		146	13	0-28

Steggerda et al. (12).

[a] All products were toasted with live steam at 100° C for 40 min.

[b] Fed at a level three times higher than that present in the defatted soy flour diet.

[c] Amount equal to that present in 146 g of defatted soy flour.

[d] One subject, otherwise four subjects per test.

In contrast, soy protein concentrate (72% protein and 25% polysaccharide) and the water-insoluble residue (25% protein and 75% polysaccharide) have low flatus activity. Soy proteinate, with a protein content of at least 92% and less than 1% oligosaccharide, is devoid of flatus activity.

A basal diet produces on the average 13 ml flatus/hr. On a navy bean diet, flatus volume increases to about 179 ml/hr. Some volunteers produce less than 5 ml/hr on a test meal of navy beans and others nearly 500 ml. Usually soy flour diets are less flatulent, but occasionally some subjects produce amounts of gas comparable to a navy bean diet.

Even though defatted soy flour and soybean meal contain about 30% total carbohydrate, its metabolic availability ranges from 14% in chicks to 40% in rats. On the basis of rat feeding, caloric value of soy carbohydrates is 1.68 Cal/g compared to a value of about 4.0 for highly digestible sugars (13). Sucrose accounts for the caloric value of the carbohydrates of soy flour. As a result, raffinose and stachyose and the polysaccharides are not metabolized by mammalian enzymes, but only the oligosaccharides are utilized for flatus production by the intestinal microflora.

Richards et al. (14) demonstrated that anaerobic bacterial cultures isolated from the dog colon can metabolize raffinose and stachyose to produce large amounts of carbon dioxide and hydrogen, the major gases in flatus. This in vitro technique was used by Rackis et al. (15) to determine the gas-producing activity of the same products used in the human studies. As shown in Table V, there is good agreement between in vitro tests and results obtained by human tests (Table IV).

Table V. Anaerobic Fermentation in vitro of Soybean Products, Anaerobic Cultures Isolated from Dog Colon Biopsies[a]

Sample	Gas volume, cc/24 hr	Composition of gas	
		% CO_2	% H_2
Soybean meal (dehulled-defatted)	40	44	51
Whey solids	40	47	48
80% Alcohol extractives	39	34	61
Water-insoluble residue	3	No gas for analysis	
Sodium soy proteinate	0	No gas for analysis	
Sodium caseinate	0	No gas for analysis	

Rackis et al. (15).

[a] To 10 cc of thioglycollate-anaerobic bacteria media, 0.5 g of sample was added.

Raffinose, when added to a soy protein isolate diet at a level equivalent to the total amount of raffinose plus stachyose in a soy grit diet (defatted soybean meal), produced just as much gas as the soy grit control diet [Figure 3 (16)]. Sucrose consumed at a level twice that found in soy grits did not cause flatulence.

Animal Tests

In a series of detailed experiments with rats, Cristofaro et al. (17) found that diets containing stachyose and verbascose exhibited the highest flatus activity. Carbon dioxide and hydrogen were the primary gases collected. Raffinose and lactose, incorporated at a level to equal the galactose level of the stachyose diet, induced an insignificant increase in flatus (Figures 4 and 5).

As shown in Figure 6, the amount of gas produced in fecal matter of dogs fed a flatulent soy grit diet was much greater than the amount formed on a nonflatulent all-meat diet (18). Heat resistant bacteria in fecal matter heated to 80° C for 20 min before incubation account for more than 75% of the total gas produced. Carbon dioxide content ranged from 76 to 85%, hydrogen content averaged about 10%, with hydrogen sulfide, nitrogen, and other gases accounting for the remaining portion (5-14%).

Relationship Between Intestinal Bacteria and Flatus

Richards and Steggerda (19) reported that 80% of the gas produced in surgically prepared intestinal segments of the dog when incubated with a navy bean homogenate occurred in the ileum and colon (Table VI). In our studies with soybean meal homogenates, almost all the gas was also produced in the ileum and colon. Carbon dioxide and hydrogen, the major constituents in flatus, were again the primary gases produced in intestinal segments. Practically no gas was produced in the intestines containing methyl cellulose. Under these conditions of little or no flatus production, nitrogen was the primary gas.

Based on studies of anaerobic cultures of the dog colon, Richards et al. (14) concluded that Clostridium perfringens, normally present in the gastro-intestinal tract in man and animals, was primarily responsible for the production of flatus in the ileum and colon. Rockland et al. (20) published data to show that the growth of Clostridia is stimulated by a substrate containing beans. Carbon dioxide and hydrogen were the major gases formed. When dejecta from human ileal and colonic segments of the intestine are cultured with stachyose, large amounts of gas are produced (21). The dominant gases were: 58-62% carbon dioxide and 28-36% hydrogen. About 12% methane was produced only

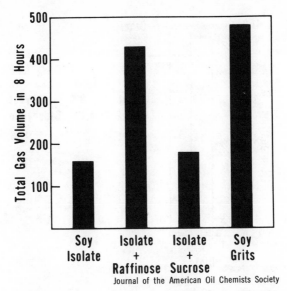

Journal of the American Oil Chemists Society

Figure 3. Flatus activity of soybean oligosaccharides in humans. Raffinose intake, 13 g/day; sucrose intake, 23 g/day (16).

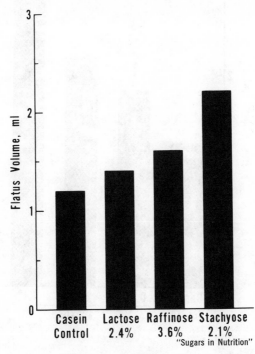

"Sugars in Nutrition"

Figure 4. Effect of various sugars on gas volume and composition in the rat intestine (17)

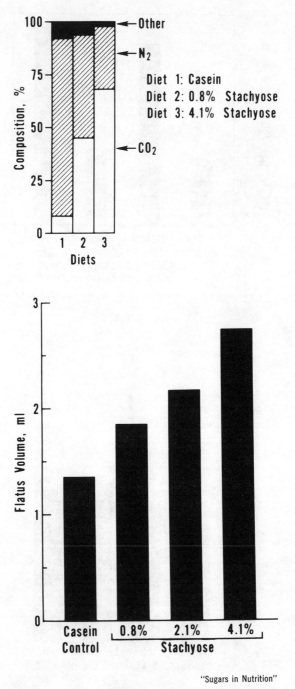

Figure 5. *Flatus activity of oligosaccharides in the rat intestine* (17)

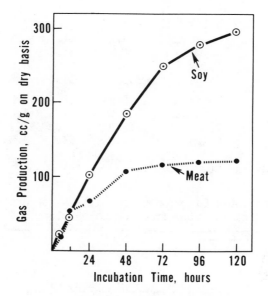

Figure 6.   Flatus activity in fecal matter of dogs fed a soy grit and an all-meal diet, incubation temperature, 37°C (18)

with colon dejecta. These data suggest that the intestinal flora may contain an α-1,6-galactosidase.

Table VI. Volume and Composition of Gas in Intestinal Segments of the Dog

Substrate	Intestinal segments	Mean gas volume, ml/3 hr	Gas composition, %			
			CO_2	O_2	N_2	H_2
Methyl cellulose[a]	Duodenum	0				
	Jejunum	1.5	9.3	13.9	76.8	0
	Ileum	1.5	9.3	13.9	76.8	0
	Colon	1.5	9.3	13.9	76.8	0
Navy bean[a]	Duodenum	5.7	21.3	6.5	38.3	33.9
homogenate	Jejunum	4.9	21.0	4.7	46.4	27.9
	Ileum	15.0	21.7	6.0	44.6	27.7
	Colon	31.9	34.3	3.8	28.7	33.2
Soy flour	Duodenum	5.9	21.5	3.8	46.7	28.0
homogenate	Jejunum	4.8	21.5	3.6	47.8	27.1
	Ileum	11.0	32.0	3.7	33.1	31.2
	Colon	12.0	33.0	3.8	26.9	36.3

[a] Richards and Steggerda (19).

Table VII. Anaerobic Gas Production with Carbohydrates. Anaerobic Cultures Isolated from Dog Colon Biopsies

Substrate[a]	Total gas produced, ml				Gas composition, %	
	1 hr	6 hr	12 hr	24 hr	CO_2	H_2
Monosaccharides						
Glucose	0	23	38	51	37	62
Maltose	0	19	38	43	38	61
Fructose	0	10	20	37	41	58
Galactose	0	8	20	36	38	61
Oligosaccharides						
Sucrose	0	19	27	30	32	68
Raffinose	0	9	25	30	35	65
Stachyose	0	10	27	31	37	63
Control	0	1.5	1.5	2.0		

Rackis et al. (15).
[a] To 10 ml of thioglycollate anaerobic bacteria medium, 0.1 g of substrate was added.

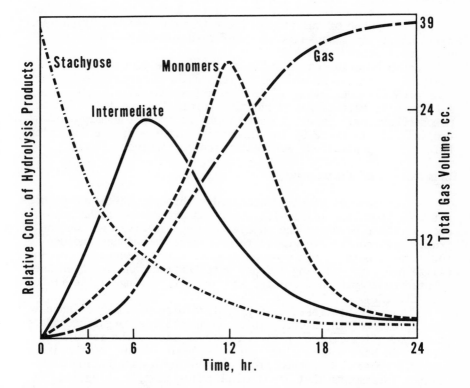

*Figure 7.   Relationship between the enzymatic hydrolyses of stachyose and gas produc-
tion.   Anaerobic culture isolated from the dog colon.   Curve A, stachyose; curve B, di-
and trisaccharides; curve C, monomer sugars; curve D, gas production.*

Rackis et al. (15) confirmed that anaerobic cultures isolated from dog colon biopsies can metabolize raffinose and stachyose to produce the characteristically high concentrations of
carbon dioxide and hydrogen. Glucose gave the most gas and at
a rate greater than for either fructose or galactose (Table VII).
With raffinose and stachyose, gas production occurred at the
slowest rate. Evidently, the oligosaccharides break down to
monosaccharides before the gas-producing mechanism can take
place. It is understandable then that a longer delay must occur
before the onset of gas production with raffinose and stachyose,
particularly if glucose is the preferred substrate (see Figure 1).

Gas production was related to the degree of enzymatic hydrolysis of stachyose and the corresponding intermediate breakdown products consisting of di- and trisaccharides (Figure 7).
As a result, rate of gas production paralleled the formation of
monosaccharides. Paper chromatography recorded the enzymatic hydrolysis of stachyose by the anaerobic cultures of the dog colon.
Relative concentrations were determined by photodensitometry.

Elimination of Flatulence

Since removal of oligosaccharides through genetic means does
not look promising (Table III), various processing techniques
such as those used for the manufacture of isolates and concen-
trates are required to remove them. These techniques include
hot water treatment and aqueous alcohol extraction which insolu-
bilize protein. Soaking and hot water extraction have been used
to prepare tempeh, a fermented soy product, having little flatus
activity (22).

Enzymatic processes that hydrolyze oligosaccharides have
been developed (23, 24, 25, 26). An immobilized α-galactosidase
continuous flow reactor has been used to reduce the raffinose
content in beet sugar molasses (27). About 70% of the raffinose
plus stachyose was removed from soybeans by a combination of
various treatments that involved pH adjustment, soaking, and
germination (28). Germinating soybeans contain an α-galactosidase since raffinose and stachyose decrease rapidly during the
first 3 days and disappear after 5 days of germination (17).
However, soybean and mung bean sprouts retain most of the
flatulence-inducing activity of the intact seed when tested in
humans (22). In contrast, autolysis of California small white
beans, as measured by the disappearance of α-oligosaccharides,
significantly reduces rat hydrogen production (29). The reason
for this anomaly is unclear and requires further investigation.
Possibly the soybean polysaccharides, which normally do not have
flatulent properties, are degraded during sprouting to form intermediate products that could then be fermented by intestinal
bacteria into large amounts of gas, whereas, the starch in white
beans would be digested and absorbed.

Literature Cited

1. Protein Advisory Group of the United Nations System, PAG Bulletin, Vol. III, No. 2, 1 (1973).
2. Beck, J. E., Ann. N.Y. Acad. Sci. U.S.A. (1968) 150, 1.
3. Calloway, D. H., Handb. Physiol. Alimentary Canal (1968) 5, 2839.
4. French, D., Advan. Carbohyd. Chem. (1954) 9, 149.
5. Kawamura, S., Tech. Bull. Fac. Agr. Kagawa Univ. (1967) 18, 117.
6. Hymowitz, T., Walker, W. M., Collins, F. I., Panczer, P., Commun. Soil Sci. Plant Anal. (1972) 3, 367.
7. Gitzelmann, R., Auricchio, S., Pediatrics (1965) 36, 231.
8. Ruttloff, H., Taeufel, A., Krause, W., Haenel, H., Taeufel, K., Nahrung (1967) 11, 39.
9. Taeufel, K., Krause, W. G., Ruttloff, H., Maune, R., Z. Gesamte Exp. Med. Einschl. Exp. Chir. (1967) 144, 54.
10. Krause, W. G., Taeufel, K., Ruttloff, H., Maune, R., Ernaehrungsforschung (1968) 13, 161.
11. Calloway, D. H., Burroughs, S. E., Gut (1969) 10, 180.
12. Steggerda, F. R., Richards, E. A., Rackis, J. J., Proc. Soc. Exp. Biol. Med. (1966) 121, 1235.
13. Liener, I. E., in "Soybeans: Chemistry and Technology," Vol. 1, "Proteins," Edited by A. K. Smith and S. J. Circle, Avi Publishing Co., Westport, Conn. (1972).
14. Richards, E. A., Steggerda, F. R., Murata, A., Gastroenterology (1968) 55, 502.
15. Rackis, J. J., Sessa, D. J., Steggerda, F. R., Shimizu, J., Anderson, J., Pearl, S. L., J. Food Sci. (1970) 35, 634.
16. Rackis, J. J., J. Amer. Oil Chem. Soc. (1974) 51, 161A.
17. Cristofaro, E., Mottu, F., Wuhrmann, J. J., in "Nutrition Monogram, Sugars in Nutrition," Edited by H. L. Sipple, International Conference Sugars in Nutrition, Vanderbilt University, Nashville, Tennessee, November 1972.
18. Shimizu, T., Steggerda, F. R., Rackis, J. J., unpublished data.
19. Richards, E. A., Steggerda, F. R., Proc. Soc. Exp. Biol. Med. (1966) 122, 573.
20. Rockland, L. B., Gardiner, B. L., Pieczarka, D., J. Food Sci. (1969) 34, 411.
21. Calloway, D. H., Colasito, D. J., Mathews, R. D., Nature (1966) 212, 1238.
22. Calloway, D. H., Hickey, C. A., Murphy, E. L., J. Food Sci. (1971) 36, 251.
23. Sherba, S. E., U.S. Patent 3,632,346 (1972).
24. Sugimoto, H., Van Buren, J. P., J. Food Sci. (1970) 35, 655.
25. Ciba-Geigy, A. G., French Patent 2,137,548 (1973).
26. Yamane, T., La Sucrerie Belge. (1971) 90, 345.
27. Reynolds, J. H., Biotechnol. Bioeng. (1974) 16, 135.

28. Kim, W. J., Smit, C. J. B., Nakayama, T. O. M., Lebensm.-
    Wiss. Technol. (1973) 6, 201.
29. Becker, R., Olson, A. C., Frederick, D. P., Kon, S.,
    Gumbmann, M. R., Wagner, J. R., J. Food Sci. (1974) 39,
    767.
30. Hardinge, M. G., Swarner, J. B., Crooks, H., J. Amer. Diet
    Ass. (1965) 46, 197.
31. Aspinall, G. O., Bigbie, R., McKay, J. E., Cereal Sci. Today
    (1967) 12, 233.

14

The Lysosomal α-Glucosidases of Mammalian Tissues

BARBARA I. BROWN, ALLEN K. MURRAY, and DAVID H. BROWN

Department of Biological Chemistry, Division of Biology and Biomedical Sciences, Washington University, St. Louis, Mo. 63110

This Symposium has focused attention on various dietary carbohydrates, their absorption, interconversions and physiological fates. As has been pointed out, one of the criteria for utilization of [^{14}C]-labeled sugars has been the extent of isotope incorporation into glycogen as well as the formation of $^{14}CO_2$. The average 70 kg adult may have stored in his tissues half a kilogram of glycogen. However, a 7 kg infant with Type II Glycogen Storage Disease (Pompe's disease), which is one of the more common forms of glycogen storage disease, also may have stored a like quantity of glycogen. This fact serves to emphasize the importance of the α-glucosidase which has an acidic pH optimum in the catabolism of glycogen in normal human tissues, since patients with Type II disease have been shown to have a congenital and generalized deficiency of this glucosidase (1). The purified enzyme has both α-1,4 and α-1,6 glucosidase activity and can convert glycogen totally to glucose (2). The activity in normal tissue homogenates is such that if the enzyme were in contact with its substrate, it would have the capacity of totally degrading the polysaccharide present in liver in 3 to 5 hours and that in muscle in 8 to 12 hours.

By comparison of its properties with those of an α-glucosidase purified to homogeneity from rat liver lysosomes (3), the human enzyme is assumed to be in lysosomes also. Electron micrographs of liver samples obtained from patients with Type II glycogen storage disease show that a large quantity of glycogen is present within membrane enclosed vacuoles and this observation is consistent with the hypothesis that the α-glucosidase has a lysosomal localization (4). Similar enzymes have been purified from a variety of sources such as rat (2,5,6) and beef liver (7), rabbit muscle (8), and human placenta (6) and liver. Most of the preparations have taken advantage of the property of the enzyme to be specifically retarded by adsorption to Sephadex as an important aid in its purification. Figure 1 illustrates the behavior of the human liver enzyme upon Sephadex G-100 chromatography. Previous steps in the purification procedure had included repeated

freezing and thawing of the liver homogenate to rupture the lysosomes, a heat treatment at 55° and ammonium sulfate fractionation
between 35 and 55% saturation. The dialyzed, concentrated ammonium sulfate fraction applied to the Sephadex column usually contained 60% of the starting units of enzyme activity and had a
specific activity of 0.15 unit per mg protein corresponding to
its being 10 to 12-fold purified at this stage. However, the enzyme recovered from the Sephadex column usually had an activity
of about 30 units per mg corresponding to an overall purification
of more than 2000-fold with a recovery of approximately 40% of
the total units. From 1 to 2 mg of enzyme could be obtained from
100 grams of human liver (9).

As indicated in Figure 1, maltose or glycogen can be used as
a substrate in measuring the activity of the enzyme. The specific activities given above refer to µmoles of maltose hydrolyzed
per minute per mg of protein at pH 4 and 37° and at a substrate
concentration of 10 mM. Usually incubations with glycogen were
carried out with 1% substrate, at pH 4.5, and the activities then
expressed as µmoles of glucose formed per minute at 37°. The placental enzyme purified by de Barsy et al. (6) had a specific activity of 7.3 units per mg when assayed at 3.7 mM maltose. However, these investigators found that the K_m for the human placental enzyme was 11 mM for maltose and 2% for glycogen.

Even though glycogen is the natural substrate for the enzyme, for convenience many investigators have used maltose as a
substrate in assaying for the α-glucosidase. We had previously
shown that the rat liver enzyme exhibited substrate inhibition by
maltose and by maltosidically linked oligosaccharides when the
initial substrate concentrations exceed 5 to 10 mM (2). Studies
with the enzyme purified from human liver have revealed no substrate inhibition at concentrations as high as 100 mM maltose.
The K_m for maltose for the human liver enzyme appears to be 9 mM,
while for isomaltose a K_m of 33 mM was found.

Polyacrylamide gel electrophoresis of the purified human
liver enzyme resulted in a single peak of activity as shown in
Figure 2. In this experiment after electrophoresis the gel was
frozen, sliced into 1 mm slices and the activity of the eluted enzyme determined in each slice. Essentially 100% of the loaded
units were recovered. Of greater interest is the fact that a good
correspondence was found between total absorbance at 280 nm, protein staining with Coomassie blue, enzymatic activity revealed by
incubation with methyl umbelliferyl glucopyranoside (another substrate of the α-glucosidase), and PAS positive material in the
same or parallel gels. Since PAS staining indicates the presence
of carbohydrate, the α-glucosidase isolated from human liver appears to be a glycoprotein (9).

In isoelectric focusing gels there always was evidence of the
presence of several isozymes as indicated in Figure 3 where the
eluted enzyme showed similar patterns of activity with the two
substrates. The pH values were obtained by measuring the pH of

water in which groups of four consecutive slices of a duplicate gel were extracted following overnight electrophoresis of a 17 cm gel cast with pH 3 to 6 ampholine. Duplicate gels were also stained for protein and PAS reactive material. The scans of the stained gels (Figure 4) indicated correspondence between protein and carbohydrate throughout the region containing the charge isozymes. Following column chromatography of the glucosidase on Biogel P-200, some difference in the isozyme pattern of individual fractions could be ascertained in isoelectric focused gels such that the more acidic isozymes were more prominent in the earlier fractions eluted from the column while the less acidic ones emerged later. The position of the main peak is compatible with a molecular weight on the order of 100,000 similar to the value of 114,000 found for the rat liver lysosomal α-glucosidase (3) and of 107,000 found for the bovine liver enzyme (7).

One of the main purposes of purifying the human liver enzyme was to make it possible to obtain an antibody to the protein to investigate whether, using such an antibody, evidence could be found for cross-reactive material in the tissues of individuals afflicted with Type II glycogen storage disease. The evidence that the α-glucosidase has an essential role in normal metabolism has been inferred from the apparent serious effects of its absence in the tissues of the infant with this disease who frequently dies at an early age with massive accumulation of glycogen particularly in the heart and skeletal muscles. However it should be pointed out that adult forms of the deficiency also exist (10) and, while these adults have essentially no demonstrable α-glucosidase activity at acid pH in extracts of their tissues, the content of glycogen may be only slightly above normal and the clinical symptoms may be confined to a mild muscular weakness. Since the activity of the α-glucosidase is demonstrable in leukocytes and cultured skin fibroblasts of normal individuals, fibroblasts may be utilized as an experimental tissue (11,12).

Rabbits were immunized by subcutaneous injection of 0.5 to 1 mg of enzyme in 1 ml of complete Freunds adjuvant in multiple sites at monthly intervals followed by 0.1 mg of enzyme intravenously. The titer of antibody obtained varied with the rabbit and the time of bleeding during the immunization schedule. A typical preparation of antibody was 5 to 10 times as effective in inhibiting the activity of the enzyme toward glycogen as toward either maltose or isomaltose when all activities were assayed at concentrations equal to the K_m of the respective substrates. Action on glycogen could be completely inhibited by antibody, while in general no more than 80% of maltose hydrolysis could be blocked even by large amounts of antibody. Similar effects were observed by deBarsy et al. (6).

In giving attention next to some of the experimental results obtained utilizing fibroblasts, it is significant to recognize that units of activity are expressed as nanomoles of maltose hydrolyzed, or glucose formed from glycogen, per minute per mg of

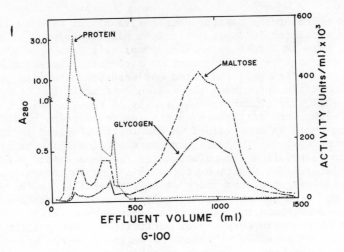

Figure 1. *Chromatography of human liver α-glucosidase on Sephadex G-100. See text for assay conditions.*

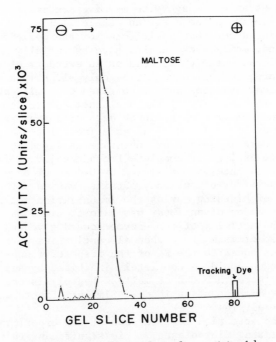

Figure 2. *Elution of α-glucosidase activity following polyacrylamide gel electrophoresis of the purified enzyme on a 6% gel (1% crosslinked) according to the method of Orr et al. (19)*

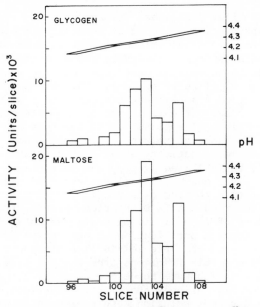

Figure 3. Elution of α-glucosidase activity following electrophoresis on an isoelectric focusing gel cast with pH 3–6 ampholine and run for 11 hrs. Gel slices extracted overnight with pH 4, 0.05M acetate buffer before assay. Measurements of pH made on water extracts of slices from gels run in parallel. The 17-cm gels were cut into 170 slices; only the area of recovered enzyme activity is shown.

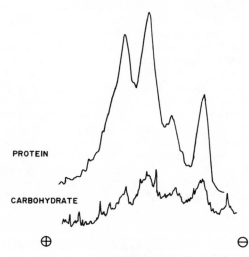

Figure 4. Coomassie Blue staining (protein) and PAS staining (carbohydrate) of other isoelectric focused gels run in parallel with the gel shown in Figure 3

protein in fibroblast sonicates. Assays usually have involved
incubation at pH 4 of about 50 µg of sonicate protein for periods
of up to 3 hours in a final volume of 0.10 to 0.15 ml. Slight inhibition of α-glucosidase activity at 200 mM maltose was sometimes
seen. Fibroblasts as well as other tissues also contain an α-glucosidase with an alkaline pH optimum. Whether the trace of activity measurable at pH 4 in fibroblasts cultured from Type II glycogen storage disease patients is due to the persistence of an
isozyme of the acid α-glucosidase or is due to a low activity of
the neutral glucosidase at this pH could not be ascertained. Although the glucosidase activity at acid pH present in fibroblast
sonicates could be inhibited by exposure to the antibody to the
purified human liver enzyme, the fibroblast sonicates contained
insufficient protein to produce a precipitin reaction in double
diffusion test carried out in Ouchterlony plates. Fractions prepared from livers of Type II glycogenosis patients, following the
steps outlined for the purification of the enzyme from human
liver, failed to produce a precipitin line although reaction was
obtained with comparable fractions from control livers.

Attempts were also made to detect cross-reacting protein in
affected tissues via antibody consumption experiments. That is,
aliquots of an antibody solution were preincubated with fractions
prepared from Type II glycogen storage disease tissues or fibroblasts and then added to purified enzyme or, in other experiments,
to tissue extracts or fibroblasts from non-Type II individuals,
prior to the addition of substrate. The inhibition curves were
not influenced by the conditions of preincubation in any of these
experiments. Fibroblast cultures were available from several
adults who were deficient in α-glucosidase activity at acid pH
and sonicates of these cells also failed to alter the antibody inhibition curves of the purified human liver enzyme.

An example of the effect of addition of increasing amounts of
antibody to a fibroblast sonicate is shown in the upper portion
of Table I. As indicated in the legend, the numbers given are
measurements of specific activity. Inhibition was found to be
proportional to the amount of antibody added. The lower portion
of the Table reports the results obtained with six different control fibroblast cultures each of which was incubated with antibody which either had or had not been preincubated with other
sonicates prepared from fibroblasts cultured from patients with
Type II glycogen storage disease. Up to 3 times as much protein
from the Type II sonicates were present as in the control sonicates. Under these conditions there was no demonstrable difference in the amount of activity inhibited by added antibody.

Table I
Glycogen Hydrolysis By Fibroblast Sonicates In The Presence Of
An Antibody Preparation

(nanomoles of glucose formed/min/mg sonicate protein)

A Control Activity	B Antibody*	C Antibody + Type II Sonicate**	A–B	A–C
8.87	5.44[a]		3.43	
	3.72[b]		5.15	
	2.39[c]		6.48	
4.79	2.36[a]	2.68[a]	2.43	2.11
5.40	4.23[d]	4.10[d]	1.17	1.27
6.69	4.86[d]	4.78[d]	1.83	1.91
7.25	3.79[a]	3.54[a]	3.46	3.71
10.77	5.58[c]	5.58[c]	5.19	5.19
10.87	7.07[a]	6.91[a]	3.80	3.96
	4.05[c]	4.00[c]	6.82	6.87

*The antibody preparation was diluted 1:250 in 0.9%
NaCl and the volumes added per 0.1 ml reaction mixture were as follows: (a) 0.01 ml; (b) 0.015 ml;
(c) 0.02 ml. Experiments labeled (d) contained
0.01 ml of a 1:300 dilution of the antibody.

**Sonicates of fibroblasts cultured from patients with
Type II glycogen storage disease preincubated with
antibody prior to addition of control sonicates.

Another approach to the problem of assessing the importance
of the α-glucosidase in the glycogen catabolism has involved the
production of glycogen storage in normal fibroblasts by growth of
the cultures in the presence of an inhibitor of the α-glucosidase.
In the course of experiments on the metabolism of the fibroblast
cell lines derived from patients with Pompe's disease, it had been
observed that the glycogen content of such cells tended to be
higher than that found in normal cell lines and that the half life
of glycogen which had been formed during culture in [^{14}C]-glucose
tended to be prolonged. Dingle, Fell, and co-workers had shown
that culture of several cell types in sucrose or other non-metab-
olizable sugars led to extensive vacuolation of the cytoplasm and
the appearance of lysosomal acid phosphatase within the vacuoles
(13,14). On the assumption that other enzymes of the primary
lysosome of the cell might also appear within such persistent
vacuoles and that some glycogen might be sequestered there as

well, we added a potential inhibitor of the α-glucosidase to the medium in which normal fibroblasts were growing. It was thought possible that a normal cell line grown in the presence of such a disaccharide inhibitor might become similar to Type II fibroblasts, in which the glucosidase is missing, in that the glycogen content of the treated cells might be significantly elevated and the turnover rate of pre-labelled polysaccharide might also be markedly affected (15).

Preliminary experiments established that the glycogen content of a given cell line was relatively constant during a number of subcultures and that it was independent of the glucose concentration of the medium within the range of 1 to 20 mM (15). Several disaccharides were considered for use in these experiments. Hers and co-workers had found that D-(+)- turanose is a specific inhibitor of the lysosomal glucosidase (16), and we had shown by kinetic analysis that this disaccharide is almost purely a noncompetitive inhibitor of glycogen hydrolysis by the purified rat liver lysosomal enzyme (2). Although these findings suggested that turanose might be well suited to produce glycogen storage in fibroblast cultures, preliminary experiments indicated that there was a significant inhibition of cell growth in its presence. We had also shown that trehalose is an inhibitor of α-glucosidase of human liver and heart acting on glycogen at pH 4 (11). When it was found that trehalose could be added to the culture media in which human fibroblasts were growing at concentration up to 0.15 M without serious effect on growth rate, its effect on the α-glucosidase of fibroblasts was investigated. Trehalose proved to be a potent, non-competitive inhibitor with a K_i of from 5 to 8 mM depending on the cell line investigated (17). When fibroblasts were grown in the presence of added trehalose, the glycogen content increased to an extent which was dependent upon both the concentration of the disaccharide in the medium and the time of exposure to it. In view of the presumed mode of action of trehalose in inducing glycogen storage mentioned previously, it was of interest to measure the total activity of some enzymes which are presumably chiefly of lysosomal origin, after the fibroblasts and any subcellular organelles which they might contain were broken by sonic treatment. Table II shows results obtained with 3 normal cell lines and includes a comparison of the action of trehalose with that of sucrose – which has also been reported to be an inhibitor of lysosomal α-glucosidase – and of lactose which is supposed to be ineffective in this respect. It is apparent that trehalose and sucrose induce glycogen storage and that lactose does not. Of interest was the finding that N-acetyl-β-glucosaminidase showed a regular and substantial increase in activity, since it has been suggested that this glucosaminidase is firmly bound to the lysosomal membrane. We have shown by growing fibroblasts in 0.06 M [^{14}C]-trehalose for three days that the intracellular content of this disaccharide becomes as great as 0.4 to 0.6 μmole per mg of protein. If this trehalose were localized within lysosomes, its concentration would be sufficient to inhibit lysosomal α-glucosidase during growth. However, in sonicates of such cells, the trehalose concentration would not exceed 5% of its K_i value as an inhibitor of glycogen hydrolysis.

Table II
Effect of Disaccharide Addition During Culture On The Ratio Of
Experimental To Control Values For Glycogen Content And
Enzyme Activity In Fibroblasts

Cell Line	Disaccharide Added	Glycogen Content	α-Glucosidase (Glycogen, pH 4.2)	N-Acetyl-β- Glucos- aminidase
1	Trehalose	1.50	1.09	1.81
	Sucrose	1.43	0.82	1.95
	Lactose	1.11	0.82	0.93
2	Trehalose	1.78	1.18	1.84
	Sucrose	2.01	1.14	1.82
	Lactose	0.68	0.86	1.14
3	Trehalose	2.0	0.68	
	Sucrose	2.2	0.75	
	Lactose	1.0	1.10	

Figure 5 compares the logarithmic rate of decline of [14C]-glycogen in normal fibroblasts maintained in the presence and absence of 40 mM trehalose added to the culture media. The fibroblasts were preloaded with [14C]-glycogen by culture of the cells to confluency in the presence of [14C]-glucose in the media. At zero time, the cells were washed with unlabelled media and culture continued in the absence of labelled glucose. The glycogen content of the control cells averaged 0.82 μmole of polymeric glucose per mg of protein and increased to 1.34 μmoles/mg in the cells maintained in trehalose. The time required for the disappearance of 50% of the radioactivity from glycogen was about tripled (from 1.4 to 4.6 days) in the cells maintained in trehalose. As previously mentioned, some cell lines from type II glycogen storage disease patients have shown a remarkable preservation of [14C]-glycogen in their cultured fibroblasts. Data from one such cell line is also shown where an apparent half-life of 7 days was measured for its glycogen. The average glycogen content of the 12 samples giving rise to this curve was 1.3 μmoles of polymeric glucose per mg of protein. Note that no trehalose was present. Other Type II fibroblasts have had apparent half-lives of their glycogen of 4 to 5 days.

In summary, the α-glucosidase active at pH 4 has been purified to homogeneity from human liver. It appears to be a glycoprotein. Antibody to the enzyme has been produced in rabbits.

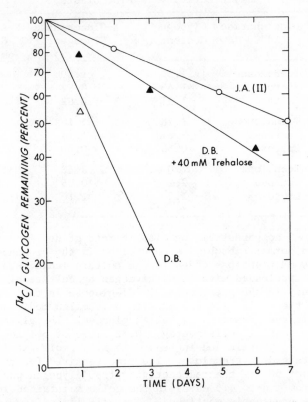

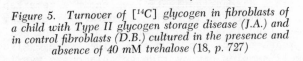

Figure 5. Turnover of [¹⁴C] glycogen in fibroblasts of a child with Type II glycogen storage disease (J.A.) and in control fibroblasts (D.B.) cultured in the presence and absence of 40 mM trehalose (18, p. 727)

No evidence for cross reactive protein has been obtained using fibroblast cultures derived from patients with either the infantile or adult forms of the deficiency. Glycogen storage and delayed turnover of this polysaccharide can be induced in normal fibroblasts by culture of the cells in the presence of an inhibitor of the α-glucosidase activity.

Acknowledgments:
    A part of this work was carried out while one of us (A.K.M.) was a Post Doctoral Fellow of the National Institutes of Health. Present address (AKM): Department of Pediatrics, California College of Medicine, University of California, Irvine, California 92664. This work has been supported in part by Grant GM-04761 from the National Institutes of Health and Grants 71-973 and 74-928 from the American Heart Association. Communications regarding this publication should be addressed to Dr. Barbara I. Brown, Department of Biological Chemistry, Washington University School of Medicine, 660 South Euclid Avenue, Saint Louis, Missouri 63110.

Literature Cited

1. Hers, H.G., Biochem. J., (1963), **86**, 11.
2. Jeffrey, P.L., Brown, D.H. and Brown, B.I., Biochemistry, (1970), **9**, 1416.
3. Jeffrey, P.L., Brown, D.H. and Brown, B.I., Biochemistry, (1970), **9**, 1403.
4. Baudhuin, P., Hers, H.G. and Loeb, H., Lab. Invest., (1964), **13**, 1139.
5. Auricchio, F., Bruni, C.B. and Sica, V., Biochem. J., (1968), **108**, 161.
6. deBarsy, T., Jacquemin, P., Devos, P., and Hers, H.G., Eur. J. Biochem., (1972), **31**, 156.
7. Bruni, C.B., Auricchio, F. and Covelli, I., J. Biol. Chem., (1969), **244**, 4735.
8. Palmer, T.N., Biochem. J., (1971), **124**, 701.
9. Murray, A.K., Brown, D.H. and Brown, B.I., In preparation.
10. Engel, A.G., Brain, (1970), **93**, 599.
11. Brown, B.I., Brown, D.H. and Jeffrey, P.L., Biochemistry, (1970), **9**, 1423.
12. Angelini, C., Engel, A.G. and Titus, J.L., New Eng. J. Med., (1972), **287**, 948.
13. Dingle, J.T., Fell, H.B. and Glauert, A.M., J. Cell Science, (1969), **4**, 139.
14. Nyberg, E. and Dingle, J.T., Exper. Cell Res., (1970), **63**, 43.
15. Brown, B.I. and Brown, D.H., Biochem. Biophys. Res. Commun., (1972), **46**, 1292.
16. Lejeune, N., Thines-Sempoux, D. and Hers, H.G., Biochem. J., (1963), **86**, 16.

17. Brown, D.H. and Brown, B.I., In "Biochemistry of the Glyco-
     sidic Linkage," PAABS Symposium, editors, R. Piras and H.G.
     Pontis, p. 687, Academic Press, New York and London, (1972).
18. Brown, B.I., In "Biochemistry of the Glycosidic Linkage,"
     PAABS Symposium, editors, R. Piras and H.G. Pontis, p. 725,
     Academic Press, New York and London, (1972).
19. Orr, M.D., Blakley, R.L. and Panagou, D., Anal. Biochem.,
     (1972), 45, 65.

Enzymes of Glycogen Metabolism and Their Control

HAROLD L. SEGAL

Division of Cell and Molecular Biology, State University of New York, Buffalo, N.Y. 14214

While there is a continual expenditure of energy in living organisms, albeit of variable degree above the basal level essential to physiological function, the dietary intake of utilizable energy is sporadic. Therefore, the ability to store energy resources and meter their release in a manner consistent with need is an attribute of living organisms essential to their survival. Thus, there must be a post-prandial flow of nutrients into storage forms, and a reverse flow out of storage forms between meals. The two major dietary energy resources are carbohydrate and fat, with protein normally comprising a significantly smaller contribution.

Carbohydrates are stored as such or converted to fat, dietary fat is stored only as such, and protein is convertible to both carbohydrate and fat (Fig. 1). It is an important point to emphasize that of the total fat and carbohydrate energy stores, the latter represents less than 10% by weight and half that by caloric content. However, carbohydrate is ubiquitously distributed and readily available, whereas fat is stored primarily at remote depots and must be mobilized, transported, and transformed before entering the catabolic pathway. Therefore, carbohydrate represents a more immediately available energy store, while fat constitutes a much larger, long term store. Since a minimal level of circulating glucose is essential to life and since the amount of stored carbohydrate is relatively small, the convertibility of protein to carbohydrate is vital for the maintenance of blood glucose levels during prolonged food deprivation or on severly carbohydrate-low diets. Consonant with the purposes of this symposium, my discussion will deal with the regulation of the formation and utilization of glycogen, the storage form of carbohydrate in animal tissues.

The predominant sugar of the diet is glucose, which is converted to glycogen without cleavage of the hexose chain. As seen in Fig. 1, this applies to galactose as well, which is epimerized to a substituted form of glucose that is on the direct pathway of glucose metabolism. Fructose, on the other hand, is for the most part not converted to a glucose derivative, except indirectly via trioses, and therefore regulation of its metabolism would be expected to resemble more closely that of glycogenic amino acids or glycerol, as well as to involve unique features of its own.

Fig. 2 shows the immediate steps in the formation and utilization of glycogen, catalyzed by glycogen synthetase a and phosphorylase a, respectively, and the interconverting systems which produce and remove these forms. Several points should be noted in these pathways.

a) At least three enzymes in this scheme exist in active and inactive forms, designated a and b, respectively. These are glycogen synthetase, phosphorylase, and phosphorylase kinase. The a and b forms differ from one another by the presence or absence of phosphate groups covalently linked to serine residues of the protein. Some evidence has been reported suggesting the existence of active and inactive forms of phosphorylase phosphatase and glycogen synthetase phosphatase as well.

b) The active form can be either the phosphorylated form, as is the case with phosphorylase and phosphorylase kinase, or the dephosphorylated form, as is the case with glycogen synthetase.

c) The active and inactive forms in a set are interconvertible by a kinase-catalyzed, ATP-dependent phosphorylation and a phosphatase-catalyzed hydrolysis of esterified phosphate.

d) The phosphorylase and glycogen synthetase systems are linked by the common cyclic AMP-stimulated protein kinase which activates the former and deactivates the latter; phosphorylase kinase is a distinct enzyme.

e) The potential for futile cycling exists between glycogen and glucose-1-phosphate (G-1-P). Each cycle costs one high energy phosphate bond; cycling is held in check by the opposite effects of the cyclic AMP-stimulated protein kinase on the two systems, as well as other factors to be discussed subsequently.

f) Conflicting reports exist regarding the identity or distinctiveness of the three phosphatases in these systems. In one case a preparation from muscle was described which possessed dephosphorylating activity toward phosphorylase kinase and glycogen synthetase, but not phosphorylase (1); i.e., that the enzymes which were common substrates for protein kinase were also common substrates for the same phosphatase. In another report, however, a preparation from heart was stated to dephosphorylate all three of the interconvertible enzymes (2).

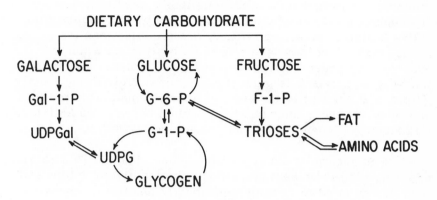

Figure 1.   *Interconversions of carbohydrates, fats, and amino acids*

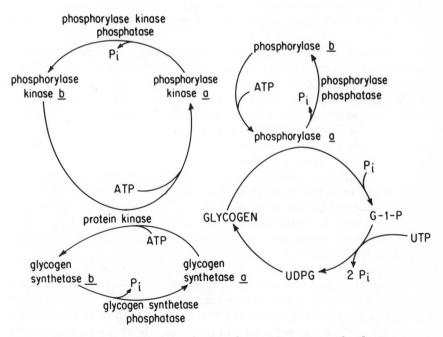

Figure 2.   *Components involved in glycogen formation and utilization*

The control of both the phosphorylase and glycogen synthetase systems is complex. Phosphorylase $\underline{a}$, the phosphorylated form, is highly active under all conditions likely to exist in tissues. The dephosphorylated form, phosphorylase $\underline{b}$, is completely inactive in liver. Muscle phosphorylase $\underline{b}$ is also inactive except in the presence of high levels of AMP, a situation which can occur $\underline{in}$ $\underline{vivo}$ under conditions of oxygen deficiency. In resting tissue phosphorylase is present mainly or entirely in the inactive $\underline{b}$ form, and, except in the state of relative anoxia referred to above, where the system can be turned on by elevated AMP levels, its activation depends upon the conversion of the $\underline{b}$ form to the $\underline{a}$ form.

This is accomplished by phosphorylase kinase. This enzyme, however, also is present primarily in the inactive or $\underline{b}$ form and must be activated to become significantly functional. As with phosphorylase itself, this can be accomplished in two ways. Phosphorylase kinase $\underline{b}$ can be stimulated by elevated Ca^{+2} levels, which occurs as a consequence of muscle stimulation and membrane depolarization. With this there is a very rapid activation of the kinase and in consequence a conversion of phosphorylase to the active form and an initiation of rapid glycolysis. Thus energy production is provided synchronously with its need to maintain muscle contraction. Alternatively, phosphorylase kinase can be activated by conversion to the active, or $\underline{a}$, form. This requires a phosphorylation and is accomplished by the cyclic AMP-dependent protein kinase. This kinase, in turn, is activated by elevation of cyclic AMP levels. Recent reviews of the phosphorylase system have been published ($\underline{3},\underline{4}$).

Regulation of the phosphorylase reaction is effected by a number of hormones which elevate cyclic AMP levels; notably glucagon in the liver, epinephrine in the muscle, and both of these plus ACTH and other hormones in adipose tissue. Thus, in response to external signals in the form of tissue-specific hormones, phosphorylase is converted to a form which is fully active, and in this way the restraints which exist to serve intracellular homeostasis are overriden to meet a more urgent need of the whole organism ($\underline{5}$).

Another regulatory factor of more direct relationship to the subject of this symposium is glucose itself. Glucose has been shown to stimulate the phosphorylase phosphatase reaction which converts phosphorylase from the fully active $\underline{a}$ form to the inactive $\underline{b}$ form ($\underline{6}$). Thus, in response to an adequate level of glucose to meet metabolic needs, the release of glucose units from glycogen is blocked and the carbohydrate stores are preserved. Glucose

also inhibits glucagon release from the pancreas, thereby reducing the cyclic AMP-mediated stimulation of the phosphorylase
kinase branch which turns phosphorylase on. Thus glucose
produces a two-pronged effect in stimulating phosphorylase phosphatase activity and reducing phosphorylase kinase activity,
both of which diminish the level of active phosphorylase and
spare glycogen utilization. These patterns of regulation are
summarized in Fig. 3.

Similar patterns of control exist with the glycogen synthetase
system, often by the same mediators as with phosphorylase,
operating in the reverse sense, and therefore in the same direc-
tion from the point of view of metabolic flow. As with phosphorylase, the a form of synthetase, which in this case is the
dephosphorylated form, is fully active under physiological
conditions. The b form, which predominates in resting tissue, is
inactive except in the presence of high levels of glucose-6-
phosphate (G-6-P) - a situation unlikely to exist in liver, but
which may occur in post-tetanic muscle. Thus activation of the
system depends primarily on conversion of the b to a form be
dephosphorylation (Fig. 2).

In this case, the effect of cyclic AMP-dependent protein
kinase is the reverse of that with phosphorylase, converting
synthetase to the inactive form. Thus the effect of cyclic AMP-
elevating hormones is to turn off synthetase synchronously with
the turning on of phosphorylase, and thereby diminishing futile
cycling of G-1-P into and out of glycogen.

Since the "off" form of synthetase is the phosphorylated form
and the reverse is true for phosphorylase, and since the "off"
forms are normally the predominant ones, it is apparent that the
kinase is a critical factor in converting phosphorylase to an
active state, but is of significance in the case of synthetase only
in promoting its return to an inactive state once activated. This
suggests that it is again the activating process, in this case
catalyzed by the phosphatase branch, which is the critical one in
regulating the tissue level of synthetase activity.

Furthermore, a number of factors which stimulate hepatic
glycogen synthesis have now been shown to be effectors of the
phosphatase branch of the glycogen synthetase system. Since
there is a close correlation in individual livers between the level
of glycogen synthetase a and the rate of glycogen synthesis, it
can be concluded that promotion of the phosphatase reaction,
with the consequent elevation of synthetase a levels and glycogen
synthesis, underlies in large measure the glycogenic effect of
these factors.

Thus the fundamental question in this case is, what are the regulatory processes of the phosphatase branch which convert synthetase to the active form and turn on glycogen synthesis? At present at least 4 factors appear to be involved in regulation of the phosphatase system, namely, glucocorticoids, insulin, glucose, and glycogen itself.

The long-known effect of glucocorticoids in promoting liver glycogen deposition can be attributed, in part at least, to a direct or indirect influence of these hormones on the phosphatase branch of the glycogen synthetase system. In adrenalectomized rats deprived of food, glycogen levels, synthetase a levels, and phosphatase activity are virtually nil. Several hours after glucocorticoid administration there is a restoration of phosphatase activity, synthetase a levels, and rates of glycogen synthesis in a sequence consistent with a causal relationship in that order. This effect, which appears to be mediated by insulin, is blocked by cycloheximide or actinomycin D, and thus may be concluded to depend upon an induction of the phosphatase or some other component which leads indirectly to an elevation of phosphatase activity (7).

A different type of glucocorticoid effect has also been observed. In this case pretreatment of animals with the hormone led to a phosphatase activity in liver extracts where the lag period which is normally observed prior to the expression of full activity was greatly reduced. Phosphorylase a is an inhibitor of synthetase phosphatase, and glucocorticoids increase the activity of phosphorylase phosphatase, which removes phosphorylase a. Therefore, it was proposed that the lag period represents the time required for removal of phosphorylase a and that the glucocorticoid response in these experiments depends on the increased rate of phosphorylase a removal (8).

Two types of effect of glucose on the phosphatase system have been observed. In the starved, adrenalectomized animals referred to above, intubation of glucose restored synthetase phosphatase activity similarly to but independently of the glucocorticoid effect (7). In this case the response was also blocked by cycloheximide, but not by actinomycin. A possible explanation for the glucocorticoid and glucose effects is that in the starved, adrenalectomized liver, a factor required for phosphatase stabilization (glycogen?) is lacking, and that this factor is restored by glucose administration, or by glucocorticoids via a process depending upon enzyme induction.

In contrast to the glucose effect referred to above, which requires a minimum of about 1 1/2 hours to become manifested, a

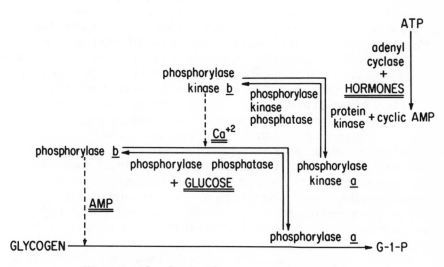

Figure 3. *The phosphorylase system and its regulation*

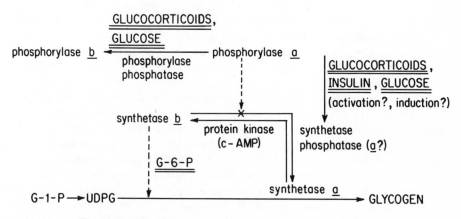

Figure 4. *The glycogen synthetase system and its regulation*

very rapid response to glucose of a different sort has also been observed. In normal animals or perfused livers therefrom, within a few minutes after glucose administration there was a rise in the levels of active synthetase (a form), together with a fall in phosphorylase a levels (9). Given the inhibition of synthetase phosphatase by phosphorylase a discussed above and the stimulatory effect of glucose on the phosphorylase phosphatase reaction which removes phosphorylase a (6), this acute glucose effect on synthetase activation appears to be explainable by its effect on the latter reaction. In livers from starved, adrenalectomized animals referred to above or in diabetic animals, where phosphatase activity has disappeared, the acute elevation of synthetase a in response to glucose does not occur.

The reduction in phosphatase activity in the diabetic state is restored several hours after insulin administration. Some evidence exists which suggests that the phosphatase exists in interconvertible forms differing in their sensitivity to Mg^{2+} and that insulin promotes conversion to the more active form (10), but the mechanism of the insulin effect still remains largely undefined.

Finally, there appears to be a type of feed-back regulation by glycogen itself, since, although low concentrations of glycogen promote the phosphatase reaction in vitro, at higher concentrations it is inhibitory. Furthermore, there is a correlation between the sensitivity of liver and muscle phosphatase to glycogen and the level of glycogen which these tissues can accumulate. That is, glycogen accumulation is cut off at a lower level in muscle than in liver, and its phosphatase is inhibited by a lower level of glycogen than is the liver phosphatase.

The foregoing regulatory elements are summarized in Fig. 4. Recent reviews of the glycogen synthetase system and its control have appeared (5, 11).

The regulation of glycogen metabolism is obviously complex and not all its intricacies have been related to the physiological role they subserve. Nevertheless, it seems clear that the key to understanding the adaptability provided by the rapid interconvertibility between active and inactive forms lies in the capability it provides to respond to external signals which override the internal restraints that maintain internal homeostasis. A number of critical aspects of the nature of the operation and control of these systems have not yet been solved. These include the specificity of the relevant phosphatases, whether the latter exist in interconvertible forms, and the mechanisms of their regulation.

Literature Cited

1. Zieve, F. J., and Glinsmann, W. H., Biochem. Biophys. Res. Commun. (1973), 50, 872–878.

2. Nakai, C., and Thomas, J. A., J. Biol. Chem. (1974), 249, 6459–6467.

3. Fischer, E. H., Pocker, A., and Saari, J. C., Essays in Biochem., ed. by P. N. Campbell and F. Dickens (1970), 6, 23–68.

4. Fischer, E. H., Heilmeyer, L. M. G., Jr., and Haschke, R. H., Current Topics in Cellular Regulation, ed. by B. L. Horecker and E. R. Stadtman (1971), 4, 211–251.

5. Segal, H. L., Science (1973), 180, 25–32.

6. Holmes, P. A., and Mansour, T. E., Biochim. Biophys. Acta (1968), 156, 275–284.

7. Gruhner, K., and Segal, H. L., Biochim. Biophys. Acta (1970), 222, 508–514.

8. Stalmans, W., De Wulf, H., and Hers, H. G., Europ. J. Biochem. (1971), 18, 582–587.

9. Glinsmann, W. H., Pauk, G., and Hern, E., Biochem. Biophys. Res. Commun. (1970), 39, 774–782.

10. Bishop, J. S., Biochim. Biophys. Acta (1970), 208, 208–218.

11. Larner, J., and Villar-Palasi, C., Current Topics in Cellular Regulation, ed. by B. L. Horecker and E. R. Stadtman (1971), 3, 195–233.

16

α-Amylase Inhibitors from Plants

J. JOHN MARSHALL

Laboratories for Biochemical Research, Howard Hughes Medical Institute and
Department of Biochemistry, University of Miami School of Medicine, Miami, Fla. 33152

Introduction

Many plants contain substances which are inhibitory to
enzyme action and among the most widespread of such compounds are
inhibitors of hydrolytic enzymes. In this article, the nature and
distribution of enzyme inhibitors in plants is reviewed, and
possible *in vivo* functions of these inhibitors are discussed.
Particular consideration will be given to the proteinaceous
inhibitors of the important digestive enzyme, α-amylase, including
the detection, assay, specificities and other properties, and
physiological effects of these inhibitors.

Distribution and Function of Hydrolytic Enzyme Inhibitors

A survey of the literature, summarized in Table 1, has revealed reports of inhibitors of proteases, ribonuclease, invertase,
polygalacturonase, cellulase and α-amylase from plant sources.
These inhibitors are of two general types - those which are
proteins and are rather specific for a particular enzyme, and
those which are non-proteinaceous, usually polyphenolic or tannin
in nature. Inhibitors of the latter type are much less specific,
often inhibiting a number of quite different enzymes.
Proteinaceous inhibitors of proteolytic enzymes have been
isolated from many plants, and their chemistry has been examined
in detail. Primary structures of many of these inhibitors are
known, credible mechanisms of action have been postulated, and the
nature of protease-inhibitor interaction has been examined by X-
ray crystallography (1-4). The role of protease inhibitors in
plants has not been established unequivocally; possible functions
include their involvement in the regulation of the activity of
plant proteases, protection of plants against microbial attack or
insect predation, or that they serve as storage proteins (3).
Inhibitors of other hydrolytic enzymes have been examined in
much less detail than the protease inhibitors and, with the
exception of α-amylase inhibitors, only brief mention of them will

TABLE 1

NATURALLY OCCURRING INHIBITORS OF HYDROLYTIC ENZYMES

Enzyme	Source of Inhibitor	Nature of Inhibitor	References
Protease	Many plants	Protein	1-3
Invertase	Potato	Protein	5-8
	Maize	Protein	9
	Ipomoea petals	Protein	10
Polygalacturonase	Bean hypocotyls, tomato stems, cultured sycamore cells	Protein	11-13
Cellulase	Many plants	Polyphenol	14-17
Ribonuclease	Lilac leaves	Probably protein	19
α-Amylase	Many plants	Polyphenol and protein	See Table 2

be made. Invertase inhibitors, which are proteins, probably serve
to regulate sucrose breakdown in plants. This can be said with
some degree of certainty because they do inhibit the corresponding
plant invertases (5-8). It has been suggested (11-13) that polygalacturonase inhibitors, which are also proteins, are involved in
protecting plants against invasion by plant pathogens, which
usually gain entry into plants by breakdown of the cell walls
under the action of pectic enzymes. Cellulase inhibitors (14-17)
are, apparently without exception, polyphenolic and may play a
role in protecting the structural material of plants against
degradation by cellulolytic micro-organisms. It is probable that
they also act to inhibit the cellulolytic enzymes of rumen microorganisms, so that such inhibitors may have an undesirable effect
on the growth characteristics of animals fed on materials rich in
such inhibitors (15,17,18). There is only one report (19) of an
inhibitor of ribonuclease in plants. It was suggested that this
inhibitor is proteinaceous; its *in vivo* function is not known.

Like the protease inhibitors, inhibitors of α-amylase appear
to be widely distributed throughout the plant kingdom, and because
of their ability to inactivate α-amylase *in vivo*, they may be of
considerable nutritional significance. For this reason, much
attention is now being focussed on these inhibitors. Their
function in plants is not yet known with certainty. However, consideration of the specificities of α-amylase inhibitors (*vide
infra*) suggests that they might serve to protect the seeds in
which they occur against predation by insects and animals, by
virtue of their inhibitory activity towards the digestive
amylases of the predators. Most α-amylase inhibitors are inactive towards microbial and plant α-amylases, indicating that they
are not antimicrobial agents, nor do they serve to regulate the
levels of α-amylase in the plants. The remainder of this article
reviews the current status of our knowledge regarding inhibitors
of α-amylase.

Detection and Assay of α-*Amylase Inhibitors*

A variety of methods for determination of α-amylase inhibitor
activities in plant extracts have been used, and virtually all
workers have expressed inhibitor activities in different ways.
However, with only a few exceptions it has been realized that it
is necessary to pre-incubate α-amylase and inhibitor for inhibition to take place, rather than simply to incorporate inhibitor
directly into a digest containing a mixture of enzyme and
substrate. For the most part, the duration, pH, temperature and
other conditions of pre-incubation appear to have been arbitrarily
chosen. After pre-incubation, uninhibited amylase activity
remaining has been determined by a variety of methods, most
usually based on the increase of reducing power [measured with
dinitrosalicylic acid (20) or an alkaline copper reagent (21)], or
by the decrease in iodine staining power (22), during action on

starch. Amylase inhibitor activities have in many instances been
expressed in units, based on the amount of inhibitor which will
inhibit a certain proportion of a fixed amount of α-amylase. It
has not usually been made clear whether the measured extent of
inhibition represents the maximum obtainable with the amount of
inhibitor used, or whether it is less than the maximum obtainable
with that amount of inhibitor. In the latter case, inhibitor
activity is being measured in terms of the rate of amylase
inhibition, rather than reflecting the stoichiometry of amylase-
inhibitor interaction.

     During recent studies (23) on the amylase inhibitor from
kidney beans *Phaseolus vulgaris*, particular attention was given to
the selection of pre-incubation conditions which express optimal
inhibitor activity. The findings highlighted the importance of
careful choice of the pre-incubation conditions. Assays based on
determination of the total amount of α-amylase which a sample of
the inhibitor can render inactive were unsatisfactory. Extended
pre-incubation times were required to achieve maximum inhibition,
and loss of α-amylase activity tended to occur during the pre-
incubation period, even in the absence of inhibitor. Measurement
of the rate of inhibition of α-amylase was found to be much more
convenient and accurate, and required only short pre-incubation
times.

     The conditions found suitable for assay of the kidney bean
inhibitor are summarized in Scheme I. A temperature of 37°C and
a pH of 5.5 are used for the pre-incubation, these conditions
being favorable for rapid inhibition of hog pancreatic α-amylase
by the kidney bean inhibitor (23). Calcium chloride and human
serum albumin are included in the pre-incubation digest, to protect the α-amylase against spontaneous inactivation. Amylase
activity is measured, after pre-incubation, by addition of starch
buffered at pH 6.9, and determination of the decrease in iodine
stain during incubation for 5 min. One unit of inhibitor activity
is defined as the amount which causes 50% inhibition of the α-
amylase during pre-incubation for 20 min. The extent of inhibition is proportional to the amount of inhibitor present and to the
duration of pre-incubation, provided the extent of incubation does
not exceed 50%. Thus the amount of inhibitor and the duration of
pre-incubation must be such as to give no more than this degree of
inhibition in order to ensure a valid assay.

     A simple method for detection of amylase inhibitors in
extracts of biological materials has recently been described (24).
A narrow cellulose strip saturated with the solution being examined for inhibitor, is placed on a buffered starch-agar gel plate
for 2 hours at 37°C. The strip is then removed and another narrow
strip saturated with amylase solution is placed on the gel at
right angles across the position occupied by the first strip.
After incubation for 6-18 hr at 37°C, the second strip is removed
and the slab is flooded with iodine solution, amylase activity
being shown by clear zones on a purple background. The presence

SCHEME I

ASSAY OF α-AMYLASE INHIBITOR ACTIVITY (23)

Pre-incubation: A 1.5 ml digest containing

hog pancreatic α-amylase (1 μg)
calcium chloride   (1.5 mg)
human serum albumin   (1.5 mg)
acetate buffer   6.7 mM, pH 5.5)
and inhibitor

is incubated at 37°C for a suitable
period of time (usually 20 min). The
amount of inhibitor present should be
sufficient to cause 10-50% inhibition of
the α-amylase during the pre-incubation
period.

Assay of Residual   Buffered soluble starch solution (1.0 ml
α-Amylase Activity: containing 10 mg starch in 100 mM
glycerophosphate buffer pH 6.9 and 20 mM
calcium chloride) is added to the pre-
incubation mixture. The resulting
digest is then incubated at 37°C for
exactly 5 min. The absorbance of the
starch-iodine complex obtained on addition of a sample of the digest (0.1 ml)
to 5.0 ml of 0.02% iodine - 0.2%
potassium iodide solution, is measured
at 680 nm. α-Amylase activity is
expressed as the difference in the
absorbance from that of a substrate
blank digest containing everything except α-amylase.

Controls: (1)   α-Amylase pre-incubated without inhibitor (gives the uninhibited activity).

(2)   In cases where the inhibitor preparation
also contains amylase activity, a sample
of the inhibitor preparation is preincubated with all the other digest
constituents except α-amylase, then
incubated with starch for the usual time.
This control is usually necessary when
crude extracts are being assayed.

Unit of Inhibitor: 1 Unit of inhibitor is the amount which
causes 50% inhibition of α-amylase in
20 min under the above conditions.

of inhibitor is indicated by interruption of the lysis zone where
the inhibitor-containing and amylase-containing strips crossed.
A variation of the method, involving measurement of the diameter
of cleared zones produced by amylase-inhibitor mixtures placed in
small wells cut in the starch-agar gel slab, was also described.
In view of the extended time required to obtain results, and their
essentially qualitative nature, there appears to be little advantage gained by the use of this method, rather than a more conventional inhibitor assay, such as that described above.

Properties of α-Amylase Inhibitors

General Properties. α-Amylase inhibitors have been known for
a considerable time, but compared with the protease inhibitors,
little is understood about their structures and mechanism of
action, their nutritional significance, or their role *in vivo*.
Proteinaceous and non-proteinaceous inhibitors of α-amylase have
been discovered (Table 2).

Insoluble α-amylase inhibitors, such as the "sisto-amylase"
described by Chrzaszcz and Janicki (30,31) may function simply by
adsorption of the enzyme, preventing its interaction with substrate, rather than by formation of a specific enzyme-inhibitor
complex. An ether-soluble substance from navy beans (54) interferes with α-amylase action on starch probably by interacting with
the substrate rather than the enzyme. Neither of these substances
can be considered a true inhibitor of α-amylase. Potato tubers
and certain varieties of sorghum contain dialyzable, non-
proteinaceous, α-amylase inhibitors (25-28). The inhibitor from
sorghum is the better characterized; it is dialyzable, heat-
stable (even on autoclaving), and organic-solvent soluble (27).
It inhibits many enzymes besides α-amylase, and appears to be a
tannin of the leucocyanidin group (28).

The properties of the inhibitor from sorghum contrast with
those of the proteinaceous α-amylase inhibitors, which are
specific for α-amylase, are non-dialyzable, and may be inactivated
by heating. Proteinaceous α-amylase inhibitors, although susceptible to heat inactivation, are generally rather heat-stable
proteins, often requiring prolonged heating at elevated temperatures, or even autoclaving, to destroy their activity completely.
Of all the proteinaceous α-amylase inhibitors which have been
isolated from plants (Table 2), the best known is that from wheat,
first studied by Kneen and his co-workers (36,37) in the 1940's,
although the inhibitors in rye (36,37), and in navy beans (51)
were first detected at about the same time.

Only those α-amylase inhibitors of the proteinaceous type
will be considered in detail. In the following sections the
specificities of inhibitors from different sources will be considered, then the properties of the two best-characterized
proteinaceous inhibitors of α-amylase, those from wheat and kidney
beans, will be discussed.

TABLE 2

NATURALLY OCCURRING INHIBITORS OF α-AMYLASE

Source of Inhibitor	Nature of Inhibitor	Characteristics	References
Potato tubers	Non-proteinaceous	Ether-soluble; dialyzable	25,26
Sorghum	Tannins of the leucocyanidin group	Organic-solvent soluble; general enzyme inactivator	27,28
Acorn	Not identified	Also inhibited β-amylase	29
Buckwheat malt	Protein	Water-insoluble; heat-labile (50°C)	30,31
Oat seeds	Protein	Non-dialyzable; heat-stable (100°C); also inhibited β-amylase; inhibition reversed by sulfhydryl compounds	32
Mangoes	Protein	Heat-labile (unspecified temperature); non-dialyzable	33
Colocasia esculenta tubers	Protein	Heat-stable (100°C); destroyed by autoclaving; non-dialyzable	34,35
Wheat	Protein	Refer to text	36-49
Rye	Protein	Heat-stable (100°C); non-dialyzable	45,50
Phaseolus vulgaris	Protein	Refer to text	23,51-53

Specificities of α-*Amylase Inhibitors.* Of the α-amylase inhibitors which are proteinaceous in nature, only two have been reported to inhibit enzymes other than α-amylase. An inhibitor preparation from navy beans also inhibited trypsin (51), but the activity towards the latter enzyme was probably due to contamination by a specific trypsin inhibitor, also known to be present in these beans (55). An inhibitor preparation from oats (32) inhibits both β-amylase and α-amylase. The ability to restore the activity of these enzymes by addition of sulfhydryl reagents, such as glutathione, indicated that the inhibition was the result of interaction of the polypeptide inhibitor with thiol groupings in the enzymes, rather than a specific protein-protein interaction as is considered to take place with other inhibitors. Thus the inhibitor from oat seeds, although apparently proteinaceous, belongs to a different class from the specific proteinaceous α-amylase inhibitors, in which we are primarily interested in this article.

α-Amylases from different sources show differences in susceptibility to inhibition by the specific proteinaceous inhibitors of α-amylase (Table 3). Furthermore, these inhibitors do not all have the same specificity. The inhibitor from *Colocasia esculenta* (34,35) has the simplest specificity; salivary α-amylase is the only enzyme it has been found to inhibit. Kneen and Sandstedt reported that the wheat inhibitor was active towards salivary and pancreatic α-amylases, and also the saccharifying type (56) of bacterial α-amylase; it was without action on the more common bacterial α-amylase, the liquefying type, or on plant α-amylase (36,37). In a more recent study of the wheat inhibitor (40,42), Shainkin and Birk separated two proteins with inhibitory action. One of these (designated Aml_2) had specificity similar to that reported by Kneen and Sandstedt (36,37), and was also found to inhibit insect (*Tenebrio molitor* larval midgut) α-amylase (57). The second form (Aml_1) inhibited only the insect α-amylase. Similar findings were reported by Silano and co-workers (47). The α-amylase inhibitor from rye (36,37,45) inhibits salivary and pancreatic α-amylases and, like that from wheat, is without action on bacterial liquefying α-amylase and plant α-amylase (50). Jaffé and co-workers reported that a partly purified inhibitor from kidney beans (*Phaseolus vulgaris*) was active towards salivary and pancreatic α-amylases, and also to a small extent against bacterial liquefying α-amylase (53). Studies in our Laboratory (23) did not support the suggestion that bacterial α-amylase is inhibited by the *Phaseolus vulgaris* inhibitor. The most likely explanation of these different findings is that the Venezuelan workers may not have included adequate controls, to correct for the spontaneous loss of α-amylase activity during pre-incubation. In the case of the bacterial enzyme, such losses are particularly large because of the presence of traces of proteolytic enzymes, even in crystalline preparations of the amylase (58). The inhibitor from kidney beans also inhibits *Helix pomatia* (snail) α-amylase, but at about only half the rate it inhibits salivary

TABLE 3

SPECIFICITIES OF INHIBITORS TOWARDS α-AMYLASES FROM DIFFERENT SOURCES

Source of Inhibitor	Reference	α-Amylase							
		Salivary	Pancreatic	Fungal	Bacterial (liquefying)	Bacterial (saccharifying)	Plant	*Helix pomatia*	Insect (*Tenebrio molitor*)
Colocasia esculenta	34,35	+	-	-	-	ND	ND	ND	ND
Rye	50	+	+	-	-	ND	-	ND	ND
Wheat	36,37	+	+	-	-	+	-	ND	ND
Aml_1	42[a]	-	-	-	-	ND	-	ND	+
Aml_2	42[a]	+	+	-	-	ND	-	ND	+
Phaseolus vulgaris	52,53	+	+	ND	+	ND	-	ND	ND
	23	+	+	-	-	-	-	+	ND

+ indicates inhibition; - indicates no inhibition; ND indicates not determined. The relative affinities of a particular inhibitor for the different α-amylases, when these are known, are discussed in the text.

[a] similar results reported in Refs. 47 and 48.

and pancreatic α-amylases, the latter two enzymes being inactivated at almost identical rates (23).   In this respect the bean inhibitor differs markedly from one cereal (rye) α-amylase inhibitor, which acts on the salivary enzyme about 10-times faster than on the pancreatic enzyme (50).   One possible explanation for the difference in rate of inhibition of these two α-amylases is that the carbohydrate present in the latter (59), but apparently absent from the former, interferes with enzyme-inhibitor interaction.   Decrease in susceptibility to inhibition by naturally occurring proteinaceous inhibitors has previously been observed after chemical attachment of carbohydrate to pancreatic α-amylase and pancreatic trypsin (60).   At the present time, the differences in susceptibility of amylases to inhibition are not clearly understood.   However the possibility does exist that studies of enzyme-inhibitor interaction will eventually be of value in examinations of the structures and active site topography of α-amylases.

α-Amylase Inhibitors from Wheat.   The α-amylase inhibitor from wheat has received more attention than any of the other α-amylase inhibitors.   Initial studies on the inhibitor (36,37), prepared by extraction of wheat flour with water, followed by boiling to destroy endogenous amylase activity, showed it to have the properties of a protein.   Thus the inhibitor was precipitated by ammonium sulfate, and by high concentrations of ethanol. Although it was quite thermostable, being little affected by prolonged storage at 70°C, or on boiling for short periods, auto-claving at 121°C for 30 min caused complete loss of inhibitor activity.   As well as being water-soluble, the inhibitor was also soluble in aqueous ethanol at concentrations up to 70% ethanol. The ethanol solubility was used to demonstrate that amylase inhibition was reversible, addition of ethanol to a final concentration of 70% precipitating α-amylase from a mixture of amylase and inhibitor, leaving the inhibitor in solution.   Kneen and Sandstedt (36,37) reported that complete inhibition of α-amylase with the wheat inhibitor could not be achieved;   this observation may indicate that amylase inhibition is partly reversible by substrate.   Treatment with pepsin rendered the inhibitor inactive.

The production of wheat inhibitor with kernel development was followed, and showed that the inhibitor was produced just as the kernels reached maturity, approximately 15 days after flowering (36,37).   It did not disappear on germination.   Since the level of inhibitor was markedly lower in wheat brans than in whole ground wheat, the suggestion was made that the majority of the inhibitor is located in the endosperm.   The inhibitor was present in similar amounts in all wheats tested, namely hard red winter wheat, soft red winter wheat, and hard red spring wheat.

Subsequent work (38) on the wheat inhibitor resulted in a 750-fold purification from wheat extracts by a 70°C heat treatment, ethanol fractionation and adsorption on alumina.   The ability to

inactivate the inhibitor by treating with nitrous acid, which
reacts with protein amino groups, and by digestion with the
proteolytic enzyme, ficin, was presented as further evidence that
the inhibitor is a protein. Papain, however, did not destroy its
activity. These later studies (39) showed some differences from
the earlier findings (36,37). Thus, purification involved precipitation with 70% ethanol; previously the inhibitor was reported
to be soluble in this concentration of alcohol, and no reason was
suggested for the apparent discrepancy. A further difference was
in the effect of dialysis on the activity of the inhibitor. While
activity was retained on dialysis against tap water or salt
solutions, the activity of the purified material was lost on
dialysis against distilled water. This observation was taken to
indicate the requirement for a dialyzable inorganic cofactor for
activity. The less-pure preparation used earlier did not lose
activity on dialysis against distilled water, and it was suggested
that contaminating proteins in that preparation in some way prevented exhaustion of cofactor during dialysis.

The heat stability properties of the purified inhibitor
preparation were examined under a variety of conditions, from
which it was found that activity was lost faster in alkaline than
in acidic solution, at any particular temperature (38).
Denaturation was achieved in 10 min at 95°C and pH 9.0. At pH 5.3,
more than 60 min was required. The stability of the inhibitor,
even in acidic solution, appeared to be lower than that reported
previously (36,37), but again the reason may have been the
stabilizing effect of contaminating proteins in the less pure
preparation.

The inhibitor was inactivated by a number of reducing agents,
i.e. sodium sulfite, hydrogen sulfide and ascorbic acid (39).
Oxidizing agents - chlorine, bromine, sodium chlorite and hydrogen
peroxide - were even more effective in causing loss of activity.
A strong positive test for tryptophan in the inhibitor preparation,
together with the knowledge that oxidizing agents readily attack
tryptophan, led to the suggestion that tryptophan plays an important part in the activity of the inhibitor (39). Further support
for the important role of tryptophan came from the observation
that aldehydes, such as acetaldehyde and benzaldehyde, which react
with indole rings, also caused inactivation.

Freshly prepared solutions of the purified inhibitor increased in inhibitory power on standing, this being explained on the
basis of dissociation to reveal the active sites responsible for
combination with α-amylase (39). It was also shown that inhibition of α-amylase did not take place instantaneously on addition of
inhibitor, but increased during a period of pre-incubation of
enzyme and inhibitor, before addition of starch. A study of the
nature of the inhibition showed this to be non-competitive. This
latter finding was considered to be in accord with the difference
in the effect of the inhibitor towards different α-amylases (*vide
supra*). If the inhibitor acted by competing with starch for the

active site of the enzyme, all amylases would have been expected
to be affected. Since the reaction is non-competitive, it follows
that certain amylases have groupings which can combine with the
inhibitor, while others do not, although all the amylases have the
catalytic groupings necessary for starch hydrolysis.

The inhibitor from wheat received little further attention
until recently; it is now being investigated by several groups of
workers. Shainkin and Birk (40-42) purified two forms of the α-
amylase inhibitor from wheat flour by ammonium sulfate fractionation, and chromatography on DEAE-cellulose and CM-cellulose.
These two inhibitors, designated AmI_1 and AmI_2, differed in
specificity (Table 3), in molecular weight (18,000 for AmI_1 and
26,000 for AmI_2), and in many other properties (42). Dilute
solutions of AmI_1 were not affected when boiled (at unspecified
pH) for 10 min, whereas AmI_2 lost 10-15% of its activity after
1 min, and 70-80% after 10 min. Treatment with 6.4 M urea for
24 hr had no affect on the inhibitory activity of AmI_1 and AmI_2,
but reduction with mercaptoethanol in the presence or absence of
6.4 M urea resulted in total loss of activity in both cases. The
differences between the two inhibitors were apparent from their
susceptibility to digestion with proteases. AmI_1 was inactivated
by trypsin and chymotrypsin, whereas AmI_2 was resistant to these
enzymes. Pronase completely destroyed AmI_1 and 60% of the AmI_2
in 3 hr; pepsin readily inactivated both forms of the inhibitor.
AmI_1 and AmI_2 also reacted in a different manner when subjected to
chemical modifications such as esterification with methanol/HCl,
and on carboxymethylation at different pH values affecting select-
ively methionine, histidine and aromatic amino acids, as well as
on cleavage with cyanogen bromide (42). On the whole, AmI_2 was
more sensitive to these treatments than was AmI_1. Cyanogen
bromide treatment, performed in a controlled manner, removed all
the activity of AmI_2 towards salivary α-amylase, but had little
effect on the activity of AmI_2, or the more specific inhibitor
AmI_1, towards *Tenebrio molitor* α-amylase. On the basis of this
finding it was suggested that AmI_2 is comprized of AmI_1 plus an
additional peptide fragment which contains the binding site for
salivary α-amylase.

Inhibition of α-amylase by the wheat inhibitors was markedly
greater after pre-incubation of enzyme with inhibitor, followed
by addition of substrate, than after pre-incubation of substrate
with inhibitor, followed by addition of enzyme (41,42). A
similar situation is observed in the case of α-amylase inhibitor
from kidney beans (*vide infra*). Although addition of substrate
cannot reverse inhibition, when α-amylase is added to a mixture
of kidney bean inhibitor and excess substrate, the enzyme acts at
the same rate as it does in the absence of inhibitor (23).
Shainkin and Birk suggested that pre-incubation of substrate and
inhibitor gives a complex in which the amylase binding site in
the inhibitor is masked. However, in the absence of any good
evidence to show that inhibitor and substrate do actually

associate, the low extent of inhibition observed when α-amylase
is added last can be explained simply on the basis of the affinity
of the enzyme for its substrate, and the high concentration of the
substrate compared with inhibitor in the mixture, so that substrate protects the enzyme from inactivation by the inhibitor.

The data on solubility, charge properties, amino acid
composition and molecular weights of the inhibitors (42) suggested
a resemblance of these proteins to the gliadins (43), wheat
proteins without any previously known biological activity. The
possible relation between wheat α-amylase inhibitor and the wheat
gliadins was also recognized by Strumeyer, who prepared the
inhibitor by water extraction of wheat flour, followed by heat
treatment at 70°C, then ammonium sulfate and ethanol precipitation
(45). Molecular-sieve chromatography gave a value of 55,000 for
the molecular weight of the inhibitor (46), this being rather
different from that reported by Shainkin and Birk (42), and others
(47-49). Recent studies in this Laboratory (50), however, support
Strumeyer's value. Disc electrophoresis of the purified inhibitor
showed two major protein bands, wiich corresponded in electrophoretic mobility to the α-gliadins (46). The amino acid
composition of the inhibitor preparation showed that it contained
high amounts of glutamine (30%) and proline (50%), but a low level
of lysine (less than 1%). None of these figures is similar to
those in the amino acid analysis of the two forms of inhibitor
isolated by Shainkin and Birk. Strumeyer and Fisher demonstrated
complex formation between inhibitor and α-amylase by gel
filtration (46).

Silano and co-workers (47), like Shainkin and Birk (42), have
separated two types of α-amylase inhibitor from wheat, by using
chromatography on columns of Sephadex G-100. They have also shown
(48) that albumins from the kernels of hexaploid wheat can be
separated electrophoretically into six fractions. Five of these
albumins had very similar properties, and were considered to
belong to a family of closely related proteins; all inhibited
Tenebrio molitor α-amylase, but no other α-amylase. The sixth
albumin, designated 0.19, was distinct from the others, and
inhibited salivary and pancreatic α-amylases in addition to
Tenebrio molitor α-amylase. The 0.19 albumin contained two non-
identical subunits (48). One subunit, responsible for the inhibitory activity towards *Tenebrio molitor* α-amylase, was considered
to be a member of the five albumin family specific for this
amylase. The nature of the second subunit, responsible for the
inhibitory activity of 0.19 albumin towards salivary α-amylase was
not clear. It was also proposed (48) that 0.19 albumin corresponded to the AmI_2 inhibitor isolated by Shainkin and Birk (42).
While these latter workers had suggested (42) that the polypeptide
chain of AmI_2 consisted of AmI_1, plus an additional peptide
segment, Silano and co-workers proposed (48) that AmI_2, like
0.19 albumin, contained two subunits, one of which was AmI_1.

The situation regarding the number of α-amylase inhibitors in

wheat, and their relationship, has become more confused following
a recent report from Saunders and Lang (49). These workers
separated two albumin proteins with inhibitory activity, termed
inhibitors I and II, by chromatography of a heat-treated wheat
extract on DEAE-Sephadex. Inhibitors I and II had almost identical physical properties (pI 6.7, molecular weight 20,000 for I;
pI 6.5, molecular weight 21,000 for II) and it is not clear
whether they are distinct proteins, or whether the fractionation
was artefactual. Inhibitors I and II were distinct from Silano's
0.19 albumin (pI 7.3, molecular weight 23,800). Each inhibitor,
I, II and 0.19 was reported to act in an uncompetitive fashion
against pancreatic α-amylase, with K_i 5 x 10^{-8}M.

Further work will be necessary to clarify the exact number of
α-amylase inhibitors present in wheat, and to define their
relationship at the molecular level.

α-Amylase Inhibitor from Phaseolus vulgaris. Although it was
first detected in the 1940's (51), the α-amylase inhibitor present
in beans did not receive further attention until recently. The
observation that rats fed on diets of raw kidney beans excreted
undigested starch (61) prompted Jaffé and his co-workers to
examine extracts of these beans for the factors responsible. They
purified an α-amylase inhibitor 3-fold from a crude extract, by
heat treatment at 60°C for 30 min (52). The partly purified
inhibitor, which was non-dialyzable and was destroyed by heating
at 100°C for 15 min, had the properties of a protein. Its
molecular weight was judged, by molecular-sieve chromatography on
Sephadex, to be greater than 50,000. The nature of the inhibition
was reported to be non-competitive. Inhibitors with apparently
similar properties are present in many varieties of beans and
other legumes (53).

Kidney bean α-amylase inhibitor has recently been prepared
in a high state of purity in this Laboratory (23), by using a
series of conventional fractionation techniques (summarized in
Table 4). The close correlation between protein and inhibitor
activity in the fraction from the CM-cellulose column (Fig. 1),
the final step in the purification scheme, was taken as indicative
of purification to homogeneity. This was confirmed by polyacrylamide gel electrophoresis and analytical ultracentrifugation.

Purification can also be achieved (23) by taking advantage of
the affinity of the enzyme for Sepharose-bound α-amylase, the
inhibitor being recovered by washing with pH 3.0 buffer - probably
as a result of destruction of the acid-labile α-amylase. This
method is, however, not used routinely because purification can
be achieved so readily by the conventional fractionation techniques.

Examination of the properties of the inhibitor (23) showed
that the inhibition was pH dependent - a phenomenon which has not
been observed, nor apparently even investigated, in the case of
studies on other α-amylase inhibitors. The maximum rate of

TABLE 4

PURIFICATION OF PHASEOLUS VULGARIS α-AMYLASE INHIBITOR (23)

Steps and procedures	Total units[a]	Total protein (mg)	Specific activity (units/mg)	Recovery (%)	Purification
Step 1 : crude extract (500g beans)	312,800	64,600	4.8	100	
Step 2 : heat treatment (70°C, 15 min)	222,600	34,000	6.5	71	1.4
Step 3 : dialysis	203,200	10,100	20.1	65	4.2
Step 4 : DEAE-cellulose chromatography	142,500	3,100	46	46	9.6
Step 5 : Sephadex G-100 chromatography	150,100	1,150	131	48	27.3
Step 6 : CM-cellulose chromatography	116,700	770	152	37	31.7

[a] Activities determined as in Scheme I.

inhibition of α-amylase is observed at pH 5.5, the rate dropping off sharply at higher pH values. Inhibitor activity is also strongly dependent on the temperature of pre-incubation; inhibition of α-amylase takes place about 20-times faster at 37°C than at 25°C, and is negligible at 0°C. However, once inhibition has occurred, it cannot be reversed by conditions which are themselves unfavorable for inhibitor activity - low temperature or alkaline pH. Neither can substrate reverse the inhibition, showing that α-amylase has greater affinity for the inhibitor than it has for its substrate. Interaction of α-amylase and inhibitor is reversed at low pH, presumably as a result of α-amylase destruction as indicated above. Investigation of the stoichiometry of interaction has shown that hog-pancreatic α-amylase and inhibitor combine in a 1:1 fashion. Complex formation has been demonstrated directly by molecular-sieve chromatography on Sephadex G-100 after pre-incubation of stoichiometric amounts of α-amylase and inhibitor (Fig. 2). *Phaseolus vulgaris* α-amylase inhibitor has a molecular weight of approximately 45,000, this being somewhat lower than the value reported by Jaffé and co-workers (52). At the present time nothing is known about the role of functional group(s) contributing to the activity of the inhibitor.

Physiological Effects and Nutritional Significance of α-Amylase Inhibitors

The presence of high levels of α-amylase inhibitors in common plant foodstuffs, particularly legumes and cereals, raises the question whether these inhibitors can have any effect on α-amylases *in vivo* and, if so, whether this results in impaired starch digestion.

Miller and Kneen (27) suggested that the polyphenolic inhibitor in sorghum is unlikely to have an effect *in vivo*, because it is rather readily rendered ineffective as a result of its ability to combine with many proteins besides α-amylase. However, brown sorghums, which contain high levels of tannins, have been shown to retard growth of chicks, and to interfere with dry matter digestibility in rats, more than does white (low tannin) sorghum (62-66). The effect on growth, and foodstuff digestibility, may be caused by the tannins, and might well explain the bird-resistant properties of brown sorghums (62). It might also be noted that Mandels and Reese (15) believe that tannin-containing plants are likely to be undesirable foods for ruminants because of the inhibition of rumen cellulase by tannins (17). Grazing animals, and even snails, avoid plants high in tannins, perhaps because of their inhibitory effect on hydrolytic enzymes (67).

The susceptibility to proteolysis of the proteinaceous α-amylase inhibitor from wheat has been mentioned above. On the basis of this finding, Kneen and Sandstedt (37) concluded that it would be inactivated by pepsin in the stomach, and that the only

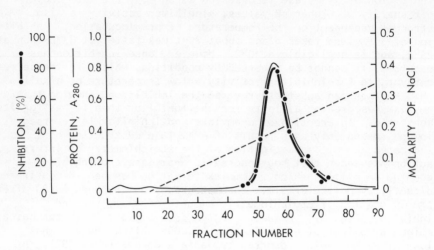

Figure 1. *Purification of* Phaseolus vulgaris *α-amylase inhibitor by chromatography on CM-cellulose* (23)

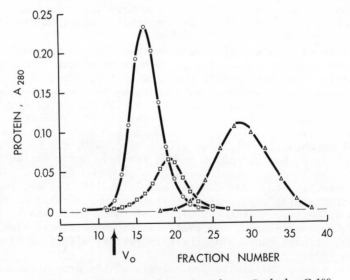

Figure 2. *Molecular sieve chromatography on Sephadex G-100 of hog pancreatic* α-amylase (△), Phaseolus vulgaris *α-amylase inhibitor* (□), *and* α-amylase/inhibitor complex (○) (23)

effect the inhibitor would have *in vivo* would be on salivary α-amylase. They therefore suggested that the wheat inhibitor would have little or no significance in normal human physiology, and that only in cases of impaired proteolysis would interference with starch hydrolysis be anticipated. Shainkin and Birk (42) came to the same conclusion.

Evidence is, however, now accumulating to suggest that the proteinaceous inhibitors of α-amylase may play an important role in modulating starch digestion *in vivo*. It has been suggested that wheat amylase inhibitors may be, at least in part, responsible for the differences in nutritional value of different varieties of wheat, as measured by the retardation of development of *Tribolium castaneum* (Herbst) larvae, compared with the optimal development achieved on a standard minimal artificial diet (68). Recent work has shown in a more convincing fashion that the α-amylase inhibitor in wheat will interfere with starch metabolism *in vivo*. In this Laboratory it has been shown that certain human and animal foodstuffs contain high levels of α-amylase inhibitor activity (69). Rats fed on a diet of one laboratory animal food-stuff (Ralston Purina rat chow) in which the inhibitor had been inactivated by autoclaving, grew at a rate 15-20% faster than did rats fed on the untreated feed. Similarly, when groups of rats were fed on a casein/starch diet in the presence and absence of purified wheat inhibitor, reduction of growth rate and increased fecal starch levels were caused by the presence of inhibitor, the magnitude of these changes being dependent on the inhibitor dosage (70). Added inhibitor did not have any effect when sucrose replaced starch as dietary carbohydrate; neither did inactivated inhibitor affect starch utilization. Strumeyer (45) has recently suggested that amylase inhibitors may be responsible for the sensitivity to wheat and rye flour in celiac disease - a gluten-induced enteropathy. Individuals with this disorder exhibit impaired ability to metabolize starch and absorb fats. These nutrients are excreted and the patients suffer from vitamin deficiency and malnutrition. According to Strumeyer (45) the cereal amylase inhibitors might be responsible for the sensitivity to wheat and rye flours by depression of an already deficient pancreatic α-amylase supply.

It is probable that bean α-amylase inhibitor is also active *in vivo*. Venezuelan workers have detected large amounts of un-digested starch, and amylase inhibitory activity, in the feces of rats fed on diets of raw kidney beans (61,71). Evans and co-workers have studied the effect of different protein fractions from *Phaseolus vulgaris* on the growth of rats. They concluded that there is present in beans a growth inhibitory factor distinct from the other toxic factors, phytohemagglutinins and protease inhibitors (72,73). Many of the properties of this growth-inhibitory protein (73) resemble those of the *Phaseolus vulgaris* α-amylase inhibitor purified and characterized in this Laboratory (23).

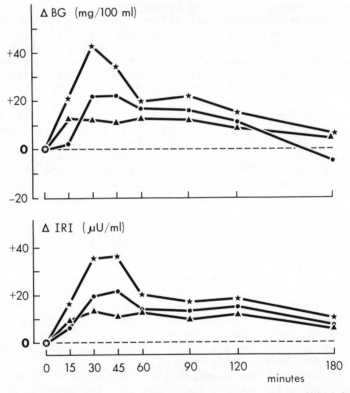

Diabetologia

*Figure 3.   Elevation of blood glucose (ΔBG) and serum insulin (ΔIRI)
levels in healthy human subjects following intake of starch (100 g) in
the absence of wheat α-amylase inhibitor (*) and in the presence of
inhibitor (●, 350 mg; ▲, 700 mg). Results shown are the mean for
seven subjects (75).*

In view of their *in vivo* action, the presence of α-amylase
inhibitors in foodstuffs prepared from plants such as wheat, rye
and beans, is clearly undesirable when maximum nutritional value
of the foodstuff is required. Wheat amylase inhibitor has been
reported to persist through bread baking, being found in large
amounts in the centers of loaves (37, 74). In this Laboratory it
has been shown that a number of common laboratory animal feeds,
of which wheat is a major constituent, contain inhibitor activity
(69). The same is true of a number of wheat-based human breakfast
cereals (69). It would seem likely that the true caloric value of
these foodstuffs will be lower than expected on the basis of their
starch contents, because of the interference with starch digestion
caused by endogeneous inhibitor. The relatively stable nature of
α-amylase inhibitors means that special attention will be required
to ensure their destruction or removal during food processing.

Finally, it is appropriate to consider α-amylase inhibitors
as possible therapeutic agents. The ability of these substances
to block starch degradation by α-amylase *in vivo* suggests their
possible use as novel dietetic agents, of use in the therapy of
obesity in subjects who find difficulty in completely eliminating
starch from their diets. A second application would be to allow
diabetic individuals to consume a moderate amount of starch, if
ingested in the presence of inhibitor. The effect of the inhibit-
or on starch digestion will help prevent the elevated blood sugar
level which normally results from starch intake, and which is
undesirable in the diabetic.

Puls and his co-workers (44) have patented a wheat α-amylase
inhibitor preparation, and have proposed its use as an antihyper-
glycemic agent. Their studies with this inhibitor provide the
most convincing evidence of the *in vivo* effect of an α-amylase
inhibitor, and support its possible use as a therapeutic agent.
On administration of the wheat inhibitor to rats, dogs and
healthy human subjects, the hyperglycemia and hyperinsulinemia
resulting from starch loading could be reduced dose dependently
by the inhibitor (75). The effect of inhibitor on the levels of
blood glucose and insulin in human subjects following ingestion
of raw starch is shown in Fig. 3. When cooked, as opposed to raw,
starch was used, the smoothing effect on hyperglycemia was somewhat reduced. The suggestion was made that this might be because
the affinity of amylase for gelatinized starch is greater than the
affinity for the inhibitor, and it was suggested that an inhibitor
with greater affinity for α-amylase might be advantageous for
therapeutic use.

Acknowledgements

Helpful discussion with Dr. W.J. Whelan is gratefully acknow-
ledged. J.J. Marshall is an Investigator of Howard Hughes Medical
Institute.

Literature Cited

1. FRITZ, H. and TSCHESCHE, H. (eds.), *Proceedings of the International Conference on Proteinase Inhibitors, Munich, Nov. 1970* , Walter de Gruyter, Berlin, 1971.
2. WERLE, E. and ZICKGRAF-RÜDEL, G., *Z. Klin. Chem. u. Klin. Biochem.* (1972) 4, 139-150.
3. RYAN, C.A., *Ann. Rev. Plant Physiol.* (1973) 24, 173-196.
4. RÜHLMANN, A., KUKLA, D., SCHWAGER, P., BARTELS, K. and HUBER, R., *J. Mol. Biol.* (1973) 77, 417-436.
5. SCHWIMMER, S., MAKAVER, R.U. and ROREM, E.S., *Plant Physiol.* (1961) 36, 313-316.
6. PRESSEY, R., *Arch. Biochem. Biophys.* (1966) 113, 667-674.
7. PRESSEY, R., *Plant Physiol.* (1967) 42, 1780-1786.
8. PRESSEY, R. and SHAW, R., *Plant Physiol.* (1966) 41, 1657-1661.
9. JAYNES, T.A. and NELSON, O.E., *Plant Physiol.* (1971) 47, 629-634.
10. WINKENBACH, F. and MATILE, P., *Z. Pflanzenphysiologie* (1970) 63, 292-295.
11. ALBERSHEIM, P. and ANDERSON, A.J., *Proc. Nat. Acad. Sci. U.S.* (1971) 68, 1815-1819.
12. ANDERSON, A.J. and ALBERSHEIM, P., *Physiol. Plant Pathol.* (1972) 2, 339-346.
13. FISHER, M.L., ANDERSON, A.J. and ALBERSHEIM, P., *Plant Physiol.* (1973) 51, 489-491.
14. MANDELS, M., HOWLETT, W. and REESE, E.T., *Can. J. Microbiol.* (1961) 7, 957-959.
15. MANDELS, M. and REESE, E.T., in REESE, E.T. (ed.), *Advances in Enzymic Hydrolysis of Cellulose and Related Materials*, pp. 115-157, Pergamon Press, Oxford, 1963.
16. MANDELS, M. and REESE, E.T., *Ann. Rev. Phytopathol.* (1965) 3, 85-102.
17. SMART, W.W.G., BELL, T.A., STANLEY, N.W. and COPE, W.A., *J. Dairy Sci.* (1961) 44, 1945-1946.
18. KING, K.W., *Va. Agric. Exp. Sta. Tech. Bull.* 127, December 1956.
19. BERNHEIMER, A.W. and STEELE, J.M., *Proc. Soc. Exp. Biol. Med.* (1955) 89, 123-126.
20. BERNFELD, P., in COLOWICK, S.P. and KAPLAN, N.O. (eds.), *Methods in Enzymology*, Vol. 1, pp. 149-158, Academic Press, New York, 1955.
21. NELSON, N., *J. Biol. Chem.* (1944) 153, 375-380.
22. HOPKINS, R.H. and BIRD, R., *Biochem. J.* (1954) 56, 86-99.
23. LAUDA, C.M. and MARSHALL, J.J., in preparation (1975).
24. FOSSUM, K. and WHITAKER, J.R., *J. Nutr.* (1974) 104, 930-936.
25. HEMBERG, T. and LARSSON, I., *Physiol. Plant* (1961) 14, 861-867.

26. SUKHORUKOV, I., KLING, E. and OVCHAROV, K., *Compt. Rend. Acad. Sci. URSS* (1939) 18, 597-602, *via Chem. Abs.* (1938) 32, 6686[4].

27. MILLER, B.S. and KNEEN, E., *Arch. Biochem.* (1947) 15, 251-264.

28. STRUMEYER, D.H. and MALIN, M.J., *Biochim. Biophys. Acta* (1969) 184, 643-645.

29. STANKOVIC, S.C. and MARKOVIC, N.D., *Glasnik Hem. Drustva, Beograd* (1960-1961) 25-26, 519-525, *via Chem. Abs.* (1963) 59, 3084d.

30. CHRZASZCZ, T. and JANICKI, J., *Biochem. Z.* (1933) 260, 354-368.

31. CHRZASZCZ, T. and JANICKI, J., *Biochem. Z.* (1933) 264, 192-208.

32. ELLIOTT, B.B. and LEOPOLD, A.C., *Physiol. Plant* (1953) 6, 65-77.

33. MATTOO, A.K. and MODI, V.V., *Enzymologia* (1970) 39, 237-247.

34. RAO, M.N., SHURPALEKAR, K.S. and SUNDARAVALLI, O.E., *Ind. J. Biochem.* (1967) 4, 185.

35. RAO, M.N., SHURPALEKAR, K.S. and SUNDARAVALLI, O.E., *Ind. J. Biochem.* (1970) 7, 241-243.

36. KNEEN, E. and SANDSTEDT, R.M., *J. Amer. Chem. Soc.* (1943) 65, 1247.

37. KNEEN, E. and SANDSTEDT, R.M., *Arch. Biochem.* (1946) 9, 235-249.

38. MILITZER, W., IKEDA, C. and KNEEN, E., *Arch. Biochem.* (1947) 15, 309-320.

39. MILITZER, W., IKEDA, C. and KNEEN, E., *Arch. Biochem.* (1947) 15, 321-329.

40. SHAINKIN, R. and BIRK, Y., *Israel J. Chem.* (1966) 3, 96.

41. SHAINKIN, R. and BIRK, Y., *Israel J. Chem.* (1967) 5, 129 p.

42. SHAINKIN, R. and BIRK, Y., *Biochim. Biophys. Acta* (1970) 221, 502-513.

43. POMERANZ, Y. (ed.) *Wheat Chemistry and Technology*, 2nd edn. American Association of Cereal Chemists, St.Paul, Minn.,1971.

44. SCHMIDT, D. and PULS, W., German Patent 2,003,934, Aug. 5, 1971, *via Chem. Abs.* (1971) 75, 91296 p.

45. STRUMEYER, D.H., *Nutr. Rep. Intern.* (1972) 5, 45-52.

46. STRUMEYER, D.H. and FISHER, B.R., *Fed. Proc.*, (1973) 32, 624.

47. SILANO, V., MINUTTI, M., PETRUCCI, T., TOMASI, M. and POCCHIARI, F., *Abs. 9th Intern. Congr. Biochem.*, Stockholm *1973*, Abs. 2p12.

48. SILANO, V., POCCHIARI, F. and KASARDA, D.D. *Biochim. Biophys. Acta* (1973) 317, 139-148.

49. SAUNDERS, R.M. and LANG, J.A., *Phytochem.* (1973) 12, 1237-1241.

50. LAUDA, C.M. and MARSHALL, J.J., unpublished work (1974).

51. BOWMAN, D.E., *Science* (1945) 102, 358-359.

52. HERNANDEZ, A. and JAFFÉ, W.G., *Acta Cient. Venezolana* (1968) 19, 183-185.

53. JAFFÉ, W.G.,MORENO, R. and WALLIS, V., *Nutr. Rep. Intern.* (1973) 7, 169-174.
54. BOWMAN, D.E., *Science* (1943) 98, 308-309.
55. PUSZTAI, A., *Europ. J. Biochem.* (1968) 5, 252-259.
56. KNEEN, E. and BECKFORD, L.D., *Arch. Biochem.* (1946) 10, 41-54.
57. APPLEBAUM, S.W., JANKOVIC, M. and BIRK, Y., *J. Insect Physiol.* (1961) 7, 100-108.
58. FISCHER, E.H. and STEIN, E.A., in BOYER, P.D., LARDY, H. and MYRBÄCK, K. (eds.), *The Enzymes*, 2nd edn., Vol. 4, pp. 313-343, Academic Press, New York, 1960.
59. BEAUPOIL-ABADIE, B., RAFFALI, M., COZZONE, P. and MARCHIS-MOUREN, G., *Biochim. Biophys. Acta* (1973) 297, 436-440.
60. MARSHALL, J.J., in preparation (1975).
61. JAFFÉ, W.G. and LETTE, C.L.V., *J. Nutr.* (1968) 94, 203-210.
62. MAXSON, E.D. and ROONEY, L.W., *Cer. Sci. Today* (1972) 17, 260.
63. FULLER, H.L., POTTER, D.K. and BROWN, A.R., *Bull. N.S. 176*, Univ. Georgia, Coll. Agr. Exp. Sta., Athens, Ga., Nov. 1966.
64. MAXSON, E.D., ROONEY, L.W., LEWIS, R.W., CLARK, L.E. and JOHNSON, J.W., *Nutr. Rep. Intern.* (1973) 8, 145-152.
65. CONNOR, J.K., HARWOOD, I.S., BURTON, H.W. and FUELLING, D.E., *Aust. J. Exp. Agr. Anim. Husb.* (1969) 9, 497-501.
66. CHANG, S.I. and FULLER, H.L., *Poultry Sci.* (1964) 43, 30-36.
67. NIERENSTEIN, M., *The Natural Organic Tannins: History, Chemistry, Distribution*, p. 287, Churchill, London, 1934.
68. APPLEBAUM, S.W. and KONIJN, A.M., *J. Stored Prod. Res.* (1967) 2, 323-329.
69. LAUDA, C.M., MARSHALL, J.J. and WHELAN, W.J., unpublished work (1974).
70. LANG, J.A., CHANG-HUM, L.E., REYES, P.S. and BRIGGS, G.M., *Fed. Proc.* (1974) 33, 718.
71. MORENO, G.R., Thesis, Central University of Caracas (1971).
72. KAKADE, M.L. and EVANS, R.J., *J. Agric. Fd. Chem.* (1965) 13, 450-452.
73. EVANS, R.J., PUSZTAI, A., WATT, W.B. and BAUER, D.H., *Biochim. Biophys. Acta* (1973) 303, 175-184.
74. BESSHO, H. and KUROSAWA, S., *Eiyo To Shokuryo* (1967) 20, 317-319, *via Chem. Abs.* (1968) 68, 113474e.
75. PULS, W. and KEUP, U., *Diabetologia* (1973) 9, 97-101.

Part C

Digestibility and Physiological Effects of Food Polysaccharides: Introduction

JOHN E. HODGE

Northern Regional Research Center, Agricultural Research Service, U.S. Department of Agriculture, Peoria, Ill. 61604

In Parts A and B of this symposium, we have discussed the metabolism and physiological effects of the smaller carbohydrate molecules. We now come to the more complex polysaccharides of much higher molecular weight which, with the exception of starch, have been less studied by food scientists. Digestibility, fermentations in the bowel, bowel functions, and the lowering of serum lipids are the main physiological topics of interest in this session.

Among the dietary polysaccharides, only cooked starch, amylodextrins, and glycogen are considered to be fully digestible. The other, largely indigestible food polysaccharides of vegetable origin are included in the group of substances called "dietary fiber." Dietary fiber is not to be confused with "crude fiber." Only a fraction of dietary fiber is fibrous, and some of it is soluble in water. It consists of amorphous as well as fibrous cellulose, along with the associated hemicelluloses, protopectin, soluble pentosans, and soluble fructans. Noncarbohydrate lignin is another component of dietary fiber. Lignin and cellulose are the main constituents of the "crude fiber" fraction of proximate analysis; i.e., the residue remaining after hot acidic and alkaline extractions of defatted foods. The natural, heterogeneously constituted and essentially indigestible food-additive gums also can be considered as dietary fiber because their various polysaccharide structures resemble those of the hemicelluloses, pectic substances, and pentosans of foods. The mammalian counterpart of dietary fiber would be the indigestible mucopolysaccharides of proteoglycans.

The literature on human digestibilities of the nonstarchy polysaccharides is sparse. The ratios determined by analyses of carbohydrate in feces vs. carbohydrate ingested have indicated an apparent digestibility; however, these analyses do not account for losses of carbohydrate by various microbial fermentations in the bowel. Microbes of the large intestine are known to utilize some of the indigestible polysaccharides, but we should know whether or not microbes operate also in absorptive regions of the alimentary canal. Adaptation of the microflora and induction of their enzymes would come into greater consideration should the microbial fermentations produce absorbable sugars and metabolites.

Salts of acidic polysaccharides can act as ion-exchange media and some acidic polysaccharides form insoluble salts and chelates with polyvalent metal ions. They also form strong complexes with proteins. The question is, do these interactions affect nutrition in any significant way? Perhaps essential mineral ions (or toxic ones) can be complexed by acidic or basic carbohydrates for man's ultimate benefit.

The merits of dietary fiber are presently being extolled. In the 1974 edition of Recommended Dietary Allowances the Food and Nutrition Board of the National Research Council, National Academy of Sciences, watchfully reports:

> More complex carbohydrates, such as cellulose and hemicellulose, are largely indigestible, as are a number of oligosaccharides certain other carbohydrates, gums, and fibrous matter found in foods of plant origin. These nondigestible substances provide bulk in the diet and aid elimination. Although there is no demonstrated requirement for fiber or bulk, their possible physiological significance has not been adequately explored. A relationship--not yet proven-- between lack of dietary "fiber" and certain chronic disorders (noninfectious disease of the bowel, some vascular diseases) has been postulated from epi- demiologic evidence.

From this statement, the need for scientific investigations on the role of dietary fiber in human nutrition is evident. It is under- standable that the indigestible polysaccharides have been slighted in favor of the digestible carbohdyrates in food research, but this practice need not be continued in view of the promising bene- fits that are presented in some of the following papers.

The Physiological Effects of Alginates and Xanthan Gum

W. H. McNEELY and PETER KOVACS

Kelco Company, San Diego, Calif.

Alginates

Algin, found in all species of brown algae where it functions as an important constituent of cell walls, was discovered by Stanford in 1881. (1) The largest source of algin for actual commercial extraction is Macrocystis pyrifera, although other species are also used. (2)

After 1935, alginates became widely used in the food industry as stabilizers, emulsifiers, and viscosity-adjusting agents. Alginates are commercially supplied to the food industry as the sodium, potassium, ammonium, and calcium salts of alginic acid, along with propylene glycol alginate. As indicated in Figure 1, alginic acid is a linear glycuronan consisting of β-$\underline{D}$-mannuronic acid and α-$\underline{L}$-guluronic acid units linked through C_1 and C_4. For Macrocystis pyrifera, the alginic acid is composed of approximately 60 percent mannuronic acid and 40 percent guluronic acid. (2) The fine structure of the alginic acid molecule has been shown by graded acid hydrolysis and p.m.r. spectroscopy to consist of blocks of polymannuronic acid units and blocks of polyguluronic acid units linked by segments in which the two uronic acid residues alternate. (3,4)

The most recent acute oral toxicity study conducted by Woodard and co-workers on rats indicated that the maximum amount of sodium alginate that could be administered by oral intubation was 5 g/kg for one day. This feeding level caused no mortalities. Gross necropsy findings, coupled with general observations, indicated that sodium alginate is non-toxic with respect to acute toxicity by the oral route. (5)

A number of acute toxicity studies have been conducted on a variety of animals by intravenous or intraperitoneal injections of alginate solutions.

Arora and co-workers reported that intraperitoneal injections of sodium alginate to rats at up to 1000 mg/kg caused no mortality, while some mortality occurred among the

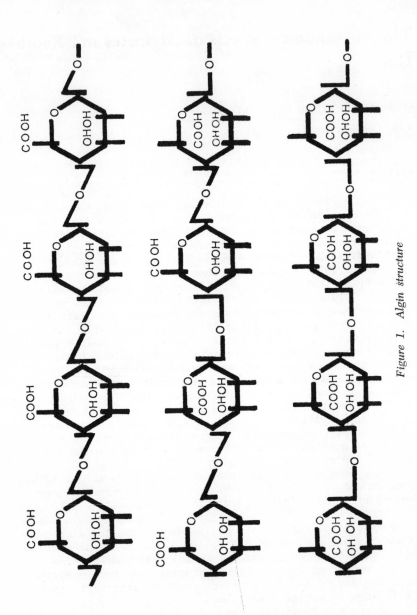

Figure 1. Algin structure

mice upon 500 mg/kg dosage administration. (6) Intravenous
injections of sodium alginate performed by Solandt to mice at
the 200-500 mg/kg level proved fatal in 1 minute to 12 hours.(7)
The LD-50 to rats by this method was determined by Sokow
as 1000 mg/kg. (8) The LD-50 of sodium alginate by the
intravenous route to rabbits was found to be 100 mg/kg. It
was postulated that the toxicity caused by the intravenous
administration of sodium alginate was due to the formation
and precipitation of the insoluble calcium alginate. (7)
Due to its known reactivity with calcium ions to form insoluble calcium alginate, algin has never been recommended
for use in intravenous injections.

The LD-50 of propylene glycol alginate determined by oral
intubation was found to be above the 5 g/kg level. No mortality occurred and no signs of toxicity or changes in the
viscera of the treated rats were found. (5) The oral administration of 10 g/kg propylene glycol alginate to rats was also
found to be harmless by Newell and Maxwell with the exception
of some transient depression. (9)

Intravenous administration of alginic acid by Thienes
and co-workers (10) and calcium alginate by Sokow (8)
produced results similar to that of sodium alginate; namely,
low LD-50 levels and significant mortality. It was suggested that the mortality was caused by embolism, as calcium
alginate as well as alginic acid is insoluble in water.

A number of short-term studies have been conducted on
sodium alginate. A 10-day study was conducted by Viola
and co-workers on rats where 0, 5, and 10 percent of the
test animals' diet consisted of sodium alginate. No apparent
effect was found at the 5 percent level, but at 10 percent
levels, depressions in calcium absorption were noted, while
the utilization of protein was not significantly affected. (11)

In a 10-week experiment, the daily diets of four groups
of rats, each consisting of six animals, were supplemented
with 5, 10, 20, and 30 percent sodium alginate. The tests
results are shown in Table I.

Table I

Short-Term, High-Level Sodium Alginate
Feeding Studies with Rats

Sodium Alginate Level	Mean Daily Weight Gain	Food Consumed Gain in Weight	Water Consumed Gain in Weight
5%	3.81 g	3.20 g	5.84 g
10%	3.47 g	3.31 g	6.28 g
20%	2.91 g	3.48 g	8.83 g
30%	2.35 g	3.87 g	13.47 g

At the highest feeding level, only two rats survived. The mortality was attributed to the low nutritional quality of the basal diet and not to any toxic effects of the sodium alginate. (12)

In an unpublished investigation by Woodard and co-workers, the effect of feeding 5 and 15 percent sodium alginate and propylene glycol alginate to purebred beagles for a period of one year was determined, After one year the animals were sacrificed, and gross histopathological examinations were made on the important organs. The results of this study indicated that the dogs tolerated levels as high as 15 percent sodium alginate and propylene glycol alginate. Animals even at the highest amount of alginate gained weight, as did the controls. Variable stool consistencies at the 15 percent feeding levels indicated the presence of unabsorbed colloid. Hemograms and blood chemistry values were generally within normal limits and showed no trends which could be related to the administration of the test materials. Based on the above, it was concluded that both sodium alginate and propylene glycol alginate were devoid of any harmful or deleterious effects. (13)

For a period of one year, propylene glycol alginate was fed to mice by Nilson and Wagner at 0, 5, 10, 15, and 25 percent by weight of the diet. No signs of toxicity were noted, but at the two highest feeding levels, smaller weight gains and increased mortality rates were noted. This was attributed to the water absorption quality of the diet limiting the essential nutrient intake. (12)   By the same workers, propylene glycol alginate was added to the diet of guinea pigs at 0, 5, 10, and 15 percent levels. After 26 weeks, no untoward effects were noted which could be attributed to the propylene glycol alginate. (12)

In a feeding study by Nilson and Wagner, cats were fed 0, 5, 10, and 15 percent propylene glycol alginate as part of their diet for up to 111 days. Although the cats receiving propylene glycol alginate in their diet had apparent problems in swallowing and eating and consequently lost weight when compared to the control animals, no indications of chronic toxicity were noted. Gross and histopathological examinations of organs of these animals revealed no lesions which could be attributed to any specific problems. (12)

Table II indicates the results of a study where, for a period of two months, alginic acid was fed to rats at 0, 5, 10, and 20 percent of their diet. As shown in this table, at up to 10 percent concentrations, no significant effect on growth or food consumption was noted. At the 20 percent level, however, a significant decrease in weight gain was observed. (10)

Table II

Short-Term Alginic Acid
Feeding Studies with Rats

Dietary Algin %	Average Weight Gain Initial	Average Weight Gain Final	Average Daily Food Consumption g/100 g.b.w.
0	66	156	10.8
5	66	154	12.6
10	64	156	12.1
20	63	116	8.8

In a detailed two-year, three-generation reproduction study by Morgan, et al., rats were placed on a diet containing 5 percent sodium alginate and propylene glycol alginate. When the animals were five to six months of age, they were mated, and the offspring, the F_1 generation, were grouped, as were the parent animals, and fed the same diets. When the F_1 generation rats were about four months old, they were also mated, and the resulting offspring, the F_2 generation, were divided, as the parent generations were, and placed on the same diet. Table III shows the body weight data for the three generations of control animals and those receiving 5 percent sodium alginate and propylene glycol alginate. As indicated in this table, there were no significant differences between the control and treated groups or between the effects of sodium alginate and propylene glycol alginate.

The conclusions of this study revealed that the feeding of sodium alginate and propylene glycol alginate to rats for the period of two years at 5 percent levels of their diets did not affect the growth rate of the parent generation and their progeny for two generations when compared to the control group. No gross pathological or hematological changes were noted in the test animals. A slight change in the bacterial flora of the gastrointestinal tract was observed, but these were not significant enough to cause changes in the digestive process or to retard the health of the animals. (15)

Pregnant mice, rats, and hamsters indicated no signs of teratogenic effects when they were administered by oral intubation propylene glycol alginate in doses of 780, 720, and 700 mg/kg during gestation. (16)

While investigating the carcinogenicity of several colloids, Epstein reported that no change in the frequency of tumors in infant mice occurred after repeated subcutaneous injections of alginic acid. (17)

Earlier publications on the digestibility of algin carried out on various animal species by Nilson and co-workers (12, 20) tended to show that algin was partially digestible.

Table III

Long-Term Sodium Alginate and
Propylene Glycol Alginate Feeding Studies with Rats

Generation	Diet Level	Day of Termination		Mean Body Weight Male		Mean Body Weight Female	
		S A	PGA	S A	PGA	S A	PGA
Parent	Control	761	761	401	401	298	298
	5% Alginate	761	761	403	402	304	291
F_1	Control	202	202	323	323	243	243
	5% Alginate	202	202	270	292	202	234
F_2	Control	212	212	287	287	204	204
	5% Alginate	212	212	272	268	236	209

Sodium Alginate (S A)

Propylene Glycol Alginate (PGA)

Analytical methods used were based on isolation of the algin
from the feces. These methods are not very reliable. Recent
studies by the more accurate radioactive C14 method by
Humphreys and Triffitt (18) for sodium alginate and by Sharratt
and Dearn (19) for propylene glycol alginate found negligible
or no absorption of the algin.

Numerous published reports dealing with the effect of
sodium alginate on the gastrointestinal absorption of radioactive strontium and several other metallic ions are listed
in a review by Tanaka and Skoryna. (21) While several
authors reported that algin inhibits the radioactive strontium
absorption, much lesser effects have been produced on the
absorption of calcium, magnesium, iron, copper, and zinc.
The current public interest created by the alleged detoxifi-
cation properties of sodium alginate with respect to lead
does not appear to be justified. In a recent study by
Harrison, et al., human volunteers were administered 5 g of
sodium alginate, which did not change the level of lead in
their systems. (22) Based on a human feeding study, Carr,
et al., reported that sodium alginate does not affect the absorption of sodium, potassium, magnesium, and phosphorous
in the gastrointestinal tract. (23) The effect of alginic
acid on the cation absorption in humans was reported earlier
by Feldman and co-workers. Four adult males were maintained
on a control diet containing 500 mg sodium per day for seven
days. After that time, 15 g of alginic acid, three times
daily, was administered for seven days. In three patients
this study was repeated with 1500 mg daily intake of sodium.
The alginic acid was well tolerated by the subjects with the
exception of mild laxative effects. (14) In a calcium-
balance experiment performed on six adult humans by Mills
and Reed, the results indicated that sodium alginate does
not interfere with the calcium absorption of the normal
varied diet. (24)

Xanthan Gum

Xanthan gum, a relatively recently developed polysaccharide produced by the bacterial fermentation of glucose
with the organism Xanthomonas campestris, was approved by
the FDA as a food additive in 1969. Since that time, xanthan
gum has been widely accepted by the food industries of many
countries as a general purpose stabilizer-thickener. The
commercial success of xanthan gum was recently manifested
by the presentation of the 1974 IFT Food Technology Industrial
Achievement Award to Kelco Company and the Northern Regional
Research Laboratory of the USDA. (25)
As indicated in Figure 2, xanthan gum is a heteropolysaccharide with main building blocks consisting of D-glucose,
D-mannose, and D-glucuronic acid residues. (26) The polymer

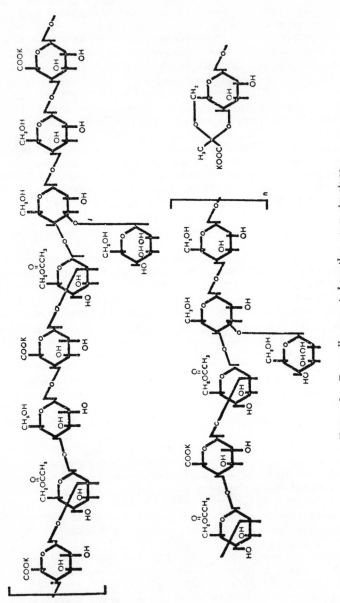

Figure 2.   Generally accepted xanthan gum structure

also contains pyruvate attached to a glucose side chain at an,
as yet, undetermined location. The molecule is a very long
linear chain with a molecular weight of 5 to 10 million.

Xanthan gum is perhaps the most extensively investigated
polysaccharide from the standpoint of toxicological and
safety properties.

The results of the acute toxicity studies are summarized
in Table IV.

Table IV

Acute Toxicity Studies with Xanthan Gum

Animal	Route	Maximum mg/kg Body Weight Administered
Mouse	Oral	1000 (27)
	Intraperitoneal	150 (27)
	Intravenous	100-250 (28)
Rat	Oral	5000 (29)
Dog	Oral	20000 (30)

In the rat and dog studies, the LD-50 levels are actually
representative of the maximum levels the animals were able
to consume within the test period. Since no mortalities or
toxic manifestations occurred, the true oral LD-50 levels
are above those shown in this table.

There were two short-term feeding studies conducted on
both rats and dogs by Booth, et al. No untoward effects
were noted upon the extensive investigation of rats when they
were fed xanthan gum for a period of 99-110 days at 7.5 percent and 10 percent as part of their daily diet. (29) In a
91-day feeding study, normal weight gains were recorded at
3 percent and 6 percent xanthan gum levels in the diet, while
some weight gain reduction was noted at 7.5 percent and
15 percent levels. No differences in organ weights, hemoglobin concentration, and white and red cell counts were
found. At the highest dosage levels, the animals did produce
abnormally high fecal pellets, but no occurrence of diarrhea
was noted. In a paired feeding test study at 7.5 percent
feeding level, no growth-inhibiting factor attributable to
xanthan gum was found. (29)

Feeding dogs 2 g/kg xanthan gum for a period of two weeks
produced diarrhea in the test group, while the same did not
occur at the 1 g/kg feeding level. Gross histopathological
examination did not reveal any organ damage attributable
to the ingestion of xanthan gum. (31) This occurrence is
not unexpected, as most hydrophilic colloids, due to their

efficient water-absorbing properties, are known to cause
diarrhea at high feeding levels.

In long-term feeding studies by Woodard, et al., a
group of 30 male and 30 female rats was fed xanthan gum at
0, 0.25, 0.5, and 1.0 g/kg as part of their daily diet for
a period of 104 weeks. No abnormalities were found which
could be attributed to the ingestion of the product. Survival
rate, body weight gain, food consumption, behavior, and appearance were normal when compared to the control group. Hematological values, organ weights, and tumor occurrence showed
no significant variation. Slightly softer stools were noted
in the middle- and high-level test animals, but the difference
from the control was not statistically significant. (32)

In a 107-week-long study on a group of four male and
four female beagle dogs, 0, 0.25, 0.37, and 1 g/kg xanthan
gum was fed to the animals as part of their daily diet. No
adverse effects were noted in the test animals with respect
to survival, food intake, body weight gain, electrocardiograms,
blood pressures, hemograms, organ weights, gross necropsy
observations, and histopathological observations. At the
highest feeding level, a dose-related increase in fecal
weights and a measurable increase in the specific gravity of
the urine and more frequent presence of urinary albumin
were noted. This test revealed no untoward effects caused
by the treatment of xanthan gum at any dosage levels. (32)

The feeding of xanthan gum was also examined in a three-
generation reproduction study by Woodard, et al., using 10
male and 20 female rats in the first generation and 20 male
and 20 female rats in subsequent generations. Dosage levels
were 0, 0.25, and 0.5 g/kg as part of the animals' diet.
The test results were evaluated for survival, body weights,
general appearance, behavior, reproductive performance,
physical condition of the offspring, and the survival of
the offspring. With respect to all criteria, no adverse
effects were noted in this study which would be attributable
to the presence of xanthan gum in the diet of the animals. (32)

According to a test conducted by the caloric availability method, the digestibility of xanthan gum was found to be zero.
This conclusion was substantiated in a report by Booth and co-
workers which found that practically all xanthan gum fed for
a period of seven days could be recovered in the stool of
the animals. (27) In another study, conducted by the more
accurate radioactive tracer method, the digestibility of
xanthan gum was found to be approximately 15 percent. The
polysaccharide constituents did not accumulate in the tissues,
and they were metabolized by the expected route as carbohydrates. In vitro tests indicated that non-enzymatic hydrolysis and the action of microorganisms were responsible for the
initial breakdown of the molecule. Based on the above studies,
the approximate caloric value of xanthan gum is 0.5 kilo-

calories per gram.

Conclusion

The foregoing, of course, is an abridged summary of
the toxicological studies conducted on alginates and xanthan
gum. There is absolutely no information available indicating that the consumption of these products at their normal
usage levels would present any health hazards. Furthermore,
it should be emphasized that the functional levels and the
per capita consumption of alginates and xanthan gum are orders
of magnitude below the feeding levels used to establish their
safety as food additives.

"Literature Cited"

1 Stanford, E. C. C., J. Soc. Chem. Ind., (1886) 5, 218.

2 McNeely, W. H. and Pettitt, D. J., in "Industrial Gums,"
   2nd Ed., pp. 49-81, Academic Press, New York, New York,
   1973.

3 Haug, A., Larsen, G., Smidsrød, O., Acta. Chem. Scand.,
   (1967) 21, 691.

4 Penman, A. and Sanderson, G., Carb. Res., (1972) 25, 273.

5 Knott, W. B. and Johnston, C. D., "Sodium and Propylene
   Glycol Alginate Acute Oral Toxicity to Rats," Woodard
   Research Corporation unpublished report, 1972.

6 Arora, C. K., Chandhury, S. K., Chanha, P. S., Indian
   J. Physiol. Pharmacol., (1968) 12 (3) 129-30.

7 Solandt, O. M., Quart. J. Exp. Physiol., (1941) 31, 25-40.

8 Sokov, L. A., Radioactivnye Izotopy Vo Vneshnei Srede i
   Organizme (Russian), (1970) 247-51.

9 Stanford Research Institute, "Study of Mutagenic
   Effects of Propylene Glycol Alginate (71-18)," PB 221 826,
   N.T.I.S., 1972.

10 Thienes, C. H., Skillen, R. G., Meredith, O. M., Fairchild,
   M. D., McCandless, R. S., Thienes, R. P., Arch. Intern.
   Pharmacodyn., (1957) 111 (2) 167-81.

11 Viola, S., Zimmerman, G., Mokady, S., Nutr. Rep. Int.,
   (1970) 1 (6) 367-76.

12 Nilson, H. W. and Wagner, J. H., Proc. Soc. Exp. Biol. Med., (1951) 76 (4) 630-5.

13 Dardin, V. J., "Feeding of KELGIN or KELCOLOID to Dogs for One Year," Woodard Research Corporation unpublished report, 1959.

14 Feldman, H. S., Urbach, K., Naegle, C. F., Regan, F. D., Doerner, A. A., Proc. Soc. Exp. Biol. Med., (1952) 79, 439-41.

15 Morgan, C. F., Farber, J. E. Jr., Dardin, V. J., "The Effects of Algin Products on the Rat," Georgetown University Medical School unpublished report, 1959.

16 Food and Drug Research Laboratories, "Teratological Evaluation of Propylene Glycol Alginate," PB 221 786, N.T.I.S., 1972.

17 Epstein, S. S., Toxicol. Appl. Pharmacol., (1970) 16, 321-4.

18 Humphreys, E. R. and Triffitt, J. T., Nature, (1968) 219, 1172-3.

19 Sharratt, M. and Dearn, P., Food Cosmet. Toxicol., (1972) 10 (1) 35-40.

20 Nilson, H. W. and Lemon, J. M., "Metabolism Studies with Algin and Gelatin," pp. 1-9, U.S. Fish and Wildlife Serv. Research Report No. 4, 1942.

21 Tanaka, Y. and Skoryna, S. C., in "Intestinal Absorption of Metal Ions, Trace Elements, and Radionuclides," pp. 101-14, Pergamon Press, New York, New York, 1971.

22 Harrison, G. E., Carr, T. E. F., Sutton, A., Humphreys, E. R., Nature, (1969) 224, 1115-6.

23 Carr, T. E. F., Harrison, G. E., Humphreys, E. R., Sutton, A., Int. J. Radiat. Biol., (1968) 14 (3) 225-33.

24 Millis, J. and Reed, F. B., Biochem J., (1947) 41, 273-5.

25 Anonymous, Food Technol., (1974) 28 (6) 18-21.

26 Sloneker, J. H., Orentes, D. G., Jeanes, A., Can. J. Chem., (1964) 42, 1261-9.

27 Booth, A. N., Hendrickson, A. P., DeEds, F., Toxicol.
    Appl. Pharmacol., (1963) 5, 478-84.

28 Hendrickson, A. P. and Booth, A. N., "Supplementary
    Acute Toxicological Studies of Polysaccharide B-1459,"
    Western Reqional Research Laboratory Research Report,
    Albany, California, 1964.

29 Jackson, N. N., Woodard, M. W., Woodard, G., "Xanthan
    Gum Acute Oral Toxicity to Rats," Woodard Research
    Corporation unpublished report, 1968.

30 Jackson, N. N., Woodard, M. W., Woodard, G., "Xanthan
    Gum Acute Oral Toxicity to Dogs," Woodard Research Cor-
    poration unpublished report, 1968.

31 Robbins, D. J., Moulton, J. E., Booth, A. N., Food
    Cosmet. Toxicol., (1964) 2, 545.

32 Woodard, G., Woodard, M. W., McNeely, W. H., Kovacs,
    P., Cronin, M. T. I., Toxicol. Appl. Pharmacol., (1973)
    24, 30-6.

18

Physiological Effects of Carrageenan

DIMITRI J. STANCIOFF and DONALD W. RENN

Marine Colloids, Inc., Rockland, Maine 04841

Abstract

Breakdown absorption and toxicity of carrageenan in the gastrointestinal tract is reviewed. Carrageenan, a linear sulfated galactan (molecular weight 250,000) derived from red seaweeds, is used as a food stabilizer, particularly in dietetic and dairy products. Breakdown in the gut appears to be insignificant and there is no evidence that it is absorbed by test animals with the possible exceptions of guinea pigs and rabbits. In large doses it inhibits pepsin activity (in vitro), depresses gastric juice secretion and reduces food absorption in rats. There is no evidence of such effects with the low levels used in food. Depolymerized carrageenan (molecular weight $< 20,000$), used in France for treatment of peptic ulcers, has shown no toxicity in man but caused mucosal erosions in the cecum of guinea pigs and at high doses also effected cell changes in the colon of rats and monkeys. Degraded carrageenan was demonstrated as being partly absorbed by the epithelial cells, deposited in the Kupffer cells of the liver and found in the urine. A broad margin of safety for food grade carrageenan in the diet is assured by low functional use levels and a minimum molecular weight of 100,000.

Introduction

Excellent reviews on the physiological effects of carrageenan have been published in the last six years: two of them by Anderson (1, 2) and the most recent by DiRosa (3). Although these reviews are very comprehensive, their emphasis is on the pharmacological properties of carrageenan administered by parenteral routes. For example, carrageenan introduced subcutaneously induces collagen proliferation with the resultant formation of a granuloma (4, 5, 6, 7, 8, 9, 10, 11, 12, 13, 14). When injected into a rodent's paw, a reproducible inflammatory edematous condition results which has been successfully used in screening compounds for anti-inflammatory activity (15, 16, 17, 18, 19, 20).

Anti-coagulant (21, 22, 23 24) and hypotensive properties (25)
have also been observed. In addition, various immunological responses have been reported which include in vitro and in vivo
complement depletion and delayed hypersensitivity (26, 27, 28,
29, 30, 31, 32, 33).

Although these physiological manifestations of carrageenan
may seem somewhat foreboding, 99.9% of the carrageenan consumed
by humans is in food rather than in drugs, and the emphasis of
this symposium is on dietary rather than pharmacological aspects
of carbohydrates. In this context the effects of parenterally
administered carrageenan is about as relevant as the effects of
an intravenous injection of beef stew. Though the latter is a
wholesome food, its physiological effect in the bloodstream
would, no doubt, be quite devastating. We will, therefore, restrict the subject of this review to carrageenan taken orally.

The use of purified carrageenan in modern food technology
dates back to the early thirties, while the use of crude preparations by Oriental and European coastal dwellers is at least several centuries old (34).

In spite of this long history of food use, or perhaps because
of it, far more has been published on its physiological effect as
an experimental drug than as a food ingredient. In fact publications are in inverse ratio to use:

        10,000,000 lbs/year used in food   -   20 papers
           10,000 lbs/year anti-ulcer drug -   70 papers
                1 lb/year parenteral use   - 150 papers

Nevertheless, we can glean enough from the literature to establish that carrageenan is not broken down or absorbed and that
at the low levels used in food has no adverse physiological effects in humans.

Source Properties and Uses of Carrageenan

But first let's say a few words about the origin, chemistry,
and physical properties of carrageenan.

Carrageenan can be obtained from about 250 species of closely
related red algae of the order Gigartinales but only about half a
dozen of them are used commercially. These include species of
Chondrus, Eucheuma and Gigartina. It is the major intercellular
constituent of these plants and represents about 60% of their
salt-free dry weight.

Carrageenan is generally prepared by hot aqueous extraction of
the seaweed, followed by filtration to remove insoluble matter,
coagulation in alcohol, vacuum drying, and grinding.

Chemically, carrageenan is a straight chain sulfated galactan
with a backbone of alternating 1-4 linked α-D-galactose and 1-3
linked β-D-galactose or its 3,6 anhydride. Commercial extracts
usually have a weight average molecular weight 100,000 to 500,000.

This simple picture is somewhat complicated by the fact that
the number and position of the ester sulfate groups and the ratio
of galactose to 3,6-anhydrogalactose may vary considerably.
Greek letter prefixes are used for categorizing the various combinations.

Two major groups of carrageenan are recognized. In the
first, the 1,3-linked units are sulfated in the 4-position while
in the second, the sulfate is in the 2-position (Figure 1).

The first group is subdivided according to the nature of the
1-4 linked units. These may be present as galactose 6-sulfate
(μ-carrageenan) or galactose 2-6 disulfate (ν-carrageenan) or as
the corresponding 3,6-anhydrides in κ- and ι-carrageenan. In
nature the 3,6-anhydrides of κ- and ι-carrageenan are formed by
enzymatic elimination of the 6-sulfate from the μ- and ν-forms,
but the conversion is not always complete. In some seaweeds
these carrageenan types can be isolated in almost pure form while
in others they exist as copolymers.

In the second group, the 1,4-linked units are sulfated in the
2-position. In λ-carrageenan the 6-position is also sulfated
while in ξ-carrageenan it is not.

Aqueous solutions of carrageenan are highly viscous. Kappa
and ι-carrageenan form heat reversible gels in the presence of
potassium and calcium ions. Carrageenans also react strongly
with large positively charged ions, notably with proteins below
their isoelectric point.

The main uses of carrageenan are as thickeners, stabilizers,
and gelling agents in food. Its strong interaction with casein
is utilized in dairy products such as chocolate milk, ice cream
and puddings. The gelling properties are useful for making
jellies, relishes, and pie fillings. The list of applications
also includes whipped topping, non-dairy coffee whiteners, and a
host of convenience foods.

The functional properties of carrageenan are highly dependent
on molecular weight. When the molecular weight is below 100,000
the stabilizing properties are almost completely lost. More detailed information on the sources, properties, and uses of carrageenan has been published in reviews by Rees (35), by Glicksman
(36), Sand and Glicksman (37), and by Towle (38).

Degraded Carrageenan

When speaking of physiological properties of ingested carrageenan we must distinguish between food grade carrageenan, which
has a molecular weight of 100,000 to 500,000 and so-called degraded carrageenan. Degraded carrageenan in which the glycosidic
linkages are hydrolized to reduce the molecular weight to less
than 20,000 is used in France for peptic ulcer treatment. It is
ineffective as a food stabilizer and also has different physiological properties. We will come back to it later, but first
let's talk about food grade carrageenan.

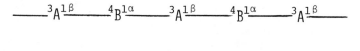

B	A	
UNITS:	UNITS:	NAME:

D-Galactose 6-sulfate	*mu*
D-Galactose 2,6-disulfate	*nu*

D-Galactose 4-sulfate

3,6-Anhydro-D-Galactose	*kappa*
3,6-Anhydro-D-Galactose 2-sulfate	*iota*

D-Galactose 2-sulfate	*xi*
D-Galactose 2,6-disulfate	*lambda*

D-Galactose 2-sulfate

3,6-Anhydro-D-Galactose 2-sulfate	*theta*

Figure 1.   Repeating units of carrageenans

Physiological Effects of Food Grade Carrageenan

Breakdown in the Intestinal Tract. Breakdown of carrageenan
in the digestive system is probably minimal, for it seems that
neither man nor the experimental animals tested so far possess
the necessary enzymes to hydrolyze it.

In the stomach, where pH is very low, a small amount of acid
hydrolysis undoubtedly does occur. However, in vitro experiments
with simulated gastric juice at pH 1.2 and 37°C showed that in
three hours (which is about the maximum residence time in the
stomach) the breakdown of glycosidic linkages was less than
0.1% (39).

Information about what happens in the lower gut is notoriously
lacking. Incubation of a carrageenan solution with the cecal contents of rats for several hours at 37°C did not alter its viscosity, which indicates that the microbial flora, of the rat gut at
any rate, will not break down carrageenan (40).

There is always the possibility that, after several months of
feeding large doses of carrageenan, the microbial flora would be
changed enough to cause some breakdown. However, there is so far
no suggestion that this might occur. In fact there seem to be
very few bacteria, other than those of marine origin, that can de-
compose carrageenan. Our own waste disposal difficulty with digesting carrageenan with activated sewage sludge attests to that.

Absorption. If carrageenan is not broken down, is it absorbed
without breakdown? In three species of monkey (41, 42, 43), dog
(44), pig (45), rat (41, 46, 47, 48, 49), mouse (41), ferret (41),
hamster (41), it apparently is not. Houck (44) obtained 100% recovery in the feces of dogs. In a 2-year feeding study by Nilson
and Wagner (48), rats received from 1 to 25% carrageenan mixed
with the dry diet. Growth rates and internal organs of the animals were normal at dose levels up to 10%. At high doses growth
was retarded, and some animals fed 25% carrageenan showed liver
abnormalities. Nilson and Wagner attributed the latter to a dietary deficiency caused by the large bulk of the ingested carrageenan. Recovery in the feces was 50% irrespective of the level
fed. This rather surprising result was, however, obtained by an
analytical method which left something to be desired. Two later
studies, also with rats, resulted in 90-100% recovery (46, 47).

In the case of guinea pigs and rabbits, results have been contradictory. Watt and Marcus (50) found that high molecular weight
carrageenan caused ulceration of the cecum and colon of guinea
pigs. Grasso, Sharratt, Carpanini and Gangoli (41) confirmed
these results and also showed that rabbits were similarly affected. Although the bulk of the carrageenan was excreted in the
feces, a certain amount was absorbed by the macrophages in the
subepithelial layers of the cecum and colon. On the other hand,
a study at the Albany Medical College showed neither absorption
nor lesions (49, 51). Anderson and Soman (52), likewise, showed

that high molecular weight carrageenan was not absorbed through
the gut of guinea pigs and could not be detected in the blood or
urine unless administered intravenously. Grasso et al. hypothe-
size that absorption by macrophages may be peculiar to guinea pigs
and rabbits, herbivorous rodents, both of which possess an unusually large cecum, and suggest that absorption may be due to incomplete neonatal cloture of the intestinal barrier to macro-
molecules.

Other Effects. Now, if carrageenan is not digested and not
absorbed, just what physiological effects does it have? So far,
several effects have been reported in the literature:

  Reduction of peptic activity
  Reduced flow of gastric secretions in the stomach
  Antilipemic activity
  Increase in water content of the gut

All these effects can be attributed to the hydrophilic and
polyanionic properties of the macromolecule, however, they all
result only from very high dosages of carrageenan and cannot be
detected at the low levels at which carrageenan is used in food.

Antipeptic activity. The first and the best documented of
these effects is the antipeptic activity. Carrageenan interferes
with the proteolytic activity of pepsin, both in vitro and in
vivo (44, 52, 53). Several researchers have concluded that the
inhibition is due to the interaction of carrageenan with the substrate and not with the pepsin. This view is supported by the
fact that the degree of inhibition depends on the ratio of carrageenan to substrate and not on the amount of pepsin (54, 55, 56).
Anderson (1, 54) has pointed out that at pH 1.3 most proteins
become positively charged and form insoluble complexes with carrageenan, whereas pepsin with an isoelectric point of 1.0 remains
anionic under these conditions and is unlikely to react. The non-
interaction of carrageenan and pepsin has also been shown electrophoretically (57).
You may ask then, if carrageenan inhibits peptic activity,
will it not then interfere with digestion and cause reduced protein intake? This certainly would have been a possibility if carrageenan interacted with the pepsin, because then, even small
doses should interfere. However, since it reacts with the substrate, the amount of protein digested depends on how much of it
remains unreacted with the carrageenan. Since the amount of pro-
ein ingested in a normal diet is considerable, very large doses
of carrageenan would be needed to inactivate all the substrate.
Indeed, such seems to be the case. Hawkins and Yaphe (47)
found that young rats gained weight more slowly only if their
diet contained more than 10% carrageenan (10,000 mg/kg). Such an
excess is, however, completely unrealistic and the work of

Vaughan, Filer and Churella (56) shows what occurs under conditions closer to reality. They examined peptic inhibition of carrageenan with several proteins in vitro and also measured in vivo digestibility of milk protein and carrageenan mixtures in rats. They found that inhibition depended on the ratio of carrageenan to protein. In all cases there was no detectable inhibition at ratios smaller than 0.1 and in some cases ratios were as high as 0.3 before interference occurred. In the in vivo studies the digestibility was 100% at ratios below 0.1. Even at the high ratio of 0.3 peptic activity was reduced only 10 to 20%.

The greatest use of carrageenan is in the dairy industry, however, the levels at which it is used are extremely low. In puddings the carrageenan to protein ratio is about 0.03, in chocolate milk it is 0.01, and in ice cream, evaporated milk and infant formulas it is about 0.005.

Products, such as relishes or low calorie jellies which may contain up to 0.7% carrageenan and in which the carrageenan exceeds the amount of protein, generally form only a minor part of the diet and are usually eaten at the same time as other foods which have a high protein content. Therefore, unless someone decided to go on a pure jelly and relish binge the likelihood of protein deficiency due to a surfeit of carrageenan is quite negligible. In fact the average per capita consumption of carrageenan in the United States is less than 0.5 mg/kg of body weight per day. The highest levels are consumed by infants receiving special dietary formulas during the first 2-3 months after birth. The daily levels average 25 to 50 mg/kg of body weight, but the ratio of carrageenan to protein is only about 0.005.

Gastric secretion. Carrageenan diminishes the volume and acidity of histamine-stimulated gastric secretion, but on the other hand, it also restores normal secretion in cases where supramaximal histamine stimulation has caused submaximal acid output.

According to Anderson (58), carrageenan complexes with mucin on the stomach wall and its ability to inhibit gastric secretion (59, 60) could be related by this interaction. Its ability to restore normal flow is, however, more difficult to explain (61). These phenomena are unlikely to take place with carrageenan that is ingested with food -- first because of the small amounts present and, second, because the carrageenan would be complexed with the food protein.

Lipemia clearing. The third effect of carrageenan is its hypocholesterolemic activity. Again, large dosages are necessary. Fahrenbach et al (62) obtained significant reduction in blood cholesterol of white Leghorn chicks which were fed 1 to 3% carrageenan in the diet. Ershoff and Wills (63) obtained a similar effect with 10% carrageenan in the diet of rats fed 1% cholesterol. Liver cholesterol remained at normal level and total liver

lipid were greatly reduced. The mechanism of lipemia clearing is
not known. Perhaps, carrageenan, like other non-digestible fiber
may interfere with cholesterol absorption. It is unfortunate
that, in order to take advantage of the anti-lipemic properties
of carrageenan, the oral dosage has to be so high.

Water content of the bowel. There is nothing unusual about
the fourth effect of carrageenan which increases the water content of the bowel and causes softening of the stool. This effect
is common to all hydrophilic polymers several of which, notably
agar, psyllium gum, and pectin, are used as mild laxatives because of their water-holding properties.

Physiological Effects of Degraded Carrageenan

Now a few words about degraded or depolymerized carrageenan.
This product, which has a molecular weight of 10-20,000 was developed as a more convenient, less viscous, dosage form for the
treatment of peptic and duodenal ulcers in humans. It is produced by partial hydrolysis of the glycosidic linkages with acid.

Carrageenan, both in the degraded and undegraded form, prevents or diminishes histamine-induced experimental peptic ulceration (44, 60) and alleviates peptic and duodenal ulcers in humans
(64). Anderson (58) attributes this effect to the ability of carrageenan to complex with gastric mucin, thus protecting the stomach wall against attack by the gastric juices.

The degraded product is as effective in protecting the stomach wall as undegraded carrageenan and is much easier for a patient to take because of its very low viscosity.

In contrast to food grade carrageenan, the degraded product
is partly absorbed through the gut. It has been detected in the
urine of baboons (42) and guinea pigs (52). The amount absorbed
was less than 1%. In Rhesus monkeys it accumulated in the lysosomes of the reticuloendothelial cells of the liver, spleen, and
lymph nodes, and could still be detected six months after treatment (43).

Degraded carrageenan also causes ulceration of the cecum and
colon of several test species. Gerbils and mice were not affected (51). Guinea pigs and rabbits were particularly susceptible
(40, 41, 50, 51, 65). Lesions were also produced in Rhesus monkeys (43) at high dose levels (3,000 mg/kg/day), but not in
squirrel monkeys (41).

Clinical tests by Bonfils (64) on 200 patients receiving 5
grams per day (100/mg/kg/day) of degraded carrageenan in peptic
ulcer treatment showed no adverse effects on the colon after six
months to two years of treatment.

The absorption and ulceration apparently are highly dependent
on dose level and molecular weight. Above a molecular weight of
50,000 no absorption can be detected (51, 52).

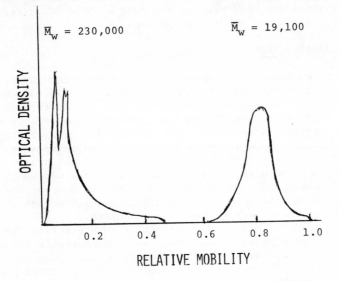

Figure 2. Gel electrophoresis densitometer curves for iota-carrageenan (mobility is measured relative to a marker dye)

Despite the apparent lack of toxicity to humans we must, nevertheless, be cautious in the event that degraded carrageenan might have adverse effects after prolonged ingestion. For this reason the Food and Drug Administration requires a minimum molecular weight of 100,000 for carrageenan in food. This is no problem because the stabilizing properties of carrageenan depend on high molecular weight. However, carrageenan is polydisperse and there is always the possibility that low molecular weight material may be present.

At Marine Colloids we have developed a rapid method for determining molecular weight and molecular weight distribution of carrageenan. The method is based on the relative electrophoretic mobility of different size carrageenan molecules in a thin film agarose gel (66). Separation is primarily according to molecular weight, with charge density exerting only a minor effect. The separated species can be quantitated by transmission densitometry. By comparing a series of progressively depolymerized carrageenans whose molecular weights had been determined by ultracentrifugation, a linear relationship was found between electrophoretic mobility and the cube root of the molecular weight.

The method has the advantage that only about 50 micrograms of sample is required, several samples can be tested at the same time, results are obtained in a day, and separation of high and low molecular weight carrageenan is very good. The densitometer scan of a pherogram of a mixture of high and low molecular weight carrageenan is shown in Figure 2.

Our work has shown that only minute amounts of low molecular weight material is present in food grade carrageenan. Currently we are testing carrageenan processed under conditions used in food processing. Our results to date show little or no change in molecular weight distribution under normal processing conditions.

Conclusion

In conclusion, the safety of carrageenan as a food additive has been the target of many in-depth studies supported by government agencies here and abroad as well as by the various carrageenan producers. From the results of these studies, we can conclude that food grade carrageenan -- an isolated component of natural food products used extensively for over two centuries -- has no adverse physiological effects and that its safety in foods is assured.

Addendum

Development since September, 1974. Recently during the course of a current three-generation feeding study, researchers at the Food and Drug Administration noted changes in the surface appearance of the livers of animals being fed 5% and 2.5% carrageenan in the dry diet (67). Liver surfaces appeared to be lumpy and irregular. At the 5% carrageenan level the frequency of this occurrence was 93% while at the 2.5% level it was 40%. Male animals fed the highest level gained less weight than normal. In other respects the rats were quite healthy and reproduction was normal.

The liver changes are difficult to explain in the light of so many previous studies, particularly since the changes were very obvious and could hardly have been missed if they had occurred before.

On the other hand, a very thorough six-month feeding study at Wyeth Labs., Inc. (68), with 4% carrageenan in the diet of rats, revealed no abnormalities whatsoever. In this case the carrageenan had been mixed into skim milk at a concentration equal to that of the protein after which the mixture was spray-dried or lyophilized. The carrageenan had no influence on growth rate, diet energy efficiency, absorption of protein, fat, or calcium, utilization of protein for growth or the utilization of iron. Gross examination of the animals' organs showed no abnormalities. Further tests are now in progress to clarify the discrepancies between the various studies.

Literature Cited

1.   Anderson, W., Can. J. Pharm. Sci., (1967), 2, 81-90.
2.   Anderson, W., Proc. Int. Seaweed Symp., (1969), 6, 627-635.
3.   DiRosa, M., J. Pharm. Pharmacol., (1972), 24, 89-102.
4.   Benitz, K.F. and Hall, L.M., Proc. Soc. Exp. Biol. Med. (1959), 108, 442-445.
5.   DiRosa, M., Giroud, J.P. and Willoughby, D.A., J. Pathol., (1971), 104, 15-29.
6.   DiRosa, M. and Sorrentino, L., Eur. J. Pharmacol., (1968), 4, 340-342.
7.   Garg, Bhagwan D. and McCandless, Esther L., Anat. Rec., (1968), 162, (1), 33-40.
8.   Hurley, J.V. and Willoughby, D.A., Pathol. (1973), 5, 9-21.
9.   Jackson, D.S., Biochem. J., (1957), 65, 277-284.
10.   Jackson, D.S., Biochem. J., (1957), 65, 459-464.
11.   McCandless, E.L., Ann. N.Y. Acad. Sci., (1965), 118, (22), 867-882.
12.   Monis, B., Weinberg, T. and Spector, G.J., Brit. J. Exp. Pathol., (1968), 49, 302-310.
13.   Robertson, W., Hiwett, J. and Herman, L.C., J. Biol. Chem., (1959), 234, 105-108.
14.   Salvaggio, J. and Kundur, V., Proc. Soc. Exp. Biol. Med., (1970), 134, 1116-1119.
15.   Winter, C.A., Risley, E.A. and Nuss, G.W., Proc. Soc. Exp. Biol. Med., (1962), 111, 544-547.
16.   Van Arman, C.G., Begany, A.J., Miller, L.M., and Pless, H.H., J. Pharmacol. Exp. Ther., (1965), 150, 328-334.

17.   Niemegeers, C.J.E., Verbrugger, F.J. and Janssen, P.A.,
      J. Pharm. Pharmacol., (1964), 16, 810-816.
18.   Bush, J.E. and Alexander, R.W., Acta Endocrinol., (1960),
      35, 268-276.
19.   Benitz, K.F. and Hall, L.M., Arch. int. Pharmacodyn., (1963),
      144, (1-2), 185-195.
20.   Schwartz, H.J. and Kellermeyer, R.W., Proc. Soc. Exp. Biol.
      Med., (1969), 132, 1021-1024.
21.   Anderson, W. and Duncan, J.G.C., J. Pharm. Pharmacol.,
      (1965), 17, 647-654.
22.   Hawkins, W.W. and Leonard, V.G., Can. J. Biochem. Physiol.,
      (1963), 41, 1325-1327.
23.   Houck, J.C., Morris, R.K. and Lazaro, E.J., Proc. Soc. Exp.
      Biol. Med., (1957), 96, 528-530.
24.   Schimpf, K., Lenhard, J. and Schaaf, G., Thrombos. Diath.
      Haemorrh., (1969), 21, 525-533.
25.   Noordhoek, J. and Bonta, I.L., Arch. Int. Pharmacodyn.
      Ther., (1972), 197, (2), 385-386.
26.   Bice, D.E., Gruwell, D.G., Salvaggio, J.E. and Hoffman, E.O.,
      Immunol. Commun. (1972), 1, (6), 615-625.
27.   Bice, D., Schwartz, H., Lake, W. and Salvaggio, J., Int.
      Arch. Allergy, (1971), 41, 628-636.
28.   Borsos, T., Rapp, H.J. and Crile, C., J. Immunol., (1965),
      94, 662-666.
29.   Davies, G.E., Immunology, (1965), 8, 291-299.
30.   Davies, G.E., Immunology, (1963), 6, 561-568.
31.   Johnston, K.H. and McCandless, E.L., J. Immunol., (1968),
      101, 556-562.
32.   Mizushima, Y. and Noda, M., Experientia, (1973), 29, (5),
      605-606.
33.   Schwartz, H.J. and Leskowitz, S., J. Immunol., (1969), 103,
      87-91.
34.   Sauvageau, C., "Utilisation des Algues Marines," 268-335,
      Gaston Doin et Cie, Paris, (1920).
35.   Rees, D.A., Structure Conformation and Mechanism in the
      Formation of Polysaccharide Gels and Networks, "Advances in
      Carbohydrate Chemistry and Biochemistry," 24, 267-332,
      Academic Press, New York, (1969).
36.   Glicksman, M., "Gum Technology in the Food Industry,"
      214-235, Academic Press, New York (1969).
37.   Sand, R.E. and Glicksman, M., Seaweed Extracts of Potential
      Economic Importance, "Industrial Gums," Second Edition,
      147-194, Academic Press, New York, (1973).
38.   Towle, G.A., Carrageenan, "Industrial Gums," Second Edition,
      83-114, Academic Press, New York (1973).
39.   Stancioff, D.J. Unpublished results.
40.   "The Biological Activity of Native and Degraded Carra-
      geenan," The British Industrial Biological Research Associa-
      tion, Carshalton, Surrey, unpublished report (1971).

41. Grasso, P., Sharratt, M., Carpanini, F.M.B., and Gangolli, S.D., Food Cosmet. Toxicol., (1973), 2, 555-564.

42. Beattie, I.A., Blakemore, W.R., Dewar, E.T. and Warwick, M.H., Food Cosmet. Toxicol., (1970), 8, 257-266.

43. Abraham, R., Golberg, L. and Coulston, F., Exp. Mol. Pathol., (1972), 17, 77-93.

44. Houck, J.C., Bhayana, J. and Lee, T., Gastroenterology, (1960), 39, 196-200.

45. Poulsen, E., Food Cosmet. Toxicol., (1973), 2, 219-227.

46. Dewar, E.T. and Maddy, M.L., J. Pharm. Pharmacol., (1970), 22, 791-793.

47. Hawkins, W.W. and Yaphe, W., Can. J. Biochem., (1965), 43, 479-484.

48. Nilson, H.W. and Wagner, J.A., Food Res., (1959), 24, 235-239.

49. Abraham, R., Golberg, L., and Coulston, F., Paper No. 192, presented at the Annual Meeting of the Society of Toxicology, March 10-14, 1974.

50. Watt, J. and Marcus, R., J. Pharm. Pharmacol., (1969), 21, Suppl. 187S.

51. "Safety Evaluation of Carrageenan," Albany Medical College, Institute Experimental Pathology and Toxicology, Albany, New York, (Unpublished report 1971).

52. Anderson, W., and Soman, P.D., J. Pharm. Pharmacol., (1966), 18, 825-827.

53. Anderson, W. and Harthill, J.E., J. Pharm. Pharmacol., (1967), 17, 647-654.

54. Anderson, W., and Baillie, A.J., J. Pharm. Pharmacol., (1967), 19, 720-728.

55. Anderson, W., Baillie, A.J. and Harthill, J.E., J. Pharm. Pharmacol., (1968), 20, 715-722.

56. Vaughan, O.W., Filer, L.J. Jr., and Churella, M., J. Agr. Food Chem., (1962), 10, 517-519.

57. Martin, F., Vagne, A.B., and Lambert, R., C.R. Soc. Biol., (1965), 159, 1582-1585.

58. Anderson, W. and Watt, J., J. Pharm. Pharmacol., (1959), 11:318.

59. Watt, J., Eagleton, J.B. and Marcus R., Nature, (1966), 211, 989.

60. Anderson, W., Marcus, R. and Watt, J., J. Pharm. Pharmacol., (1962), 14, 119-121.

61. Anderson, W. and Soman, P.D., Nature, (1967), 214, 823-824.

62. Fahrenbach, M.J., Riccardo, B.A. and Grant, W.C., Proc. Soc. Exp. Biol. Med., (1966), 123, 321.

63. Ershoff, B.H. and Wills, A.F., Proc. Soc. Exp. Biol. Med., (1962), 110, 580-582.

64. Bonfils, S., Lancet, (1970), 2, 414.

65. Watt, J. and Marcus, R., J. Pharm. Pharmacol., (1970), 22, 130-131.

66. Stanley, N.F. and Renn, D.W., Proc. Int. Seaweed Symp.,
     8th, (1974), Bangor, Wales (In press).
67. Food Chemical News, (1974), 16, (29), 3-5.
68. Tomarelli, R.M., Tucker, W.D. Jr., Bauman, L.M., Savini, S.
     and Weaber, J.R., J. Agr. Food Chem., 22, 819-824.

19

Physiological Effects of Mannans, Galactomannans, and Glucomannans

S. E. DAVIS and B. A. LEWIS

Division of Nutritional Sciences, New York State College of Human Ecology, Cornell University, Ithaca, N. Y. 14850

Galactomannans in the form of the ground endosperm of certain leguminous seeds have been consumed as foodstuffs since ancient times. In the last two decades these gums together with konjac glucomannan and the yeast mannans have come to be associated with certain physiological activities which have stimulated nutritional and physiological research. Many of the studies are contradictory and several questions remain unanswered. This paper attempts to review the recent literature on the nutritional value of the mannans and the physiological activities which they possess.

Occurrence in Foods

Few natural foods have been subjected to complete analysis for their component carbohydrates. For the most part, analyses have been directed toward the soluble low molecular weight sugars, starch, pectin and crude fiber (consisting of cellulose and smaller amounts of associated but usually unidentified cell wall hemicelluloses). Thus, the infrequent reports of mannans in foods could reflect their rarity or merely that they have been overlooked.

Pure mannans (homopolymer) are particularly rare in nature. The most familiar sources are the yeasts, where in Saccharomyces cerevisiae, for example, mannose occurs as the branched α-(1→3, 1→6)-linked yeast mannan (1).

Galactomannans are much more common since they are important as industrial gums for a variety of uses (1-3). Found most frequently in the endosperm of seeds of leguminous plants, these gums find their way into processed foods as additives for control of texture, rheological behavior and as binders. The basic structure (Figure 1) is that of an essentially linear β-mannan with single unit branches of α-galactopyranose units. The galactomannans from different sources vary in molecular weight and in the ratio of the two sugars. Thus in guaran (guar gum) the ratio of mannose to galactose is 2:1; whereas in locust bean

$$\begin{array}{c} \alpha\text{-D-Gal}_p \\ 1 \\ \downarrow \\ 6 \\ -\beta\text{-D-Man}_p\text{-}(1{\rightarrow}4)\text{-}\beta\text{-D-Man}_p\text{-}(1{\rightarrow}4)\text{-}\beta\text{-D-Man}_p\text{-} \end{array}$$

Figure 1.   Guar and locust bean galactomannans

gum (carob gum) it is variously reported as 3:1 to 6:1. This
difference in degree of branching is reflected in the physical
properties of the gums; guar galactomannan readily hydrates in
cold water to form a colloidal solution while locust bean gum
dispersions must be heated to develop maximum viscosity.

Historically the guar plant (Cyamopsis tetragonolobis) has
been grown for centuries in India and Pakistan as a food crop for
humans as well as animals. The plant was introduced into the
United States for agricultural production in the southwest and
the galactomannan became commercially available in the 1950's.
Commercial guar gum, which is milled free from the hull and germ,
consists of about 78-82% galactomannan, 4-5% protein, 1.5-2.0%
crude fiber, and a small amount of ash and ether-soluble
material.

Food usage of the pods of the locust bean tree (Ceratonia
siliqua L.) probably dates back for thousands of years. Since
Biblical times the locust bean or carob has been immortalized as
St. John's bread. Like guar, the commercial gum is obtained from
the seeds of the pods by removing the germ and husk. The composition of the typical gum of commerce is not unlike that of guar
and is dependent on the efficiency of separation of the galacto-
mannan-containing endosperm.

Other mannose-containing heteropolysaccharides include the
glucomannans which occur most commonly in woody plants in association with cellulose. One of the few identified food sources is
konnyaku powder obtained by grinding the tubers of the plant
Amorphophalis konyac. Extraction of konnyaku powder with water
affords konjac mannan, a β-1→4-linked glucomannan (Figure 2) with
sequences of at least three mannose units.

$$-\beta\text{-D-Man}_p\text{-}(1{\rightarrow}4)\text{-}\beta\text{-D-Man}_p\text{-}(1{\rightarrow}4)\text{-}\beta\text{-D-G}_p\text{-}(1{\rightarrow}4)\text{-}\beta\text{-D-Man}_p\text{-}(1{\rightarrow}4)\text{-}$$

Figure 2.   Konjac mannan

Mannose is also a common constituent of glycoproteins where
it occurs in variable amounts from less than 1% in some proteins
to a significant proportion of other proteins. Thus, glycoproteins such as the soy globulins contain up to 5% carbohydrate.
The carbohydrate moiety of glycoproteins most frequently consists
of chains of varying length of α-linked D-mannopyranose units
attached successively through β-D-mannosyl and β-D-glucosaminyl

(usually N-acetylated) units to the protein chain. Linkage to
the protein occurs through an N-glycosidic bond to the β-amide of
asparagine or less frequently by an O-glycosidic bond to the
hydroxyl of serine or threonine. For a number of proteins including ovalbumin, ribonuclease B and taka amylase the inner core
of the glycoprotein has the following structure (4,5):

$$\beta\text{-D-Man-}(1{\rightarrow}4)\text{-D-GNAc-}(1{\rightarrow}4)\text{-}\beta\text{-D-GNAc}{\rightarrow}\text{L-ASN}$$

Little is known of the significance of the mannan moiety of
glycoproteins or of its effect on the digestibility of proteins.
Intracellular mannose-containing glycoproteins are catabolized
by lysosomal α- and β-mannosidases which display maximal activity
at slightly acid pH (5-8). However, it should be noted that
non-lysosomal α-mannosidases are known (5, 9, 10).

Digestion of Mannans

Although little is known about the fate of dietary mannans
and mannose-containing glycoproteins, it is possible that some
mannose might be released by action of mannosidases in the gastrointestinal tract (11). McMaster et al. (12) reported an α-D-
mannosidase in canine pancreatic juice. The acidic pH optimum of
this enzyme, however, suggests its probable origin in pancreatic
tissue lysosomes. While the activity of pancreatic juice α-mannosidase was low compared to trypsinogen or amylase, the output
of all these enzymes increased similarly in response to pancreatic stimulation by secretin-cholecystokinin or by secretin-pen-
tagastrin (13).

α-Mannosidase activity has been detected also in the pancreas of sheep and ox, in the wall of the stomach, ileum, and colon of sheep, ox, pig, rabbit and rat (14), and in the small
intestine of monkey. The enzyme from monkey small intestine is
dependent on Zn^{++} (15), a characteristic of α-mannosidases from
several sources (16, 17). The role of gastrointestinal α-mannosidases in vivo is not known. Mannans (including gluco- and galactomannans) are relatively resistant to mannosidase attack but
are degraded readily by exo- (5, 18) and endo-mannanases (19-22).

Reports of in vivo digestion of mannans are contradictory.
It is generally assumed that digestion does not occur to a significant extent, yet some studies in animals suggest that partial
digestion occurs (23-26).

Hypocholesterolemic Activity of Mannans

Plasma cholesterol levels in experimental animals respond to
supplemental dietary cholesterol in a manner that is remarkably
sensitive to the specific dietary carbohydrate. With sucrose as
the sole carbohydrate in the diet, plasma cholesterol levels in
chickens were shown to be double those displayed when glucose

was the source of carbohydrate (27). However, galactomannans and glucomannans, like a number of other mucilaginous polysaccharides (28), elicit a significant hypocholesterolemic response when incorporated at low levels (o.5-3% of diet) into cholesterol-supplemented diets; an effect that has been noted in chickens and rats (29). Of the 16 crude polysaccharides evaluated by Fahrenbach et al., guar gum (galactomannan) and carrageenan were most effective in lowering plasma cholesterol, while pectin was much less effective.

Guar gum, incorporated at 2% of diet, also lowered endogenous plasma cholesterol in chickens fed a basal casein-sucrose diet without cholesterol supplementation. Similar results have been obtained with rats although much higher dietary levels (5-10%) of guar gum or pectin were required to significantly lower serum and liver cholesterol (29). Total rat liver lipids were also lowered by these high levels of guar.

Supplementation of a powdered commercial basal diet with 1% cholesterol did not cause the dramatic increases in serum and liver cholesterol and total liver lipids in the rat compared with the levels observed with the casein-sucrose diet. Nevertheless dietary guar gum lowered liver cholesterol and total lipid levels (29) and was more effective in this respect than pectin.

Studies to determine the mechanism of this hypocholesterolemic activity of mannans have been limited to konjac mannan (glucomannan), an important foodstuff of the Japanese. The mechanism and the structural requirements, however, probably apply as well to the galactomannans and other polysaccharides which show such activity.

In *vivo* studies with rats (30) demonstrated that konjac mannan decreases intestinal absorption of bile salts by interference with the active transport mechanism. Bile acid transport in everted sacs prepared from rat ileum, the site of active transport, was decreased up to 50% by the presence of 0.25% konjac mannan in the mucosal medium (Table I). Active transport of cholic acid is very low in the proximal jejunum of the rat intestine and passive diffusion of cholate through everted sacs prepared from this region was not altered by konjac mannan.

In *vitro* studies (30) also fail to give evidence of binding of bile salts by konjac mannan. Thus the diffusion rate of cholate and taurocholate across a cellophane membrane was not altered by either the glucomannan or pectin.

With adult rats on a hypercholesterolemic diet, 4-^{14}C-cholesterol transport into the plasma and liver was significantly lowered by dietary konjac mannan (31). Infusion studies with anesthetized rats demonstrated the same effect. Thus the hypocholesterolemic activity of konjac mannan in the rat appears to be due to an inhibition of cholesterol absorption in the jejunum and bile salt absorption in the ileum. Inhibition of bile salt absorption is reversed when the konjac mannan concentration drops below a minimum level.

Table I

Effect of Konjac Mannan on ^{14}C-Cholic Acid Transport in Everted Sacs from the Distal One-fourth of the Small Intestine of Male Rat (30)

Sac no.	Addition[a]	No. of sacs	Total radioactivity transported to the serosal fluid (A) (dpm)	(A)/100 mg sac (dpm)	Total radioactivity remaining in mucosal fluid (dpm)
1 Male	Control	6	1132 + 96	378 + 22	9285 + 1162
2	+KM	6	403 + 86	161 + 36	11268 + 238
3	Control	6	1241 + 302	402 + 41	8900 + 473
4	+KM	6	613 + 97	216 + 37	10183 + 678
1 Female	Control	5	2970 + 210	1300 + 130	10550 + 790
2	+KM	5	930 + 80	470 + 30	13120 + 640
3	Control	5	2340 + 520	1140 + 110	11030 + 590
4	+KM	5	1360 + 180	680 + 80	11070 + 1620

[a]0.25% Konjac mannan (KM) added to mucosal medium. Mucosal fluid (5ml) was labeled with 0.01 μCi of ^{14}C-cholate. Incubation time, 40 min.

Journal of Nutrition

Certain structural and physical characteristics of the polysaccharide are required for cholesterol-depressing activity.
Native konjac mannan is a water-soluble high molecular weight
glucomannan and both features are required for activity (32).
Hypocholesterolemic activity was increased by purification, demonstrating that the polysaccharide and not a contaminant is the
active agent (33). Hydrolysis of the glucomannan with cellulase
or acid completely eliminated the hypocholesterolemic effect;
this effect was evident even when cellulase was incorporated in
the diet containing the native konjac mannan (33).
     Hypocholesterolemic activity is also lost by irreversibly
coagulating native water-soluble polysaccharide with lime water
(32).   Konnyaku, a popular food in Japan, is prepared by such
an alkaline treatment. Edible water-insoluble konnyaku has no
hypocholesterolemic activity in rats. It has also been shown
with locust bean gum preparations (29) that viscosity and water
solubility influenced the cholesterol-depressing activity in that
high viscosity preparations were more effective.
     Thus the variations in hypocholesterolemic activity of cer-
tain crude gums reported by different investigators may reflect
differences in the molecular weight, water-solubility and amount
of polysaccharide in the crude gum as affected by plant species,
growing conditions or processing methods.
     From studies with konjac glucomannan and guar and locust
bean galactomannan, it is apparent that certain high molecular
weight, water-soluble polysaccharides incorporated into hypercholesterolemic diets have the effect of lowering serum and
liver cholesterol in certain experimental animals (rat, chicken,
rabbit). In the rat konjac glucomannan activity derives from an
as yet unexplained interference with active transport of
cholesterol in the jejunum and bile acids in the ileum.

Growth Inhibition and Toxicity

     Early studies showed that growth of chickens was inhibited
when their diet contained locust bean or guar meal (34-36).
Vohra and Kratzer (36) reported growth in chicks of only 61-68%
of the controls after 20 days on a diet containing 2% guar gum,
and growth of 75% of the controls on diets containing 2% locust
bean gum. No growth depression was observed when the guar gum
was predigested with enzymes before feeding.
     Although other investigators have also noticed some reduc-
tion in body weight gain of chicks on diets containing mucilaginous polysaccharides, Fahrenbach et al. (28) were unable to
repeat the results of Vohra and Kratzer. In these studies (28)
chicks fed 2% guar flour incorporated into diets similar to those
used previously (36) showed an insignificant increase in body
weight compared with controls. However, levels of 5-10% guar in
either a 1% cholesterol-supplemented casein-sucrose or commercial basal diet did cause a reduction in weight gain in rats (29).

Ershoff and Wells (37) found no significant depression in growth
of rats fed a casein-sucrose basal diet containing 10% guar or
locust bean gum and 1% cholesterol for 28 days.

In summary, some depression of growth is observed in animals
fed high levels of guar and locust bean gum but the results are
widely variable (25, 38, 39). This is a general phenomenon,
however, which is typical of a wide variety of mucilaginous polysaccharides.

With increased interest in nutrition and the safety of food
additives the pertinent literature on guar (25) and locust bean
gum (38, 39) have been reviewed and animal studies have been
carried out to evaluate the toxicological status of guar (40-43)
and locust bean gum (44-46).

Ninety-day toxicity studies were conducted with rats fed
diets containing 1, 2 and 5% guar gum (40). Gross and microscopic examination did not reveal pathological changes which could
be attributed to ingestion of the gum, and the general condition
and survival of the rats were not adversely affected. Serum
enzyme activities (glutamic-oxaloacetic transaminase, glutamic-
pyruvic transaminase and alkaline phosphatase), hematology values, blood sugar levels and urine composition were unaltered compared with controls. Blood urea nitrogen was slightly elevated.
At all levels of dietary guar, the relative weight of the caecum
was increased. This appears to be a phenomenon common to most
mucilaginous polysaccharides as well as some starches and can be
attributed to the hydration properties of the gums. As in previous studies, body weights tended to be somewhat lower in the
guar-fed animals compared with the controls.

A similar ninety-day toxicity study of locust bean gum was
also conducted (44). The results were generally the same as
with guar. The only significant changes in the test animals
compared with the controls were in the increased caecum weight
and the somewhat lower body weights of females on the 1 and 5%
locust bean diets.

Other Physiological Effects

Polysaccharides when injected into the body elicit various
physiological effects. Two such activities are interferon-stimulation and tumor inhibition. Previous studies (47, 48) have
shown that various agents such as bacteria and their endotoxins
stimulate interferon release from leucocytes. Since both the
bacteria and their endotoxins contain polysaccharides, it has
been suggested that the constituent polysaccharides are responsible for the stimulation.

In vitro studies with mouse peritoneal cells demonstrated
that purified mannans and mannan-protein complexes from Candida
albicans when incorporated into the medium stimulated interferon
release. However, the mannan from S. cerevisiae was inactive
(49). Lower molecular weight mannans (MW 20,000) showed the

greatest activity which could explain why the higher molecular weight Saccharomyces mannan was inactive. Interferon-stimulation also occurred in in vivo studies although the results were less reproducible than with in vitro studies. The mechanism by which interferon release is activated by the mannans has not been established.

The role of a variety of polysaccharides in tumor inhibition has been a subject of continuing interest. Mannans from baker's yeast (50) and from Candida utilis (51, 52) injected intraperitoneally inhibited growth of implanted tumor cells such as sarcoma-180 in mice. More recently baker's yeast mannan has been shown to inhibit development of 3-methylcholanthrene-induced epithelial tumors in mice when daily intraperitoneal injections of mannan were started 10 days prior to application of the carcinogen to the skin (53).

Acute toxicity, which was evident in intravenous but not in intraperitoneal injection of mannans, was eliminated by preparation of the carboxymethyl derivative of the mannan (54). Enhancement of the cellular antibody response of the host animal has been considered to be the general mechanism by which the mannans act. Labeled carboxymethyl mannan accumulated to some extent in the solid tumor (sarcoma-180) and in various organs but was most strongly accumulated by the liver and spleen (52).

Mannose Absorption and Metabolism

Absorption and Reabsorption. When mannose was administered to rats by stomach tube, it was absorbed at only 12.3% the rate of glucose (55). Mannose was weakly accumulated in everted hamster intestinal slices and accumulation was not stimulated by Na^+, indicating that mannose is passively absorbed rather than actively transported by the Na^+-dependent carrier. Presumably the failure of mannose to be actively transported can be attributed to its deviation from the D-glucopyrano configuration at C-2 (56). In a study with everted sacs of rat intestine it was also found (57) that mannose was not actively transported but it was metabolized in the serosal fluid.

In contrast to the low absorption of mannose from the small intestine, its reabsorption by the luminal membrane of the proximal tubule of dog kidney was comparable to that of glucose, which is well conserved. The evidence suggests the presence of two separate sets of binding sites on the luminal surface, one for glucose and a different one for mannose (58).

Mannose Metabolism. It appears that mannose is metabolized almost as readily as glucose. Indeed, mannose has even been shown (59) to be a suitable substrate for metabolism by isolated rat brain, an organ which is usually thought to have an absolute requirement for glucose. The metabolism of mannose has been reviewed by Herman (11, 60). Pathways of mannose metabolism are outlined in Figure 3.

Mannose is phosphorylated to mannose 6-phosphate (Man-6-P) by hexokinase in an ATP-requiring reaction. Phosphorylation coefficients for mannose by rat brain (61) and rat adipose tissue (62) hexokinases were 0.65 and 1.0, respectively, compared to glucose as 1.0, indicating that the affinity of hexokinase for mannose is high. In human erythrocytes (63) mannose is phosphorylated by an enzyme that is electrophoretically indistinguishable from the glucose-phosphorylating enzyme. Mannose phosphorylation is competitively inhibited by glucose, and glucose phosphorylation is competitively inhibited by mannose. Furthermore, Man-6-P (1 mM) noncompetitively inhibits the phosphorylation of mannose. This finding is interesting in view of the earlier report (64) that Man-6-P (8.5 mM), unlike glucose 6-phosphate (G-6-P), had no inhibitory effect on mannose phosphorylation by rat brain hexokinase. Recently, Arnold et al. (65) noted that bee hexokinase was inhibited by G-6-P but not by Man-6-P. They suggested that the failure of Man-6-P to inhibit bee hexokinase, which resulted in a severe reduction in the ATP level, accounts for mannose toxicity in honeybees.

Man-6-P is converted to fructose 6-phosphate (Fru-6-P), an intermediate in glycolysis, by phosphomannose isomerase. This enzyme has been shown (66, 67) to be distinct from phosphoglucose isomerase. Interestingly, phosphomannose isomerase is a Zn^{++}-metalloenzyme and inhibited by EDTA (68-70). There is evidence that the enzyme may play an important role in the regulation of glycolysis. Thus, when isolated rat brain was perfused with either mannose or glucose, there was a build-up of Man-6-P relative to Fru-6-P (59). When human erythrocytes were incubated with mannose, Man-6-P also accumulated (Figure 4), indicating that phosphomannose isomerase rather than hexokinase is the rate limiting enzyme (63).

Conversion of Man-6-P to mannose 1-phosphate (Man-1-P) is catalyzed by phosphomannomutase, which is apparently distinct from phosphoglucomutase. Either glucose 1,6-diphosphate or mannose 1,6-diphosphate must be present for the reaction to occur (71). Man-1-P is transformed into guanosine diphosphate mannose (GDP-Man), a sugar nucleotide, by reaction with guanosine triphosphate. GDP-Man is of physiological importance since (a) it serves as substrate for mannosyl transferase and (b) it can be transformed into guanosine diphosphate fucose, the substrate for fucosyl transferase (72). It appears that mannosyl transferases from several sources require a divalent cation, particularly Mn^{++} or Mg^{++}, for their activity (73-76). Glycosyl transferases, which are probably located along the endoplasmic reticulum, are responsible for the incorporation of glycosyl residues, one at a time, into various glycoprotein, glycolipid and mannan acceptors (77).

There is considerable evidence that polyprenyl mannosyl phosphates are involved as intermediates in the transfer of mannose

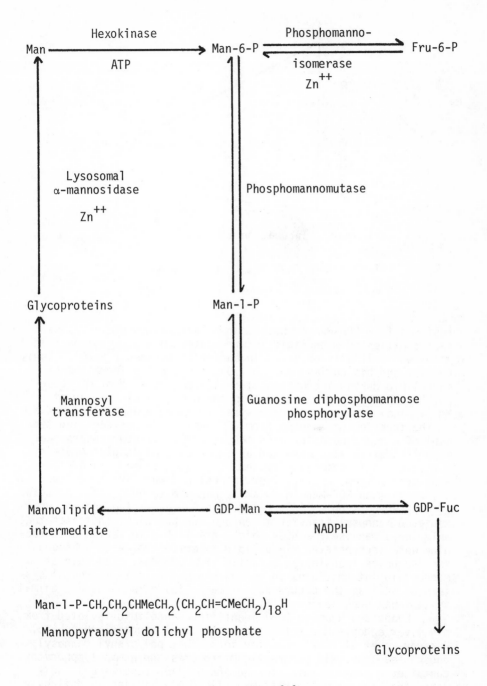

Figure 3. Mannose metabolism

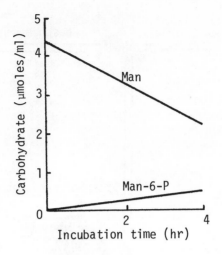

Figure 4. Incubation of human erythro-cytes with 10 mM mannos (63)

residues from GDP-Man to both mannans and glycoproteins. The participation of mannolipid intermediates in glycosylation reactions was initially observed in bacterial systems (78-80). Thus, Lennarz and his colleagues (78, 79) reported the formation of mannolipid during incubation of cell-free extracts of Micrococcus lysodeikticus with GDP-Man in the presence of Mn^{++} or of Mg^{++}. They subsequently demonstrated its role as an intermediate in the transfer of mannose from GDP-Man to the non-reducing termini of a membrane-associated mannan (80). It now appears that mannolipids are also involved as intermediates in glycoprotein biosynthesis in mammalian systems (81-84). Indeed, in a cell-free system from hamster liver, mannolipid was five times more effective than GDP-Man in donating mannose to endogenous proteins (84). Recent studies (85, 86) with a S. cerevisiae enzyme, which mediated mannosyl transfer to endogenous proteins, indicated that only those mannose residues which were linked to serine or threonine were incorporated via a lipid intermediate, with subsequent mannose units transferred directly from GDP-Man. The role of mannolipid intermediates in mannan biosynthesis in microbial systems as well as the occurrence of mannolipids in plant and animal systems has been reviewed (87).

Evans and Hemming (88) identified mannolipid isolated from pig liver endoplasmic reticulum as dolichyl mannosyl phosphate. Herscovics et al. (89) recently found that polyprenyl mannosyl phosphates from calf pancreatic microsomes and human lymphocytes contained a β-mannosidic linkage. An earlier report (90) indicated that the calf pancreas mannolipid was similar to dolichyl α-mannosyl phosphate, but at that time synthetic dolichyl β-mannosyl phosphate was not available for comparison. The preparation of the latter was recently described (91).

Effect of Mannose on Glycogen Formation. The glycogenic ability of mannose was first noted by Deuel et al. (92) in 1938. They reported a small increase in liver glycogen following oral administration of mannose to rats. However, glucose was more efficiently converted into glycogen even when it was given in an amount comparable to the rate of mannose absorption. Bailey and Roe (93) also showed that mannose was much less glycogenic than glucose when given orally to rabbits but that when given parenterally the rate of conversion was similar to that of glucose. Incorporation of label from ^{14}C-mannose into glycogen by rat adipose tissue has been demonstrated in vitro (94, 95).

Effect of Mannose on Blood Sugars. In 1944, it was reported (93) that oral administration of mannose led to elevated blood glucose and the appearance of mannose in the peripheral venous blood of the rabbit. However, data for only one animal were given. More recently, it was found (96) that following oral infusion of mannose in rabbits there was no elevation in blood glucose and only a slight increase in the blood mannose level. Intravenously injected mannose also failed to produce an elevation in blood glucose.

Effect of Mannose on Insulin Secretion. The ability of mannose to stimulate release of insulin from the pancreas in vitro is well known. Grodsky et al. (97) claimed that mannose was as effective as glucose in stimulating insulin secretion in isolated rat pancreas. However, in studies with fetal rat pancreatic explants (98) and with pieces of rabbit pancreas (99), the stimulatory effect of mannose was only half that of glucose. Using fragments of rat pancreas, Malaisse et al. (100) found that mannose at various concentrations induced insulin secretion to an extent that was somewhat less marked than that produced by glucose. Recently it was shown (101) that insulin release from isolated rat pancreas during a 60-minute period of constant mannose infusion was diphasic, with an initial spurt in insulin output followed by a gradual decline. This suggested that mannose triggers insulin secretion but not its biosynthesis. Fructose increased the insulin response elicited by mannose. In an in vivo study with rabbits, Nijjar et al. (96) found that the serum insulin level was greatly elevated immediately following an intravenous injection of mannose. Furthermore, it appears that orally administered mannose elicited a slow, very slight, and probably insignificant insulin response despite the authors' conclusion that oral mannose failed to stimulate insulin release. In support of the hypothesis that only metabolizable sugars stimulate insulin secretion, Jarrett and Keen (102) reported that ^{14}C-mannose was readily metabolized by isolated rat islets of Langerhans as determined by $^{14}CO_2$ recovery.

Several studies have shown that insulin exerts a stimulatory effect on mannose utilization in vitro by rat adipose tissue. Thus, Wood et al. (94) reported that insulin increased the incorporation of radioactivity from either ^{14}C-labeled mannose or glucose into fatty acids, glyceride-glycerol, and glycogen to a similar extent. Goodman (103) found that the uptake of ^{14}C-mannose by adipose tissue, the incorporation of ^{14}C into fatty acids, and the production of $^{14}CO_2$ was enhanced by insulin and, to a lesser extent, by growth hormone. Finally, Kuo and Dill (95) showed that insulin as well as several proteolytic enzymes that mimic certain of its effects stimulated the incorporation of label from ^{14}C-mannose into CO_2, fatty acids, glyceride-glycerol, protein and glycogen.

Literature Cited

1. Smith, F. and Montgomery, R. "The Chemistry of Plant Gums and Mucilages," Reinhold, New York (1959).
2. Glicksman, M. "Gum Technology in the Food Industry," Academic Press, New York (1969).
3. Whistler, R. L., ed. "Industrial Gums," 2nd ed., Academic Press, New York (1973).
4. Lee, Y.C. Fed. Proc. (1971) 30, 1223.
5. Snaith, S.M. and Levvy, G.A. in Advan. Carbohyd. Chem. Biochem. (1973) 28, 401.
6. Conchie, J. and Hay, A.J. Biochem. J. (1963) 87, 354.
7. Sukeno, T., Tarentino, A.L., Plummer, Jr., T.H., and Maley,F. Biochemistry (1972) 11, 1493.
8. LaBadie, J.H. and Aronson, Jr., N.N. Biochim. Biophys. Acta (1973) 321, 603.
9. Marsh, C.A. and Gourlay, G.C. Biochim. Biophys. Acta (1971) 235, 142.
10. Dewald, B. and Touster, O. J. Biol. Chem. (1973) 248, 7223.
11. Herman, R.H. Am. J. Clin. Nutr. (1971) 24, 488.
12. McMaster, W., Desbaillets, L., and Menguy, R. Proc. Soc. Expt. Biol. Med. (1970) 135, 87.
13. Desbaillets, L., McMaster, W.C., and Menguy, R. Proc. Soc. Expt. Biol. Med. (1971) 136, 597.
14. Conchie, J. and Macdonald, D.C. Nature (1959) 184, 1233.
15. Seetharam, B. and Radhakrishnan, A.N. Indian J. Biochem. Biophys. (1972) 9, 59.
16. Snaith, S.M. and Levvy, G.A. Biochem. J. (1968) 106, 53P.
17. Snaith, S.M. and Levvy, G.A. Nature (1968) 218, 91.
18. Jones, G.H. and Ballou, C.E. J. Biol. Chem. (1968) 243, 2442.
19. Eriksson, K.-E. and Winell, M. Acta Chem. Scand. (1968) 22, 1924.
20. Emi, S., Fukumoto, J., and Yamamoto, T. Agr. Biol. Chem. (1972) 36, 991.

21. Tsujisaka, Y., Hiyama, K., Takenishi, S., and Fukumoto, J. Nippon Nogei Kagaku Kaishu (1972) 46, 155.
22. Sugiyama, N., Shimahara, H., Andoh, T., and Takemoto, M. Agr. Biol. Chem. (1973) 37, 9.
23. Krantz, J.C., Carr, C.J. and de Farson, C.B. J. Am. Diet. Assoc. (1948) 24, 212.
24. Wisconsin Alumni Research Foundation, Assay Rept. No. 3110860 and 3110861 (1964).
25. Battelle Columbus Laboratories, NTIS Rept. No. PB-221216 (1972).
26. Bains, G.S. Food Sci. (1963) 12, 344.
27. Grant, W.C. and Fahrenbach, M.J. Proc. Soc. Expt. Biol. Med. (1959) 100, 250.
28. Fahrenbach, M.J., Riccardi, B.A. and Grant, W.C. Proc. Soc. Expt. Biol. Med. (1966) 123, 321.
29. Riccardi, B.A. and Fahrenbach, M.J. Proc. Soc. Expt. Biol. Med. (1967) 124, 749.
30. Kiriyama, S., Enishi, A.,and Yura, K. J. Nutr. (1974) 104, 69.
31. Kodama, T., Nakai, H., Kiriyama, S., and Yoshida, A. J. Jap. Soc. Food Nutr. (1972) 25, 603.
32. Kiriyama, S., Morisaki, H., and Yoshida, A. Agr. Biol. Chem. (1970) 34, 641.
33. Kiriyama, S., Ichihara, Y., Enishi, A., and Yoshida, A. J. Nutr. (1972) 102, 1689.
34. Bornstein, S., Alumot, E., Mokadi, S., Nachtomi, E., and Nahari, V. Israel J. Agr. Res. (1963) 13, 25.
35. Vohra, P. and Kratzer, F.H. Poultry Sci. (1964) 43, 502.
36. Vohra, P. and Kratzer, F.H. Poultry Sci. (1964) 43, 1164.
37. Ershoff, B.H. and Wells, A.F. Proc. Soc. Expt. Biol. Med. (1962) 110, 580.
38. GRAS Food Ingredients: Carob Bean Gum (Locust Bean Gum), NTIS Rept. No. PB-221203 (1972).
39. Evaluation of the Health Aspects of Carob Bean Gum as a Food Ingredient, NTIS Rept. No. PB-221952 (1972).
40. Sub-chronic Toxicity Study with Guar Gum in Rats, Rept. No. 4095, Centraal Instituut Voor Voedingsonderzoek (1974).
41. Study of Mutagenic Effects of Guar Gum (71-16), NTIS Rept. No. PB-221815 (1972).
42. Teratologic Evaluation of FDA 71-16 (Guar Gum), NTIS Rept. No. PB-221800 (1972).
43. Teratologic Evaluation of FDA 71-16 (Guar Gum), NTIS Rept. No. 223819 (1973).
44. Sub-chronic Toxicity Study with Locust Bean Gum in Rats, Rept. No. 4093, Centraal Instituut Voor Voedingsonderzoek (1974).
45. Study of Mutagenic Effects of Locust Bean Gum (FDA 71-14), NTIS Rept. No. PB-221819 (1972).
46. Teratologic Evaluation of FDA 71-14 (Carob Bean Locust Gum), NTIS Rept. No. PB-221784 (1972).

47. Borecky, L., Lackovic, V., Blaskovic, D., Masler, L., and Sikl, D. Acta Virol. (1967) 11, 264.
48. Feingold. D.S., Youngner, J.S., and Chen, J. Biochem. Biophys. Res. Comm. (1968) 32, 554.
49. Lackovic, V., Borecky, L., Sikl, D., Masler, L., and Bauer, S. Proc. Soc. Expt. Biol. Med. (1970) 134, 874.
50. Suzuki, M., Chaki, F., and Suzuki, S. Gann (1971) 62, 553.
51. Oka, S., Kumano, N., Sato, K., Tamari, K., Matsuda, K., Hirai, H., Oguma, T., Ogawa, K., Kiyooka, S., and Miyao, K. Gann (1969) 60, 287.
52. Kumano, N., Kurita, K., and Oka, S. Gann (1972) 63, 675.
53. Kumano, N., Kurita, K., and Oka, S. Gann (1973) 64, 529.
54. Oka, S., Kumano, N., and Kurita, K. Gann (1972) 63, 365.
55. Deuel, Jr., H.J., Hallman, L.F., Murray, S., and Hilliard, J. J. Biol. Chem. (1938) 125, 79.
56. Barnett, J.E.G., Ralph, A., and Munday, K.A. Biochem. J. (1970) 118, 843.
57. Barry, R.J.C., Eggenton, J., and Smyth, D.H. J. Physiol. (London) (1969) 204, 299.
58. Silverman, M., Agánon, M.A., and Chinard, F.P. Am. J. Physiol. (1970) 218, 743.
59. Ghosh, A.K., Mukherji, B., and Sloviter, H.A. J. Neurochem. (1972) 19, 1279.
60. Herman, R.H. Am. J. Clin. Nutr. (1971) 24, 556.
61. Sols, A. and Crane, R.K. J. Biol. Chem. (1954) 210, 581.
62. Hernandez, A. and Sols, A. Biochem. J. (1963) 86, 166.
63. Beutler, E. and Teeple, L. J. Clin. Invest. (1969) 48, 461.
64. Crane, R.K. and Sols, A. J. Biol. Chem. (1954) 210, 597.
65. Arnold, H., Seitz, U., and Löhr, G.W. Hoppe-Seyler's Z. Physiol. Chem. (1974) 355, 266.
66. Slein, M.W. J. Biol. Chem. (1950) 186, 753.
67. Noltmann, E. and Bruns, F.H. Biochem Z. (1958) 330, 514.
68. Gracy, R.W. and Noltmann, E.A. J. Biol. Chem. (1968) 243, 3161.
69. Gracy, R.W. and Noltmann, E.A. J. Biol. Chem. (1968) 243, 4109.
70. Gracy, R.W. and Noltmann, E.A. J. Biol. Chem. (1968) 243, 5410.
71. Glaser, L., Kornfeld, S. and Brown, D.H. Biochim. Biophys. Acta (1959) 33, 522.
72. Ginsburg, V. J. Am. Chem. Soc. (1958) 80, 4426.
73. Behrens, N.H. and Cabib, E. J. Biol. Chem. (1968) 243, 502.
74. Letoublon, R.C.P., Comte, J., and Got, R. Eur. J. Biochem. (1973) 40, 95.
75. Levrat, C. and Louisot, P. Can. J. Biochem. (1973) 51, 931.
76. Arnold, D., Hommel, E., and Risse, H.-J. Biochem. Biophys. Res. Comm, (1973) 54, 100.
77. Spiro, R.C. New Eng. J. Med. (1969) 281, 991.
78. Scher, M., Lennarz, W.J., and Sweeley, C.C. Proc. Natl. Acad. Sci., U.S.A. (1968) 59, 1313.

79. Lahav, M., Chiu, T.H., and Lennarz, W.J. J. Biol. Chem. (1969) 244, 5890.
80. Scher, M. and Lennarz, W.J. J. Biol. Chem. (1969) 244, 2777.
81. Baynes, J.W., Hsu, A.-F., and Heath, E.C. J. Biol. Chem. (1973) 248, 5693.
82. Waechter, C.J., Lucas, J.J., and Lennarz, W.J. J. Biol. Chem. (1973) 248, 7570.
83. Behrens, N.H., Carminatti, H., Staneloni, R.J., Leloir, L. F., and Cantarella, A.I. Proc. Natl. Acad. Sci., U.S.A. (1973) 70, 3390.
84. Maestri, N. and DeLuca, L. Biochem. Biophys. Res. Comm. (1973) 53, 1344.
85. Babczinski, P. and Tanner, W. Biochem. Biophys. Res. Comm. (1973) 54, 1119.
86. Lehle, L. and Tanner, W. Biochim. Biophys. Acta (1974) 350, 225.
87. Lennarz, W.J. and Scher, M.G. Biochim. Biophys. Acta (1972) 265, 417.
88. Evans, P.J. and Hemming, F.W. Fed. Eur. Biochem. Soc. Lett. (1973) 31, 335.
89. Herscoviçs, A., Warren, C.D., Jeanloz, R.W., Wedgwood, J.F., Liu, I.Y., and Strominger, J.L. Fed. Eur. Biochem. Soc. Lett. (1974) 45, 312.
90. Tkacz, J.S., Herscovics, A., Warren, C.D., and Jeanloz, R.W. Biochem. Soc. Trans. (1973) 1, 1174.
91. Warren, C.D., Liu, I.Y., Herscovics, A., Wedgwood, J.F., and Jeanloz, R.W., Am. Chem. Soc. Abstracts, Atlantic City (1974).
92. Deuel, Jr., H.J., Hallman, L.F., Murray, S., and Hilliard, J. J. Biol. Chem. (1938) 125, 79.
93. Bailey, W.H. and Roe, J.H. J. Biol. Chem. (1944) 152, 135.
94. Wood, Jr., F.C., Leboeuf, B., Renold, A.E., and Cahill, Jr., G.F. J. Biol. Chem. (1961) 236, 18.
95. Kuo, J.F. and Dill, I.K. Biochim. Biophys. Acta (1969) 177, 17.
96. Nijjar, M.S. and Perry, W.F. Diabetes (1970) 19, 155.
97. Grodsky, G.M., Batts, A.A., Bennett, L.L., Vcella, C., McWilliams, N.B., and Smith, D.F. Am. J. Physiol. (1963) 205, 638.
98. Lambert, A.E., Junod, A., Stauffacher, W., Jeanrenaud, B., and Renold, A.E. Biochim. Biophys. Acta (1969) 184, 529.
99. Coore, H.G. and Randle, P.J. Biochem. J. (1964) 93, 66.
100. Malaisse, W., Malaisse-Lagae, F., and Mahy, M. Ann. Endocrinol. (Paris) (1969) 30, 595.
101. Curry, D.L. Am. J. Physiol. (1974) 226, 1073.
102. Jarrett, R.J. and Keen, H. Metabolism (1968) 17, 155.
103. Goodman, H.M. Endocrinology (1967) 80, 45.

20

Metabolism and Physiological Effects of Pectins

WANDA L. CHENOWETH and GILBERT A. LEVEILLE

Food Science and Human Nutrition, Michigan State University,
East Lansing, Mich. 48824

Non-digestible dietary carbohydrates recently have received much attention. Although most of this attention has focused on the importance of cereal sources of dietary fiber, poorly digested pectic substances derived primarily from fruit and vegetable sources likewise may be of significance in relation to human health.

Pectic substances are complex, colloidal carbohydrate derivatives which occur in or are isolated from plants. They contain a large proportion of anhydrogalacturonic acid units, most likely combined in a chain-like arrangement. The carboxyl groups of the polygalacturonic acids may be partly esterified or may form salts with various cations (1, 2). Pectin is a general term usually employed to designate water-soluble pectinic acids of varying methyl ester content and degree of neutralization capable of forming gels with sugar and acids (1).

The amount of pectic substances in several common fruits and vegetables is shown in Table I. Estimation of the total amount of pectic substances in an average diet is not possible because data are available only for a limited number of foods. Comparison of the content of pectic substances in various foods is further complicated by differences in analytical methods and incomplete descriptions of the foods. In addition to pectic substances found naturally in plant foods, pectin may be added to foods during processing. The most common use of pectin is in making jams and jellies; however pectin is an acceptable additive in a number of other foods. Pectins also have found numerous uses in the preparation of various pharmaceutical products.

Much of what is known about the physiological effect of pectin has evolved as a consequence of interest in the use of pectin for therapeutic purposes. Pectin and combinations of pectin with other colloids have been used extensively to treat diarrheal diseases, especially in infants and children (3 - 6).

Journal Article No. _____7046_____, Michigan Agricultural Experiment Station.

This use of pectin had its origin in the treatment of diarrhea
with a diet of scraped apples, a home-remedy practiced for hundreds of years in Europe and introduced into this country in 1933
by Birnberg (7).

The effectiveness of pectin in treating diarrhea subsequently
led to investigations to determine the mechanism of its effect and
its fate in the alimentary tract. Experiments in dogs showed that
when 20g pectin was fed in combination with a mixed diet, only 10
percent of the pectin could be recovered in the feces; however, if
the same amount was fed during fasting an average of 50 percent
was excreted (Table II). Results obtained with humans fed 50g of
pectin daily with a mixed diet were similar to those in dogs with
approximately 90 percent apparent decomposition of pectin taking
place (8, 9). The degree of decomposition appears to be influenced by the retention time in the intestine, adjustment of the
animal to the diet, and the degree of esterification of the pectin
(9, 10).

Tests made with human subjects and dogs indicated a lack of
enzymes in saliva and gastric juice which could act on pectin.
Likewise, trypsin, pepsin and rennet had no effect on pectin in
vitro; however pectin incubated with feces was rapidly decomposed
(11). Results of studies in animals and humans with ileostomies
indicated that the breakdown of pectin occurs chiefly in the colon
most likely by the action of bacterial enzymes (9). Isolation of
the microorganisms which are capable of decomposing pectin revealed that the most active groups were Aerobacillus, Lactobacillus, Micrococcus and Enterococcus (12, 13). The chief products
formed during bacterial fermentation are carbon dioxide and formic
and acetic acid. If galacturonic acid is produced it apparently
is broken down rapidly since only a small amount is present in
incubation mixtures. Although a bactericidal action of pectin
has been proposed to explain the effectiveness of pectin in
treating diarrhea, most experimental results do not support this
theory (14, 15). However, recent evidence suggests that under
certain in vitro conditions, pectins may have a slight antimicrobial action toward E. coli (16).

Most of the recent interest in pectin has been in relation to
its effect on lipid metabolism. In 1957 Lin and coworkers (17)
first reported that in rats the addition of pectin to a basal diet
containing cholesterol increased the excretion of fecal saponifi-
able and non-saponifiable lipids and decreased the absorption of
exogenous cholesterol. About the same time Keys and coworkers
(18) proposed that the lower incidence of atherosclerosis associated with "Italian-type diets" might be related to the amount of
complex carbohydrates such as pectin, hemicellulose and fiber
present in the fruits and vegetables abundant in these diets.
Subsequent investigations have thus focused on the effect of
pectin on serum and liver cholesterol concentrations and the fecal
excretion of lipid and sterols.

Numerous experiments in rats (Table III) have shown that

TABLE I

PECTIN CONTENT OF VARIOUS FOODS

Food		Pectic substances
		%
Apples	fresh basis	0.5 - 1.6
Bananas	" "	0.7 - 1.2
Peaches	" "	0.1 - 0.9
Strawberries	" "	0.6 - 0.7
Cherries	" "	0.2 - 0.5
Green peas	" "	0.9 - 1.4
Carrots	dry matter basis	6.9 - 18.6
Orange pulp	" " "	12.4 - 28.0
Potato	" " "	1.8 - 3.3
Tomato	" " "	2.4 - 4.6

Adapted from "The Pectic Substances" (2).

TABLE II

RECOVERY OF PECTIN FROM FECES BY URONIC ACID ESTIMATION

	Per Cent
Pectin fed with basal diet:	
dogs	8.9
humans	8.7
Pectin fed during fasting:	
dogs	51.2
humans	13.8

Adapted from Am. J. Dig. Dis. (9).

TABLE III

Effect of Pectin on Plasma and Fecal Lipids in Rats[1]

Dietary Cholesterol	Dietary Pectin	No. Days on diet	Plasma Cholesterol	Liver Cholesterol	Liver Total Lipids	Fecal Total Lipids	Fecal Sterols	Fecal Bile Acids	Ref
50 mg/day	500 mg/day	6				↑	↑		(17)
0	5%	42	0	0	0				(19)
1%	2.5%	28	↓	↓	0				
1%	5%	28	↓	↓	↓				
1%	5%	28	↓(NS)[2]	↓	↓				(20)
1%	10%	28	↓(NS)	↓	↓				
1%	5%	28	↓	↓	↓(NS)				(22)
1%	5%	21	↓	↓	↓				
1%	5%	28	↓(NS)	↓	↓		0	↑	
1%	5%	28	0	↓	0				(23)
1%	10%	28	↓(NS)	↓	↓(NS)				
1%	5%	28	↓	↓	↓				(25)
0	3%	18	0						(36)
1%	3%	18	↓						
0	10%	12	↓(NS)			↑	↑		(33)

[1] Results expressed as increase or decrease compared to results in rats on same diet without pectin

[2] NS = no statistically significant difference

addition of 3 to 10% pectin to a diet containing 1% cholesterol
counteracts the increase in liver cholesterol and liver total
lipid induced by cholesterol feeding (19-25). A decrease in serum
cholesterol is usually observed as a result of pectin supplementation although in some experiments the decrease has not been
statistically significant. Protopectin and pectins with a low
methoxy content do not appear to be effective in lowering serum
or liver cholesterol. Supplements of tomato pectin have been
reported to produce a smaller decrease in liver cholesterol than
citrus pectin (25); however citrus pectin N.F. and apple pectin
apparently are equally effective (19).

An anti-hypercholesterolemic action of pectin has also been
reported in chickens (26-28) and swine (29). In chickens the
addition of 3 to 5% pectin to the diet caused a marked increase
in fecal excretion of cholesterol and total lipids irrespective
of the cholesterol content of the diet (26, 27). In guinea pigs
and hamsters pectin apparently does not have a cholesterol-
lowering effect (30). Although long-term feeding of pectin led
to a significant decrease in plasma cholesterol in male, but not
female, rabbits (31), short-term feeding had no effect (30).

In most experiments pectin has been found to produce an
effect on cholesterol and lipid concentrations only in animals
receiving added dietary cholesterol (19, 29, 32). However,
Mokady (33) has recently reported that in short term feeding experiments in rats, substitution of 10% pectin for starch in a
cholesterol-free diet caused a five-to ten-fold increase in fecal
total lipids and doubled or tripled sterol excretion. A small
decrease in serum cholesterol was observed but results were significant for only one of the pectins tested, a high molecular
weight citrus pectin (Table IV).

Few investigations have been conducted in humans to evaluate
the effect of pectin supplementation. Keys and coworkers (18) fed
middle-aged men controlled diets of natural foods with and without
addition of 15g daily of either cellulose or pectin. A three-week
period of pectin supplementation resulted in a fall in the mean
concentrations of serum cholesterol to levels approximately 5%
below the level on the same diet without pectin (Table V). Cellulose supplementation, however, failed to show any significant
effect on serum cholesterol concentrations. In a study by Palmer
and Dixon (34) an attempt was made to determine the effective dose
of pectin which is required to reduce blood cholesterol concentrations. Sixteen men were fed varying amounts of pectin during six
4-week test periods. Other dietary variables and risk factors
associated with atherosclerosis were not controlled. Although not
all subjects responded equally well to pectin supplementation,
daily doses of 8 to 10g pectin caused a significant decrease in
serum cholesterol of these men, all of whom had initial values
which were either normal or only slightly elevated.

Evaluation of the effect of dietary pectin on plasma and
fecal lipids in humans was made in an investigation conducted at

TABLE IV

EFFECT OF PECTIN ON BLOOD CHOLESTEROL AND FECAL LIPIDS
IN RATS FED A CHOLESTEROL-FREE DIET

	Relative[1] values for		
	Blood Cholesterol	Fecal Lipids	Total Fecal Sterols
	%	%	%
Control	100	100	100
Low MW Pectin[2]	91	458	278
High MW Pectin	76	735	372
Low M Pectin	86	390	222
Pectin S	83	553	270
Pectin MR	83	478	293

[1]Average values for 8 rats/group expressed as a percentage of
control values (for animals fed a pectin-free diet)

[2]MW = molecular weight; M = methoxy; S = slow setting; MR =
medium-rapid setting

Adapted from Nutr. Metabol. (33).

TABLE V

MEAN SERUM CHOLESTEROL CONCENTRATIONS IN 24 MEN FED 15gPECTIN/DAY

Major source of dietary carbohydrate	Serum cholesterol, mg %		
	No Pectin	+ Pectin	Δ
Legumes	202.4	192.7	−9.7
Sucrose	221.5	211.3	−10.2

Adapted from Proc. Soc. Exper. Biol. and Med. (18).

the University of Iowa (35). During an initial period of 4 weeks
three healthy male subjects were fed controlled diets having a
composition similar to that of the average American diet. During
a second 5-week period the men received the same diet plus 20 to
23g pectin N.F. which was incorporated into the foods in the diet.
The final 5 weeks represented a second control and recovery
period. Results showed that after pectin feeding there was a
significant decrease of 13% in the mean plasma cholesterol compared to the value for the control period (Table VI). No appreciable effect on the plasma triglyceride level was observed.
During the period of pectin ingestion the men showed an increase
in total fecal fat, stool volume, fecal sterol and fecal digito-
nide precipitable sterols.

Several mechanisms have been proposed by which dietary pectin
may lower plasma and liver concentrations of cholesterol in various species. Possible mechanisms would include: 1) reduction in
cholesterol absorption; 2) alteration in intestinal microflora and
3) depression of bile acid absorption or recirculation. Experimental results reported by Leveille and Sauberlich (22) indicate
that the most important effect of pectin in the rat appears to be
its influence on bile acid absorption. In cholesterol-fed rats
the addition of pectin increased fecal bile acid excretion by 32%,
whereas fecal neutral sterol excretion was not altered (Table VII).
Additional experiments with inverted intestinal sacs demonstrated
that pectin decreased in vitro taurocholic acid transport by 50%.

Further support for the importance of the inhibition of bile
acid absorption was provided by the similarity in response of
cholesterol-fed rats to pectin and cholestyramine, a known inhibitor of bile acid absorption (Table VIII). More recently, however, Phillips and Brien (36) suggested that there may be different mechanisms for the action of pectin and cholestyramine since
in their experiments pectin did not affect vitamin A absorption
whereas cholestyramine is known to limit absorption of the vitamin.

Dietary pectin somewhat decreases absorption of cholesterol-
4-^{14}C in cholesterol-fed rats, as evidenced by decreased deposition of radioactive cholesterol in the liver and increased fecal
excretion of cholesterol-4-^{14}C (22). However, impaired cholesterol absorption induced by dietary pectin apparently is only
partially responsible for the hypocholesterolemic effect of
pectin. Since pectin effectively lowers liver cholesterol even
when cholesterol and pectin are fed separately on alternate days
(19, 22), impaired absorption of the added cholesterol would not
appear to be the most critical means by which pectin exerts its
effect. In rats fed a cholesterol-free diet Mokady (37) recently
reported that hepatic biosynthesis of cholesterol, as measured by
conversion of acetate-1-^{14}C to cholesterol, was substantially
higher in rats fed 10% pectin. In vitro incorporation of label
into triglycerides, phospholipids and total lipids in the liver
was also significantly higher in the pectin-fed animals. The

TABLE VI

CHANGES IN PLASMA AND FECAL LIPIDS OF THREE MEN IN RESPONSE TO
PECTIN SUPPLEMENTATION

	Periods		
	I	II	III
	Basal Diet	Basal Diet + 20–23 g Pectin	Basal Diet
Plasma cholesterol, mg %	226 ± 6.8[1]	196 ± 9.9[2]	211 ± 8.4
Plasma, triglycerides, mg %	84 ± 12.8	90 ± 10.9	98 ± 9.5
Total fecal fat, g/24 hr	3.4 ± 0.31	5.1 ± 0.41[2]	3.2 ± 0.41
Fecal sterols, g/24 hr	1.06 ± 0.12	1.23 ± 0.12[3]	0.82 ± 0.15
Fecal digitonide precipitate, mg/24 hr	69 ± 8.3	126 ± 12.4[2]	91 ± 18.5

[1] Mean ± standard deviation for 3 subjects.

[2] Differs significantly from mean values for Periods I and III (p < 0.05).

[3] Differs significantly from mean value for Period III (p < 0.05).

Unpublished data adapted from (35).

TABLE VII

EFFECT OF PECTIN SUPPLEMENTATION IN CHOLESTEROL–FED RATS

	Cholesterol (1%)	Cholesterol (1%) + pectin (5%)
Plasma cholesterol, mg/100 ml	128 ± 3^{1}	116 ± 5
Liver fat, %	7.4 ± 0.3	6.6 ± 0.3
Liver cholesterol, mg/g	10.3 ± 0.5	7.5 ± 0.3
Fecal sterols, mg/day	142 ± 5^{2}	141 ± 8
Fecal bile acids, mg/day	17.9 ± 2.4^{2}	23.6 ± 3.3

[1]Mean ± SE of mean for 10 rats.

[2]Values are means for 5 animals.

Adapted from J. Nutr. (22).

TABLE VIII

COMPARISON OF THE EFFECT OF PECTIN AND CHOLESTYRAMINE IN
CHOLESTEROL–FED RATS

Dietary treatment	Liver		Plasma Cholesterol
	Total Lipid	Cholesterol	
	%	mg/g	mg/100 ml
1% cholesterol	7.9 ± 0.3	10.3 ± 0.5	128 ± 14
1% cholesterol + 5% pectin	7.1 ± 0.4	7.2 ± 1.1	91 ± 4
1% cholesterol + 1% cholestyramine	5.8 ± 0.2	4.0 ± 0.2	86 ± 4

[1]Mean for 5 rats ± SE of mean

Adapted from J. Nutr. (22).

author suggested that the higher rate of hepatic lipogenesis observed in the pectin-fed rats might be due to a reduction in the absorption of dietary fat, since absorbed lipid is known to inhibit hepatic fatty acid synthesis.

The effect of dietary pectin on the number and types of intestinal microorganisms has not been thoroughly investigated; however, the failure of antibiotics to prevent the lowering of blood cholesterol by pectin (19, 22) indicates that intestinal microflora do not contribute significantly to its effect.

The effect of pectin on the absorption of nutrients other than lipids has received little attention. In rats the utilization of β-carotene and absorption of vitamin A was not impaired by pectin supplementation (36). Addition of 12 or 24% pectin to diets of rats has been found to decrease the digestibility of protein (38). Viola and coworkers (39) reported that slow setting pectin (55% esterified) decreased the apparent digestibility of protein but did not impair its utilization. However, addition of 10% medium-rapid-acting pectin (65% esterified) led to an impairment of protein utilization as shown by a decrease in weight gain per gram of digested protein. Both pectin preparations decreased the apparent retention of calcium by approximately 30%.

In summary, experimental results in various species indicate that ingested pectin is nearly completely broken down in the colon most likely by bacterial enzymes. The products formed apparently are not extensively utilized since pectin makes a neglible contribution to the energy value of the diet (39). The digestibility and utilization of pectin, however, needs to be re-evaluated using more sensitive and specific methods. The lowering of plasma and liver cholesterol concentrations by pectin supplementation appears to be related primatily to its effect on bile acid absorption. Results showing an increased excretion of bile acids would suggest the possibility of an increased hepatic conversion of cholesterol to bile acids thus reducing serum and liver cholesterol concentrations. By removing the feedback inhibitor of cholesterol on HMG-CoA reductase these changes would explain the increase in hepatic biosynthesis of cholesterol which has been observed. Further investigations are needed to evaluate cholesterol synthesis and turnover as well as the activity of enzymes important in the regulation of cholesterol synthesis.

Literature Cited

1. Baker, G.L., G.H. Joseph, Z.I. Kertesz, H.H. Mattern and A.G. Olsen. Chem. Eng. News (1944) 22, 105-106.

2. Kertesz, Z.I. "The Pectic Substances", pp. 281-329. Interscience Publishers, Inc., New York, 1951.

3. Howard, P.J. and C.A. Tompkins. J. Amer. Med. Assoc.(1940) 114, 2355-2358.

4. Hunt, J.S. Arch. Ped. (1936) 53, 736-739.

5. Washburn, G. J. Am. Dietet. Assoc. (1938) 14, 34-38.

6. Kutscher, G.W. and A. Blumberg. Am. J. Dig. Dis. (1939) 6, 717-720.

7. Birnberg, T.L. Am. J. Dis. Child. (1933) 45, 18-24.

8. Werch. S.C. and A.C. Ivy. Proc. Soc. Exper. Biol. Med. (1940) 44, 366-368.

9. Werch, S.C. and A.C. Ivy. Am. J. Dig. Dis. (1941) 8, 101-105.

10. Gilmore, N.M. "Effect of 5 percent pectin N.F. or 5 percent pectin L.M. upon growth, excretion, serum proteins and mineral contents in liver and kidney tissues of weanling male rats", Ph.D. Dissertation, Michigan State University, 1965.

11. Kertesz, Z.I. J. Nutr. (1940) 20, 289-296.

12. Werch, S.C., A.A. Day, R.W. Jung and A.C. Ivy. Proc. Soc. Exper. Biol. (1941) Med. 46, 569-572.

13. Werch, S.C., R.W. Jung, A.A. Day, T.E. Friedemann and A.C. Ivy. J. Infect. Dis. (1942) 70, 231-242.

14. Erschoff, B.H. and H.B. McWilliams. Am. J. Dig. Dis. (1945) 12, 21-22.

15. Prickett, P.S. and N.J. Miller. Proc. Soc. Exper. Biol. Med. (1939) 40, 27-28.

16. El-Nakeeb, M.A. and R.T. Yousef. Planta Med. (1970) 18, 201-209.

17. Lin. T.M., K.S. Kim, E. Karvinen and A.C. Ivy. Am. J. Physiol. (1957) 188, 66-70.

18. Keys, A., F. Grande and J.T. Anderson. Proc. Soc. Exper. Biol. Med (1960) 106, 555-558.

19. Wells, A.F. and B.H. Ershoff. J. Nutr. (1961) 74, 87-92.

20. Ershoff, B.H. and A.F. Wells. Exper. Med. Surg (1962) 20, 272-276.

21. Ershoff, B.H. and A.F. Wells. Proc. Soc. Exper. Biol. (1962) Med. 110, 580-582.

22. Leveille, G.A. and H.E. Sauberlich. J. Nutr. (1966) 88, 209-214.

23. Riccardi, B.A. and M.J. Fahrenbach. Proc. Soc. Exper. Biol. Med. (1967) 124, 749-752.

24. Karvinen, E. and M. Miettinen. Acta Physiol. Scand. (1968) 72, 62-64.

25. Anderson, T.A. and R.D. Bowman. Proc. Soc. Exper. Biol. Med. (1969) 130, 665-666.

26. Fisher, H., P. Griminger, H.S. Weiss and W.G. Siller. Science (1964) 146, 1063-1064.

27. Fisher, H., W.G. Siller and P. Griminger. J. Atheroscler. Res. (1966) 6, 292-298.

28. Griminger, P. and H. Fisher. Proc. Soc. Exper. Biol. Med. (1966) 122, 551-553.

29. Fisher, H., G.W. van der Noot, W.S. McGrath and P. Griminger. J. Atheroscler. Res. (1966) 6, 190-191.

30. Wells, A.F. and B.H. Ershoff. Proc. Soc. Exper. Biol. Med. (1962) 111, 147-149.

31. Fisher, H., P. Griminger and W.G. Siller. J. Atheroscler. Res. (1967) 7, 381-386.

32. Fisher, H., P. Griminger, E.R. Sostman and M.K. Brush. J. Nutr. (1965) 86, 113-119.

33. Mokady, S. Nutr. Metabol. (1973) 15, 290-294.

34. Palmer, G.H. and D.G. Nixon. Am. J. Clin. Nutr. (1966) 18, 437-442.

35. Hopson, J.J. "Studies on the effect of dietary pectin on plas-

ma and fecal lipids." M.S. Thesis, University of Iowa, 1967.

36. Phillips, W.E.J. and R.L. Brien. J. Nutr. (1970) 100, 289–
    292.

37. Mokady, S. Nutr. Metabol. (1974) 16, 203–207.

38. Gadeken, D. Archiv. Tierenahrung (1960) 19, 409–420.

39. Viola, S., G. Zimmerman and S. Mokady. Nutr. Rep. Internat.
    (1970) 1, 367–375.

The Physiological Effects of Dietary Fiber

JAMES SCALA

Thomas J. Lipton, Inc., Englewood Cliffs, N. J.

In the last century consumption of cereal fiber has decreased more dramatically than either fat or sugar consumption has increased. The 90% decline in consumption of cereal fiber compares to a 30% increase in fat and a 50% increase for sugar. Part of the decline in fiber is probably due to a shift from "crude" sources of carbohydrate such as whole grain cereal, and bread to the "more refined" modern counterparts. Table 1 summarizes the consumption dietary fiber obtained from cereal, potatoes, legumes and fruits and vegetables, as calculated by H. C. Trowell (1) and the author (2). An analysis of the data indicates the change in fiber consumption is largely confined to cereals which have decreased by 75 to 90%; fiber from potatoes has decreased by about 40%; from legumes about 20%, while fiber from fruits and vegetables has changed very little.

Table 1
Estimates of Daily Fiber Consumption in The U.S.
in 1880, 1964, and 1974

Fiber Source	1880 (1)	1964 (1)	1974 (2)
Cereals	3.2	0.3	0.8
Potatoes	1.1	0.5	0.6
Legumes	1.0	1.0	0.6
Fruits and Vegetables	2.8	3.3	2.0
Total Fiber	8.1	5.1	3.0

These changes, brought to the fore by British epidemiologists Drs. Dennis Burkitt, Hugh Trowell and the surgeon Dr. Neil Painter, raise the question of what has been sacrificed by eliminating so much cereal fiber from our diet (3). Is fiber a forgotten nutrient?

Dietary fiber is defined as plant material which is resistant to digestion by the secretions of the human gastrointestinal tract. However, nutritionists usually speak of crude fiber. "Crude fiber" is the material left after treatment with hot acid and alkalie, a method of fiber analysis developed to test animal feeds for undigestable material. In short, to protect the farmer against poor feed purchases. Consequently, we are left with a value that has little, if any, quantitative meaning in terms of human nutrition. Processed grains contain various amounts of cellulose, hemicellulose, pectin and lingins, all of which are defined as fiber; their quantities vary with variety, processing, climate and other factors. Consequently, dietary fiber, the undigestible plant carbohydrates, is from 2 to 6 times the crude fiber content of food (4). This impreciseness is a challenge to food technologists, and speaks for the need to find a method which will accurately identify the amount of "dietary fiber" in food.

I will review the major physiological effects of dietary fiber.

Transit Time

Fiber increases stool frequency and decreases transit time of materials passing through the large intestine. These two effects are indirect results of the water binding ability of fiber and have been demonstrated by comparing stool transit times to those on a refined, low fiber diet; for example, an English or U. S. diet. Table 2 summarizes data taken from studies by Burkitt in which transit time was evaluated as a function of diet.(5) These comparisons of population groups have been clinically evaluated and demonstrate that a diet high in fiber increases both stool weight and frequency. The increased weight is due to the water binding capacity of fiber which carries 4 to 6 times its weight through the large intestine. This water is "bound" in the solid phase (7) and; consequently, a high fiber diet will result in larger and more frequent elimination - or in lay terms- regularity (7).

Table 2
Transit Time as a Function of Diet

Subject	Diet	Transit Time
Ugandan Villagers and Students	Unrefined	33 - 35 hours
English Vegetarians, South African Pupils and Indian Nurses	Mixed	42 - 47 hours
English Students and Navy Personnel	Refined	69 hours

Transit times reported in Table 2, were evaluated by the method of Hinton (6) in which radiopaque pellets (rice grain in size) are fed to volunteers and are observed by X-ray of the passed, collected, stools. Hinton defines transit time as the time required to pass 80% of the pellets.

Diverticular Disease

Diverticular disease affects about 20% of adults in the United States - and with increased longevity, its numbers increase every year. Estimates by Burkitt and Trowell indicate that it is growing at a rate of 16% per year (1). This rate can be questioned because it is not age and longevity compensated. Table 3 summarizes health statistics in the U. S. which demonstrate the age relationship of diverticular disease (8). Other epidemiological surveys have shown correlations of diverticulosis with appendicitis, (9) varicose veins, (10) and hemorrhoids.

Table 3
Diverticular Disease as a Function of Age

Age	Incidence
Under 35	1%
45 - 54	10%
60 - 70	25%
over 70	40%

Diverticulosis is characterized by small defects which develop as bulges in the wall of the colon; they are similar in appearance to the bubble which appears at a weak point on an inflated rubber tube. Clinically, they are saccular outpouchings of the mucosa and submocosa which extrude through defects in the muscularis. As these evaginations fill with intestinal contents or gas, they become infected and in extreme cases, gangrenous. In all cases, they are painful and usually require surgery, in which the diseased portion of the intestine is removed - a process which often includes a temporary colestomy.

In 1967 Dr. Neil Painter found that a high fiber diet would relieve the symptoms of diverticulosis and could, in some cases, obviate the need for surgery (11). Of the 70 cases he treated with a high fiber diet, 62 could be spared from surgery. Data from Dr. Painter's original 62 patients (table 4) show that previous to the high fiber regimen the diverticular patients had irregular, infrequent, hard stools, and the simple procedure of taking about 15 grams of bran daily in three servings of two tablespoons each, produced regularity and eliminated the symptoms.

The means by which fiber relieves the symptoms of diverticulosis has been more clearly shown by Eastwood who studied diverticular patients on a high fiber diet and compared them to a group of normal healthy volunteers (7).

Table 4
Bowel Habits of 62 Patients Before
and After Taking Bran(12)

Bowel Habit (Frequency of Eliminations)	Before Bran	After Bran
Irregular	13	
Every 3 days	7	
Every 2 days	8	
Once daily	28	31
Twice daily	3	25
Three times daily	none	6
Frequent stools	3	none

The diverticular patients on Eastwood's high fiber diet confirmed Painter's findings and exhibited: 1) more normal waste transit times when put on a bran diet verifying Painter's observations, 2) their intracolonic pressure was reduced to more normal values similar to the observations of Hodgson, (13) and 3) the ratio of bound water to liquid water in the feces becomes more similar to the normal patients. These observations suggest that fiber is efficacious by transporting a larger volume of water stools into the large intestine. These softer, bulkier stools reduce the intracolonic pressure preventing distention of the diverticula.

However, it is more important that fiber probably prevents the development of high intracolonic pressures which lead to the formation of diverticula. In addition, a high fiber diet may induce a much stronger intestinal musculature containing fewer weak spots which are potential sites of diverticula. This preventive potential for fiber could be tested by animal studies.

Cardiovascular Disease

The low incidence of ischaemic heart disease and low serum cholesterol among population groups on an unrefined, high residue diet has been attributed, in part, to the hypocholesterolemic effect of nondigestible carbohydrate (14). The diet of these people is often, but not always, low in fat; long term studies with South African White and Bantu prisoners on controlled diets has confirmed the hypocholesterolemic effect of fiber (15). Comparative studies of population groups are summarized on Table 5.

Table 5
Serum Cholesterol in Population Groups Where
Diet Differs in Fiber Content (14) (15) (16)

Group	Diet	Blood Cholesterol
New Guinea (Male)	Unrefined Native	109mg%
New Guinea (Female)	Unrefined Native	134
New Guinea (Male)	Western Refined	183
New Guinea (Female)	Western Refined	187
Non Vegetarians	Western	291
Lacto Vegetarians	Vegetarians (Dairy)	256
Vegan Vegetarians	Strict Vegetarian	206
Trappist Monks	Lacto Vegetarian	180
Benedictine Monks	Mixed	225

Other studies have been performed directly to evaluate the hypocholesterolemic of dietary fiber. In general, these studies indicate that addition of fiber to the diet reduces serum cholesterol by preventing absorption of dietary cholesterol and by increasing the elimination of bile acids; thereby, the removal of hepatic synthesized cholesterol. These findings have been confirmed by extensive animal studies (33), (34). These studies are summarized in Table 6. In general, these studies have been done over short periods and have utilized fiber as refined cellulose, or from natural sources.

Table 6
The Effect of Dietary Fiber
on Serum Cholesterol on Man

Subjects	Control Diet	Experimental Diet
Young Girls (19)		(Cellulose)
	226	170
Male Volunteers (20)		(Oats)
	251	223
		(Bengal Gram)
Male Volunteers (21)	206	160

Although the hypocholesterolemic aspects of fiber has not been quantified, these studies demonstrate its effectiveness as inferred from serum cholesterol. Fiber helps in eliminating both dietary and hepatic cholesterol thereby reducing, to some extent, one major risk factor of cardiovascular disease - serum cholesterol.

Colonic Cancer

Since fiber increases the speed of material through the gut and the volume which is passed, it would be expected to reduce the exposure time of the gut tissues to any non digestible component. Therefore, duductive reasoning leads us to expect it to reduce the likelihood of colonic toxicity derived from any ingested or physiologically produced toxic agent. Toxic agents of greatest concern in the gut are carcinogens.

Although studies to relate fiber, in general, to the reduction of cancer have been unsuccessful, the recent epidemiological evaluation of Drs. Irving and Drasar have shown a significant albiet small, negative correlation with colonic cancer and cereal consumption (22). Although the correlations account for a small portion of colonic cancer, intuition and epidemiology are in such obvious agreement that the trend is significant and a milestone in epidemiology. These correlations are summarized in Table 7.

Table 7
Corelation of Cancer of the Colon With Consumption
of Various Fiber Containing Foods (22)

Source of Fiber	Correlation Coefficient	Statistical Significance
Cereals	-0.30	$0.10 < P < 0.05$
Potatoes and Starches	-0.07	N.S.
Pulses Nuts and Seeds	+0.07	N.S.
Vegetables	+0.05	N.S.
Fruit	+0.22	N.S.

Colonic cancer is second only to lung cancer as a killer among cancers. It occurs least frequently in populations with a high residue unrefined diet such as in Central Africa (23). This has been observed by epidemiologists who have evaluated blacks living in Africa against blacks in the U. S. or Japanese in Japan to those in the U. S. These data presented in Table 8 are taken from evaluations by Dr. Robert Doll at Oxford, and have been confirmed by other epidemiological surveys (24).

Table 8
Colon-Cancer Incidence in Males by Race and Country

Country	Race	Incidence
U. S. (California)	Black	69.8
U. S. (Hawaii)	Caucasian	68.0
U. S. (Hawaii)	Japanese	66.4
Rhodesia	Black	18.2
Japan (Rural)	Japanese	11.8
South Africa	Black	10.8
Nigeria	Black	5.8

Colonic cancer is highest in countries which exhibit a high incidence of cardiovascular disease and the two are highly correlated (25). Therefore, since cholesterol is the most widely accepted risk factor in cardiovascular disease, it is a common basis on which to compare the two diseases. Rose observed 5 groups of people with high risk for cardiovascular disease by their high serum cholesterol; then searched for the differences among those who had colonic cancer (26). As Table 9 indicates, the colonic cancer patients exhibited lower than expected serum cholesterol levels for a group at risk, as compared to other cancers of the alimentary system.

Table 9
Serum Cholesterol Deviations in Men
Who Died of Alimentary Carcinoma*

Site	Mean Deviation (Standard Units)	
All cancer except colon	+0.20	(Whitehall Study)
Colon	-0.13	(Whitehall Study)
Colon	-0.512	(General Electric Study)

*Adapted from Rose (26).

Dr. Erik Bjelke had conducted a retrospective and prospective study on the interrelationship between diet and cholesterol (27). The group exhibited an elevated cholesterol; however, those with lower cholesterol exhibited the higher incidences of colonic cancer. As Table 10 indicates, this relationship tested out consistently over the five year period during which the group was followed confirming the findings of Rose and adding the valuable dimension of prospective epidemiology.

Table 10
Relative Risk for Colonic Cancer
As a Function of Serum Cholesterol*

Mean Cholesterol	Retrospective Relative Risk	Prospective Relative Risk
291	1.0	1.0
287	1.4	2.3
271	2.1	2.0

*Adapted from Bjelke (27).

Other forms of suspected diet related cancer did not exhibit this same pattern - adding more confirmation to the finding; that is, colonic cancer among high serum cholesterol cardiovascular disease risk patients is inverse with serum cholesterol.

These studies raise an obvious question, "What do these people pass into their large intestines which will reduce serum cholesterol below its expected value?" One component is obvious- bile acids, dietary sterols and fat.

Since 1940, it has been known that deoxycholate, a bile acid by-product is a weak carcinogen (28). High fiber unrefined diets produce a spectrum of bile salts which are substantially different from those observed on a refined low residue diet. This is illustrated by comparing the bile acid by-products in rural Africans to Europeans, as done by Dr. James Falaiye of Nigeria (29). His data (Table 11) shows that there is more deoxycholate in the feces of people on low residue than on high residue diets.

Table 11
Bile Salt Ratios and Diet*

Population Group	Diet	Cholate	Cheno- Deoxycholate	Deoxy- Cholate
Nigerian Adults	Unrefined	1.5	1.0	0.4
English Adults	Refined	1.4	1.0	0.9

Data adapted from Falaiye (29).

These bile acid by-products are produced by the anaerobic microflora. People on a refined diet have a much greater population of anaerobes in their large intestine (29). This is apparent by contrasting the ratio of intestinal aerobes of Black Ugandins to Blacks in the U. S. (30), (31)

Along with the bile acid hypothesis, components of the food itself should be considered. Nitrogen metabolites ranging from ammonia, nitroso compounds and other amines have been implicated (32). Their production similarly depends upon transformations by the intestinal flora and the logic of development follows a pattern similar to the one considered for bile acids. A virus hypothesis is similar except that transit time and volume are the cogent factors. In each hypothesis, fiber emerges as a preventive agent.

Conclusions

The role of fiber in the diet is emerging as a preventive agent for problems of the alimentary and vascular system. This conclusion is supported by epidemiology, direct experimentation, and inferences from dietary patterns in ethnic and socio-economic groups.

More research is required by food scientists on fiber as a food component and by biomedical scientists on the long term effects of fiber in the diet. In view of the complexity of the dietary relevance such studies should be long term and cover several age groups. Much work remains to be done on animals; especially feeding studies on primates.

Literature Cited

[1]Burkitt, D.P., Walker, A.R.P., Painter, N.S., Effect of Dietary
    Fiber on Stools and Transit Times and Its Role in the Cau-
    sation of Disease. Lancet, (1972), 1408, ii.

[2]Revelle, R., Food and Population. Scientific American, (1974),
    160, 231. Increases in Food Can Help to Create Conditions
    That Stabilize Population Levels.

[3]Painter, N.S. and Burkitt, D.P., Diverticular Disease of the
    Colon: A Deficiency Disease of Western Civilization.
    British Medical Journal (1971), 2, 450-454.

[4]Williams, R.D. and Olmsted, W.H., A Biochemical Method for Det-
    ermining Indigestible Residue in Feces. Lingin, cellulose,
    and non-water-soluble hemicelluloses. J. Biol. Chem. (1936)
    108, 653-666.

[5]Burkitt, D.P., Walker, A.R.P. and Painter, N.S., Dietary Fiber
    and Disease. J.A.M.A. (1974) 229, 1068-1074.

[6]Hinton, J.M., Lennard-Jones, J.E. Young, A.C., A New Method for
    Studying Gut Transit Times Using Radio-Opaque Markers.
    J. Br. Soc. Gastroentrol, (1969), 10, 842-847.

[7]Eastwood, M.A., Findlay, J.M., Mitchell, W.D., Smith, A.N. and
    Anderson, A.J.B., Effects of Unprocessed Bran on Colon Fun-
    ction in Norman Subjects and in Diverticular Disease. Lancet
    (1974), 146-149, i.

[8]Brown, J. W., Colonic Diverticulosis in the Aged. J. Am. Geri-
    atrics Soc. (1969), 17, 366-370.

[9]Burkitt, D.P. The Aetology of Appendicitis. Br. J. Surg. (1971)
    58, 695-699, i.

[10]Latto, C., Gilmore, O.J.A. and Wilkinson, R.W., Diverticular
    Disease and Varicose Veins. Lancet, (1973) 1089.

[11]Burkitt, D.P., James, P.A., Low-Residue Diets and Hiatus
    Hernia. Lancet (1973), 128-130, 2.

[12]Painter, N.S., Almeida, A.Z., and Colebourne, K.W., Unprocessed
    Bran in Treatment of Diverticular Disease of the Colon.
    British Medical Journal, (1972), 729-731, 3.

[13]Hodgson, J., Effect of Methylcellulose on Rectal and Colonic
    Pressures in Treatment of Diverticular Disease. British
    Medical Journal, (1972),729-731,3.

[14]Lyken, R. and Janse, A.A.J., The Cholesterol Level in Blood
    Serium of Some Population Groups in New-Guinea. Trop.
    Geogr. Med., (1960), 145-148, 12.

[15]Hardinge, M.G., Chambers, A.C., Crooks, H. and Stare, F.J.,
    Nutritional Studies of Vegetarians III Dietary Levels of
    Fiber, Am. J. Clin. Nutr., (1958), 523-525, 6.

[16]Groen, J.J., Tijong, K.B., Koster, M., Willebrands, A.F.,
    Verdonck, G., and Pierloot, M., The Influence of Nutrition
    and Ways of Life on Blood Cholesterol and the Prevalence of
    Hypertension and Cornary Heart Disease Among Trappist and
    Behedictine Monks. Amer. J. Clin., (1962), 456-470, 10.

[17]Keys, A., Anderson, J.T., and Grande, F., Diet-Type (fats constant) and Blood Lipids in Man. J. Nutr., (1970), 257-266, 70.

[18]Antonis, A. and Bersohn, I., The Influence of Diet on Fecal Lipids in S. Afr. White and Bantu Prisoners. Am. J. Clin. Nutr., (1962), 142-155 ,11.

[19]Shurpaleakar, K.S., et. al., Effect of Cellulose in an Athrogenic Diet on the Blood Lipids of Children. Nature, (1971), 554-555, 232.

[20]de Groot, A.P., Luyken, R., and Pikaar, N.A., Cholesterol-Lowering Effect of Rolled Oats. Lancet, (1963), 303-304, 2.

[21]Mathur, K.S., Khan, M.A. and Sharma, R.D., Hypocholesterolaemic Effect of Bengal Gram; a Long Term Study in Man. Brit. Med. J., (1968), 30-31, 1.

[22]Irving, D., Drasar, B.S., Cancer. Br. J., (1973), 462, 28.

[23]Burkitt, D.P., Epidemiology of Cancer of the Colon and Rectum. Cancer, (1971) 3-13, 28.

[24]Doll, R., Cancer. Br. J., (1969), 1, 23.

[25]World Health Organization Statistics. Vol. 1, (1969).

[26]Rose, G. et. al., Lancet, (1974), 7850, i.

[27]Bjelke, E., Lancet, (1974), 1116, i.

[28]Cook, J. W., Kennaway, N.M., Production of Tumors by Deoxycholic Acid. Nature, (1940), 627, 145.

[29]Hill, M.J. et. al., Bacteria and the Etiology of Cancer of the Large Bowel. Lancet, (1971), 95-100, 1.

[30]Aires, V., et. al., Bacteria and Etiology of Cancer of the Large Bowel. Gut, (1969), 334-335, 10.

[31]Hill, M.J. et. al., Bacteria and Etiology of Cancer of the Large Bowel. Lancet, (1971), 95-100, i.

[32]Visek, W.J., Some Biochemical Considerations in Utilization of Non-specific Nitrogen. Agr. Food Chem., (1974), 174-184, 22.

[33]Trowell, H., Ischemic Heart Disease and Dietary Fiber. The Am. J. of Clin. Nutr., (1970), 926-932, 25.

[34]Bruns, P., Nutritional, Microbiological and Physicochemical Studies on Chemically Modified Tapioca Starch Thesis, (1974), Cornell University.

22

Digestibility of Food Polysaccharides by Man:
A Review

ALLENE JEANES

Northern Regional Research Laboratory, Agricultural Research Service,
U.S. Department of Agriculture, Peoria, Ill. 61604

Introduction

Polysaccharides that are commonly ingested by man but are
not digested have been indicated in this symposium to be significant in the human diet. Nondigestible polysaccharide constituents of foods are beneficial in providing bulk, binding water
and certain toxic substances (1), and in exerting hypocholesterolemic action (1, 2, 3). Polysaccharide food additives such as
carrageenan (4) and the alginates and xanthan (5) serve advantageous functions in food products through their specific physical
and colloidal properties without regard to digestibility.

In this review, further consideration is given to the digestibility of the great variety of other polysaccharide food additives that serve to impart aesthetic appeal and processing and
marketing advantages to foods. Since these substances usually
suffice in low concentrations, the question of their digestibility
has more import physiologically than nutritionally. Included in
this consideration are polysaccharides that have been proposed
for use in foods but do not now have significant application as
well as several types that are present naturally in foods but are
poorly utilized. Attention is given first, however, to the food
polysaccharides that are digested and to the basis for their
differentiation from those that are nondigestible. Review of
these facts discloses areas where information is lacking and
further research is needed. Before discussing the individual
polysaccharides it is necessary to define digestion and to evaluate the postulated role of microflora in the small intestine.

Digestion: Origin of Depolymerases

Digestion consists in depolymerization of large molecules
into their monomeric units which may be absorbed into the circu-
latory system for distribution to the body tissues. Several
aspects of the digestive process have been considered already
in this symposium. Crane (6) depicted the generally recognized

principle that, in the small intestine, digestion and absorption
of carbohydrates occur, whereas in the large intestine (colon)
sugars are not absorbed but undergo fermentation by the indigenous microbial flora. Hehre (7) has pointed out that microflora
may exist also in the small intestine and would be a potential
source of digestive depolymerases, especially for nonamylaceous
polysaccharides. Rackis (8) has correlated data on anaerobic
fermentation of indigestible soybean oligosaccharides (raffinose,
stachyose and verbascose) in the human intestinal tract with the
findings of other investigators that established the identity,
distribution and action of the effective microflora in test animals. Thus, in the small intestine of the dog, the greatest
bacterial metabolic activity occurred in the ileum and much less
in the duodenum and jejunum (8).

The microbial flora indigenous to the alimentary canal may
vary from species to species and to some degree within a species
(9). Conventional laboratory mice and rats possess an extensive
microflora throughout their alimentary canal. Microorganisms of
several types are localized, often in thick layers, on specific
mucosal surfaces of the stomach, caecum and colon, and long
chains of gram-negative rod- or coccal-shaped bacteria have been
found on the villous epithelium of the ileum (10). In the
normal healthy human, biopsied tissue or fluid from the lumen of
the small intestine was found to contain only small numbers of
microorganisms such as nonpathogenic streptococci or lactobacilli
(11) which apparently were not growing (12).

Comparisons of germ-free and conventional rats support the
conclusions that the maltase, invertase (sucrase), lactase, cellobiase and trehalase activities of small intestinal tissue
homogenates come from the animal itself and that the intestinal
microorganisms do not contribute to any major extent to their
production (13, 14, 15). Isomaltase, which was not measured specifically, characteristically accompanies sucrase. The same
conclusions resulted from comparable studies on oligo-1,6-
glucosidase activity from intestinal homogenates of the rat (13)
and hog (13, 16).

From his experimentation on the conventional pig, Dahlqvist
concluded that the dextran-degrading activity (dextranase[1]) found
in homogenates of ileal mucosa did not originate in contaminating,
adhering microflora. When mucosa from the colon was tested in the
same way, dextranase activity from the colon as compared with that
from the ileum was in the ratio of 1 to 5.5 (17).

As is detailed later in this review, dextranase activity in
homogenates of small intestinal mucosa has been found consistently
in close association with sucrase and isomaltase. Extensive

---

[1] In this review dextranase designates dextran-degrading
activity rather than a specific enzyme since the identity of the
enzyme has not been established.

research by numerous investigators has established the location, origin and development of the cells of the small intestinal brush-border membrane in which the disaccharidases sucrase-isomaltase, maltase, lactase and several others occur. The sucrase-isomaltase complex has been visualized in situ in biopsy specimen of human small intestinal mucosa by immunofluorescence staining (18). Among reviews on the disaccharidases of the brush border are those of Gray (19) in this symposium and of Prader and Auricchio (20).

Digestion of polysaccharides is dependent upon the presence of the requisite specific hydrolytic enzymes(s) and the absence of specific inhibitors or chemical or physical aspects of the polysaccharide that could interfere with enzyme action. The only digestive polysaccharidases that have been established in man are the α-amylases of saliva and pancreatic juice and a particle-bound (21) glucoamylase (6, 19) of small intestinal mucosa which is designated γ-amylase by some investigators (21, 22).

Polysaccharides Known to Be Digestible

Amylaceous Polysaccharides. Salivary and pancreatic α-amylases hydrolyze 1,4-α-D-glucopyranosidic linkages in amylaceous polymers with formation of maltose and α-limit dextrins. These fragments are hydrolyzed to glucose by saccharidases of the intestinal brush-border membrane (19) for transport through the absorptive cells of the intestinal mucosa (6). α-Amylase acts on starch when both are free in the intestinal cavity (23). As to its specificity, Whelan (24) has stated that "There is no evidence contrary to the belief that α-amylase is entirely specific for the hydrolysis of 1,4-α-D-glucopyranosidic bonds". The report of α-amylase action on salep mannan (a water-soluble 1,4-β-D-mannan) was shown by Allen and Whelan (25) to be erroneous. Action of salivary and pancreatic α-amylases is blocked by the 1,6-α-D-glucopyranosidic branch points or by substituent groups such as the phosphate of potato starch. Thus, the smallest fragment from α-amylolysis that contains a branch point or phosphate group is a tetrasaccharide (24).

Experimental animals usually are fed raw starches either as the granules or ground whole grain. Raw starches from various plant sources differ in their susceptibility to in vitro action of salivary and pancreatic α-amylases (26, 27) and to in vivo digestiblity (28). In general, root or tuber starches are much more resistant than are the cereal starches. Two types of non-tuberous starches are, however, also unusually resistant to α-amylolysis. These starches have amylose contents in the range of 60-75% (as compared with about 25% in most ordinary starches) and gelation temperatures in the range of about 130-150° C (as compared with about 75-80° C for most ordinary starches). These resistant starches are from (a) a wrinkle-seeded variant of the common garden pea, Pisum sativum, and (b) hybrids from genetically selected lines of Zea mays which produce good yields of an

industrially useful high-amylose starch (29). This high-amylose
corn starch is, however, finding increasing application in convenience foods because of its different physical properties (30).
Starch (63% amylose) and the corresponding ground whole grain
from high-amylose corn, when tested by pancreatin in vitro, were
42% and 37% as digestible, respectively, as normal starch controls. Under the same conditions, wrinkle-seeded pea starch (65%
amylose) was about 85% as "digestible" as the normal corn starch
control (26). When tested in the rat, the ground high-amylose
corn was found to be 77% as digestible as normal corn (31). Resistance of these novel starches to gelation and α-amylase action
appears to result from a combination of factors which includes
unusual granule morphology, strong micellar structures, and abnormally low molecular weight of both the amylose and amylopectin
fractions (29).

The effects of granule disruption and gelatinization on the
susceptibility of high-amylose corn and wrinkle-seeded pea
starches to α-amylolysis apparently have not been studied, but
might be expected to be favorable. Walker and Hope (27) showed
that the action of α-amylases is much more rapid and extensive on
starch pastes than on the raw granules. Partial gelatinization
increases the nutritional availability of starch and wheat bran
for chickens (32) and flaking and steaming improves the utilization of sorghum by cattle (33). Cooking under suitable conditions is necessary to raise the digestibility of dry-bean starches
up to about 87% (34).

Cooking provides the added benefit of diminishing or de-
stroying the activity of glycoprotein-type inhibitors of mammalian
α-amylases which occur in certain wheats, sorghum, legumes and
other plant products (32, 35). Heat-stable polyphenolic inhibitors of mammalian α-amylases also occur in numerous plant products
(35). In contrast to the action of these inhibitors, the neutral
α-D-glucan dextran increases the rate of reaction in vitro of α-
amylase on an insoluble starch substrate by enhancing the interaction between the enzyme and its substrate (36).

Modified food starches (37, 38), such as the acid-converted
or dextrinized, are utilized less completely than most natural
starches because non-1,4-glucosidic linkages are introduced by
the processing (39). Chemically derivatized starches, such as
the phosphorylated or hydroxyalkylated, are attacked by α-amylases
in inverse relation to their degree of substitution (39, 40). An
apparent anomaly to this principle reported for hydroxyethyl
starch was resolved by Banks et al. (41).

Dextran. A dextran having 95% 1,6-α-D-glucopyranosidic
linkages (42) produces a rapid increase in blood sugar and liver
glycogen when ingested by man (43) or the rat (43, 44). Digestibility and caloric availability assays in the rat indicated that
this dextran was highly digestible (90%) and was utilized for

growth (45). The 5% α-1,3-linkages at branch points are believed to prevent complete digestion (42).

Dextran-hydrolyzing activity has been demonstrated in small intestinal mucosa of man (46, 47), the rat (22, 48) and the pig (17). This activity was distinct from that of α-amylase but closely associated with "invertase" (46) and with isomaltase (48). Ruttloff et al. (22) differentiated dextranase and isomaltase and considered both to be particle-bound. The dextran used by Bloom, Wilhelmi and Adrouny (43, 46), Booth et al. (45) and Dahlqvist (17, 47) was the same structurally, and has been described by Jeanes (42).

Dahlqvist (17), using homogenates of pig tissues, showed that dextranase activity was absent in the stomach and pancreas and present to a low degree in the colon. Although of no import for digestion, dextran-degrading enzymes do occur in lysosomes, liver, spleen and kidney tissues of man and other mammals (49, 50).

Little further attention has been given to hydrolysis of dextran by intestinal enzymes. Resolution of, and establishment of the substrates for, the intimately occurring mixture of α-glucosidases of the brush-border membrane that shows isomaltase, sucrase and maltase activities, however, constitutes progress towards eventual clarification of how dextran is depolymerized in the small intestine. Isomaltose, the major disaccharide repeating unit of the dextran used in research reviewed here, is split by the isomaltase-sucrase complex of the brush-border membrane (19, 51) and also by the isomaltase subunit after separation as an independent entity (52, 53). The isomaltase-sucrase complex shows weak activity on high molecular weight dextran (51). Gray (19, 54) indicates that in intestinal digestion α-amylase limit dextrins are the natural substrate for the isomaltase (α-dextrinase)-sucrase complex. He equates this complex (54) with the oligo-1,6-glucosidase isolated from hog small intestinal mucosa by Larner and McNickle (16). This oligo-1,6-glucosidase hydrolyzed the α-1,6-linkages of isomaltose, panose and α-limit dextrins but, under the test conditions used, did not degrade a dextran (95% α-1,6-linkages) of molecular weight 75,000 (16).

Hehre and Sery (55) showed that large numbers of dextran-splitting anaerobic bacteria belonging to the Bacteroides genus occur in the human colon. Pure cultures of these enteric bacteria growing anaerobically in the presence of dextran appear to depolymerize the dextran and then metabolize the liberated glucose. The soluble dextranase system produced when a strain isolated from human feces was grown anaerobically in dextran broth was precipitated by half-saturated ammonium sulfate at 4° and found to show two major, pH-dependent activities (56). At pH 7.0-7.5 exolytic-type action occurred with liberation of glucose from a variety of structurally different dextrans and also from the long outer chains of amylopectins; at pH 5.0-5.5, endolytic-type action predominated with rapid lowering of dextran viscosity.

In contrast to these properties of the bacteroides dextranases, the dextran-degrading system isolated by Bloom and coworkers (46) from duodenal and jejunal intestinal mucosa of the rat showed a pH optimum of 6.0-6.2 and solubility in half-saturated ammonium sulfate. Other strains of Bacteroides, growing in other environments, would not necessarily produce dextranases with the same pH dependencies found by Sery and Hehre (56). Bacteroides, however, are reported to colonize only the large bowel of mice (9). In the small intestine of the normal human, Bornside et al. (12) found Bacteroides in very low numbers and Gorbach et al. (57) found them in the ileum of only 4 out of 13 normal humans. Bacteria of other genera, however, cannot be excluded arbitrarily as the possible dextranase producers. Nonpathogenic lactobacilli and anaerobic streptococci occur sparsely in the human small intestine (11) and in the stomach and small intestine of the mouse (10). Although many members of these genera produce extracellular dextran, only a few strains are known to produce extracellular dextranase, namely Lactobacillus bifidus from bovine rumen and from feces of an infant (58).

Other Polysaccharides

Plant Polysaccharides. Many variously constituted polysaccharides are utilized in food preparations, usually as additives (37, 59). Some are simply constituted, having only one or two types of constituent sugar such as cellulose and its hydrophilic derivatives, and the galacto- and glucomannans (2). The pectins are more complexly constituted (3). Numerous other polysaccharides such as the plant gums and mucilages and the hemicelluloses are heterogeneous in both composition and linkages. From among all these heteropolysaccharides, experimental data on feeding tests have been found only for gum arabic. This plant exudate gum, which is extensively used in food preparations (37) under the GRAS classification (60), has been shown to be 71% digested by the rat and to be utilized for growth (45). Several other studies, but not all, support these observations (60). Guinea pigs (60, 61) and rabbits (60) also appear to utilize gum arabic for energy. As part of a comprehensive review of information on the suitability of gum arabic for use in human food, the Food and Drug Administration has concluded that "gum arabic is capable of being digested to simple sugars in herbivores, and to some extent in omnivores, such as man" (60).

The main structural feature of gum arabic is a backbone chain of 1,3-β-D-galactopyranose units, some of which are substituted at the C-6 position with various side chains. These side chains are composed mainly of L-arabinofuranose and L-rhamnopyranose units, the glycosidic linkages of which are acid labile (62). Current concepts of depolymerization of such a heterogeneous macromolecule indicate that a combination of specific enzymes would be required, none of which are known to occur in the rat or man.

The only related intestinal enzyme known is the β-galactosidase, lactase, which appears to have cellobiase and gentiobiase activity also (47, 63) or to be closely associated with these other enzymes. Enzymic depolymerization of gum arabic would be simplified, however, if the acid-labile groups on the periphery of the molecule had already been removed by gastric acidity. If microflora of the rat small intestine are responsible for the depolymerization of gum arabic, similar activity might be expected also on other heteropolysaccharides such as hemicelluloses or, even more likely, on the more simply constituted galactomannans (2). These expectations, however, are not confirmed by observations. Obviously, definitive experimentation is necessary to resolve the enigma of gum arabic digestibility.

Inhabitants of coastal regions have always used seaweeds or their polysaccharide extracts for food purposes (59, 64). Many of these polysaccharides resemble agar or carrageenan in composition and, apparently, are not digestible. Carrageenan is known to be indigestible (4); agar has been shown to be 21% digestible in the rat (45) and to provide some growth in the guinea pig (65). The exceptional seaweed, Rhodymenia palmata, however, is reported (without documentation) to be completely digestible by man (64, 66, 67) and to have been an important food in coastal regions, especially in northern latitudes. This alga, commonly called dulse or red kale, contains about 22% protein, 3-4% fat, and 45% polysaccharide. The polysaccharide consists mainly of a 1,3- and 1,4-linked β-D-xylan and, to lesser extent, of starch- and cellulose-like materials. The claim of digestibility of this xylan, which is not supported by controlled experimentation, is included in order to complete the coverage of this review.

Glycoproteins. Mucopolysaccharides and other types of glycoproteins enter man's diet from animal products such as milk, eggs, connective tissue and tendons of meat, and organs such as liver. Glycoproteins occur also in plant seeds (68). The carbohydrate components of glycoproteins, which are covalently bound to the peptide moieties, may consist of amino sugars and one to six other sugar types and constitute from 1% up to 80% of the weight of the molecule (69). Glycosidic digestion of glycoproteins is very difficult to effect. The protein moiety, however, is acted upon by gastrointestinal proteases, some of which are specific for certain glycoproteins, until obstructed by the attached carbohydrate (68) as has been demonstrated for a soybean hemagglutinin (70). The peptide-bound oligo- or higher saccharides left would not be expected to be attacked by intestinal carbohydrases since they probably would be heterogeneous in composition as well as linkages.

Fructans. Inulin, a relatively low-molecular-weight polymer of (2→1)-linked β-D-fructofuranose, occurs as a reserve material in the tubers of certain plants such as the sunflower called

Jerusalem artichoke. The tuber apparently is not metabolized by cattle. Man does not metabolize inulin (71) either from the artichoke tuber when it is used in pickles and relishes (72) or when the extracted fructan is used in bread for diabetics (73). Levans, in which β-$\underline{D}$-fructofuranose units are linked predominantly by (2→6)-bonds, occur in many plant tissues and are produced extracellularly by many types of microorganisms. Levan from Aerobacter levanicum, when reduced to suitable molecular size, serves effectively as a nontoxic, nonantigenic blood volume expander which is slowly eliminated from the body (74). Data on digestibility have not been found.

β-(1→3)-Glucans. Two structurally different 1,3-β-$\underline{D}$-glucans have been proposed as food additives. The polysaccharide class of which these glucans are members is widely distributed in nature and includes the seaweed product laminarin and the intra- and extracellular products of many fungi and other microorganisms (75). These two microbial glucans have a backbone structure of 1,3-β-$\underline{D}$-glucopyranosidic residues; the curdlan-type is unbranched (76). The Polytran®-(or scleroglucan-) type has a glucose side-chain attached by a β-1,6-bond to every third linear chain residue (77). These glucans are essentially insoluble in cold water. When heated, the unbranched type forms a gel of unusual properties (78). The branched type swells greatly in water and forms tactily distinct gels. In the rat, this branched β-1,3 glucan has caloric value equivalent to starch and, after a period of apparent adaptation, dogs utilized this glucan well (77). These results are unexpected on the basis of currently available information on the digestibility of polysaccharides. Tests of human digestibility have not been reported.

Conclusions

From among the many and varied plant polysaccharides, man's utilization for nutrition is restricted almost exclusively to the amylaceous substances. Depolymerization of these substances to glucose in the small intestine is accomplished by man's own enzymes.

Man and the rat derive high caloric value also from the predominantly α-(1→6)-linked bacterial glucan dextran. A dextran-degrading enzyme, which has been demonstrated frequently in homogenates of the small intestinal mucosa, has not yet been identified and isolated.

The rat and the dog derive high caloric value from a predominantly β-(1→3)-linked bacterial glucan.

Definitive experimentation is needed to establish the origin, either mammalian or microfloral or both, of the small intestinal enzymes that make possible the high nutritive utilization of dextran and β-(1→3)-glucan.

The reported high caloric utilization of the heteropolysaccharide gum arabic in some rat-feeding tests and not in others, indicates need for further experimentation.

Dextran, β-(1→3)-glucan and gum arabic are not important nutritionally to man. It is important, however, to obtain through use of these polysaccharides information now unknown on digestive processes that occur in the small intestine of man, the rat and other laboratory test animals.

Literature Cited

1. Scala, J. This Symposium (1975), Part C, Chapter 21.
2. Lewis, Betty A. This Symposium (1975), Part C, Chapter 19.
3. Chenoweth, Wanda and Leveille, G. A. This Symposium (1975), Part C, Chapter 20.
4. Stancioff, D. J. and Renn, D. W. This Symposium (1975), Part C, Chapter 18.
5. McNeely, W. H. and Kovacs, P. This Symposium (1975), Part C, Chapter 17.
6. Crane, R. K. This Symposium (1975), Part A, Chapter 1.
7. Hehre, E. J. This Symposium (1975), Part B, Introductory Remarks.
8. Rackis, J. J. This Symposium (1975), Part B, Chapter 13.
9. Savage, D. C. Amer. J. Clin. Nutr. (1970) 23, 1495.
10. Savage, D. C. J. Bacteriol. (1969) 97, 1505.
11. Plaut, A. G., Gorbach, S. L., Nahas, L., Weinstein, G., Spanknebel, G. and Levitan, R. Gastroenterology (1967) 53, 868.
12. Bornside, C. H., Welsh, J. S. and Cohn Jr., I. J. Amer. Med. Ass. (1966) 196, 1125.
13. Larner, J. and Gillespie, R. E. J. Biol. Chem. (1957) 225, 279.
14. Dahlqvist, A., Bull, B. and Gustafsson, B. E. Arch. Biochem. Biophys. (1965) 109, 150.
15. Reddy, B. S. and Wostmann, B. S. Arch. Biochem. Biophys. (1966) 113, 609.
16. Larner, J. and McNickle, C. M. J. Biol. Chem. (1955) 215, 723.
17. Dahlqvist, A. Biochem. J. (1961) 78, 282.
18. Dubs, R., Steinmann, B. and Gitzelmann, R. Helv. Paediat. Acta (1973) 28, 187.
19. Gray, G. M. This Symposium (1975), Part B, Chapter 11.
20. Prader, A. and Auricchio, S. Ann. Rev. Med. (1965) 16, 345.
21. Dahlqvist, A. and Thomson, D. L. Biochem. J. (1963) 89, 272.
22. Ruttloff, R., Noack, R., Friese, R., Schenk, G. and Proll, J. Acta Biol. Med. Ger. (1967) 19, 331. Chem. Abstr. (1968) 68, 111, 599a.
23. Gray, G. M. Gastroenterology (1970) 58, 96.

24. Whelan, W. J., in "Methods in Carbohydrate Chemistry," Vol. 4, Whistler, R. L., Ed., Academic Press, New York, N.Y., 1964, p. 252.
25. Allen, P. Z. and Whelan, W. J. Biochem. J. (1963) 88, 69.
26. Sandstedt, R. M., Strahan, D., Ueda, S. and Abbott, R. C. Cereal Chem. (1962) 39, 123.
27. Walker, Gwenn J. and Hope, Pamela. Biochem J. (1963) 86, 452.
28. Booher, Lela E., Behan, Ida, McMeans, Evelyn and Boyd, H. M. J. Nutr. (1951) 45, 75.
29. Senti, F. R. and Dimler, R. J. Food Technol. (1959) 13, 663.
30. Hullinger, C. H., Van Patten, E. and Freck, J. A. Food Technol. (1973) 27, 22.
31. Borchers, R. Cereal Chem. (1962) 39, 145.
32. Saunders, R. M. Cereal Science Today (1975), in press.
33. Osman, H. F., Theurer, B., Hale, W. H. and Mehen, S. M. J. Nutr. (1970) 100, 1133.
34. Hellendoorn, E. W. Food Technol. (1969) 23, 795.
35. Marshall, J. J., Lauda, Carmen A. and Whelan, W. J. This Symposium (1975), Part B, Chapter 16.
36. Ceska, M. Experientia (1971) 27, 767.
37. Glicksman, M. "Gum Technology in the Food Industry," Academic Press, New York, N.Y., 1969, pp. 590.
38. Wurzburg, O. B., in "Handbook of Food Additives," Furia, T. E., Ed., The Chemical Rubber Co., Cleveland, Ohio, 1968, p. 377.
39. Reussner, Jr., G., Andros, J. and Thiessen, Jr., R. J. Nutr. (1963) 80, 291.
40. Parrish, F. W. and Whelan, W. J. Staerke (1961) 13, 231.
41. Banks, W., Greenwood, C. T. and Muir, D. D. Staerke (1972) 24, 181.
42. Jeanes, Allene. Food Technol. (1974) 28, 34.
43. Bloom, W. L. and Wilhelmi, A. E. Proc. Soc. Exp. Biol. Med. (1952) 81, 501.
44. Parkinson, T. M. Nature (London) (1967) 215, 415.
45. Booth, A. N., Hendrickson, A. P. and DeEds, F. Toxicol. Appl. Pharmacol. (1963) 5, 478.
46. Adrouny, G. A., Bloom, W. A. and Wilhelmi, A. E. Fed. Proc. (1957) 16, Abstr. 618.
47. Dahlqvist, A. J. Clin. Invest. (1962) 41, 463.
48. Dahlqvist, A. Biochem. J. (1963) 86, 72.
49. Fischer, E. H. and Stein, E. A., in "The Enzymes Vol. 4, Part A," 2nd ed., Boyer, P. D., Lardy, H., Myrback, K., Ed., Academic Press, New York, N.Y., 1960, p. 306.
50. Ammon, R. Enzymologia (1963) 25, 245.
51. Kolínská, J. and Semenza, G. Biochim. Biophys. Acta (1967) 146, 181.
52. Cogoli, A., Eberle, A., Sigrist, H., Joss, Christine, Robinson, Etheria, Mosimann, H. and Semenza, G. Eur. J. Biochem. (1973) 33, 40.

53. Conklin, K. A., Yamashiro, K. M. and Gray, G. M. J. Biol. Chem. (1975), in press.
54. Gray, G. M. Fed. Proc. (1967) 26, 1415.
55. Hehre, E. J. and Sery, T. W. J. Bacteriol. (1952) 63, 424.
56. Sery, T. W. and Hehre, E. J. J. Bacteriol. (1956) 71, 373.
57. Gorbach, S. L., Banwell, J. G., Jacobs, B., Chatterjee, B. D., Mitra, R., Sen, N. N. and Mazumder, D. N. G. Amer. J. Clin. Nutr. (1970) 23, 1545.
58. Bailey, R. W. and Clarke, R. T. J. Biochem. J. (1959) 72, 49.
59. Whistler, R. L., BeMiller, J. N., "Industrial Gums: Polysaccharides and Their Derivatives," 2nd ed., Academic Press, New York, N.Y., 1973, numerous contributed chapters.
60. Food and Drug Administration, "Food Additives and GRAS Substances," Federal Register (1974) 39 (185, Part II), 34203.
61. Hove, E. L. and Herndon, J. F. J. Nutr. (1957) 63, 193.
62. Glicksman, M. and Sand, R. E., in "Industrial Gums: Polysaccharides and Their Derivatives," 2nd ed., Whistler, R. L. and BeMiller, J. N., Ed., Academic Press, New York, N.Y., 1973, p. 197.
63. Semenza, G., Auricchio, S. and Rubino, A. Biochim. Biophys. Acta (1965) 96, 487.
64. Chapman, V. J., "Seaweeds and Their Uses," Methuen and Co. Ltd., London, 1950, p. 186; 2nd ed., 1970, p. 118.
65. Booth, A. N., Elvehjem, C. A. and Hart, E. B. J. Nutr. (1949) 37, 263.
66. Swartz, M. D. Trans. Conn. Acad. Sci. (1911) 16, 000.
67. Sand, R. E. and Glicksman, M., in "Industrial Gums: Polysaccharides and Their Derivatives," 2nd ed., Whistler, R. L. and BeMiller, J. N., Ed., Academic Press, New York, N.Y., 1973, p. 185.
68. Yamashina, I., in "The Amino Sugars," Vol. II B, Balazs, E. A. and Jeanloz, R. W., Ed., Academic Press, New York, N.Y., 1966, p. 81.
69. Spiro, R. G. Ann. Rev. Biochem. (1970) 39, 599.
70. Lis, Halina, Sharon, N. and Katchalski, E. Biochim. Biophys. Acta (1969) 192, 364.
71. Schanker, L. S. and Johnson, J. M. Biochem. Pharmacol. (1961) 8, 421.
72. Encyclopedia Britannica, Vol. 2, Wm. Benton, Publisher, Chicago, Ill., 1964, p. 525.
73. The Merck Index of Chemicals and Drugs, 7th Edition. Merck & Co., Inc., Rahway, N.J., 1960, p. 557.
74. Avigad, G., in "Encyclopedia of Polymer Science and Technology," Vol. 8, Bikales, N., Ed., 1968, p. 711.
75. Bull, A. T. and Chesters, C. G. C. Advan. Enzymol. (1966) 28, 325.
76. Harada, T., Misaki, A. and Saito, H. Arch. Biochem. Biophys. (1968) 124, 292.

77. Rodgers, N. E., in "Industrial Gums: Polysaccharides and Their Derivatives," 2nd ed., Whistler, R. L. and BeMiller, J. N., Ed., Academic Press, New York, N.Y., 1973, p. 499.
78. Harada, T. Proc. Biochem. (January 1974) page 21.

INDEX